AF597349

OSTEOPOROSIS

OSTEOPOROSIS

Diagnosis and Treatment

edited by

David J. Sartoris

University of California, San Diego, School of Medicine
and University of California, San Diego, Medical Center
San Diego, California

Marcel Dekker, Inc. New York • Basel • Hong Kong

Library of Congress Cataloging-in-Publication Data

Osteoporosis : diagnosis and treatment / edited by David J. Sartoris.
p. cm.
Includes bibliographical references and index.
ISBN 0-8247-9507-5 (hardcover : alk. paper)
1. Osteoporosis. I. Sartoris, David J. [DNLM: 1. Osteoporosis—diagnosis. 2. Osteoporosis—therapy. 3. Osteoporosis—physiopathology.
WE 250 085123 1996]
RC931.0730773 1996
616.7'16—dc20
DNLM/DLC
for Library of Congress 96-2683
CIP

The publisher offers discounts on this book when ordered in bulk quantities. For more information, write to Special Sales/Professional Marketing at the address below.

This book is printed on acid-free paper.

Marcel Dekker, Inc.
270 Madison Avenue, New York, New York 10016

Current printing (last digit):
10 9 8 7 6 5 4 3 2 1

PRINTED IN THE UNITED STATES OF AMERICA

Preface

This book is the culmination of the initial and most rewarding clinical and research interest of my medical career. Although my interest in the problems of aging began when I was a child, my experience with noninvasive bone-mass measurement commenced in 1980, during my radiology residency, under the precious mentorship of William Brody, Henry Jones, and Graham Sommer.

During the past fifteen years, I have witnessed dramatic improvements in both bone densitometry and osteoporosis therapy. Simultaneous changes in population demographics and health care delivery have brought the disorder to the forefront of public awareness as the millennium approaches. This book is thus timely because it arrives at a point when mankind finally is in a position to reduce the future incidence of osteoporotic fractures and their associated morbidity and mortality.

Osteoporosis is the only medical condition that affects virtually every member of our species who lives beyond the age of 35. It is the most common form of low bone mass, and is a major medical problem with rising medical, social, and economic consequences. Over 8 million Americans suffer from osteoporotic fractures, although the number of affected individuals is conservatively estimated at 14 million using the newer definitions of osteoporosis, which include those who have not yet experienced fractures but have sufficiently low bone mass to place them at risk for fractures. Other estimates for this population have been as high as 25 million. The lifetime cumulative fracture risk for a 50-year-old Caucasian woman without intervention approaches 60%. Worldwide, the number of hip fractures is increasing in both women and men. As many as 21% of nursing home patients are admitted with a diagnosis of hip fracture. Hip fracture is associated with an excess mortality of up to 20%, and vertebral fracture with an excess mortality of 4%. Survivors of both hip and vertebral fractures have a severely compromised quality of life.

The National Osteoporosis Foundation has estimated that the cost of treating osteoporosis in 1990 was $10 billion. With the aging of the population, the increasing prevalence of osteoporosis, and the current patterns of inflation, the total direct medical cost alone is predicted to reach $30–45 billion before the year 2020. Prevention of osteoporotic fractures, with the attendant reductions in health care costs and excess morbidity and mortality, depends on identification of individuals at risk for fractures, so that proper intervention (e.g., lifestyle decisions, exercise, hormone or drug therapy) can be initiated. Historical risk factors have been shown to be inadequate for the prediction of low bone mass or fracture risk. However, several prospective studies have now shown that the relative risk of fracture increases exponentially with incremental reductions in bone mass, clearly establishing the utility of bone-mass measurement in predicting a patient's future risk of fracture.

The identification of younger asymptomatic individuals who are at risk for osteoporotic fractures is imperative if the morbidity, mortality, and economic consequences of osteoporosis are to be reduced. Prevention of the first fracture is an important concept for several clinical reasons. First, asymptomatic nonfractured individuals with low bone mass (due to either low peak bone mass or bone loss of whatever etiology) have an increased fracture risk compared with individuals with normal bone mass. Second, identification of high-risk nonfractured individuals leads to discovery of possible secondary etiologies and initiation of appropriate intervention strategies. Third, once the first fracture occurs, the relative risk of a second fracture increases fivefold, independent of bone mass, and the combination of low bone mass and just one vertebral fracture increases the relative risk of a second fracture 25-fold. Lastly, once these high-risk patients are identified and intervention strategies are initiated, bone mass can be maintained, and prevention of the first fracture can be achieved in many patients. If these individuals are not identified, bone loss may continue unrecognized. Therefore, there should be a consensus to broaden the utilization of bone-mass measurements to identify those individuals with low bone mass and an increased risk of fracture.

A comprehensive understanding of osteoporosis requires insight into the pathophysiology, biochemistry, and histology of the condition. These concepts are eloquently discussed in Chapters 1 and 2 by Drs. Gary W. Edelson and Erik Fink Eriksen, respectively. The epidemiological aspects of osteoporosis and its complicating fractures are next covered in detail by a recognized authority on the subject, Dr. L. Joseph Melton, III. Chapters 4 and 5 examine the important biomechanical and orthopedic concepts of the disease, which are understandably presented by Drs. Joseph M. Lane and Earl Brien, respectively.

The focus of the book then shifts toward the imaging and densitometric aspects of osteoporosis. Chapter 6 presents an incomparable explanation of how the gross pathology of the condition translates into diagnostic radiological findings. Since quantitative computed tomography and dual-energy X-ray absorptiometry are currently the most widely utilized clinical methods for noninvasive bone-mass measurement, Chapters 7, by Dr. Dexter Wong, and 9, by Dr. Heinz Wahner, one of the pioneers in the field, are devoted to these techniques. Chapter 8, by Dr. Harry Genant and colleagues, provides a detailed overview of additional densitometric tests that presently find widespread application in research situations, many of which have potential for future clinical use. Finally, and perhaps most importantly, Chapter 10 is a lengthy treatise covering the numerous therapeutic breakthroughs that have occurred in recent years, offering substantial hope for a future reduction in the morbidity and mortality of osteoporosis.

This book will be of definite utility to trainees and practicing physicians from a broad spectrum of medical subspecialties, since osteoporosis interfaces with many aspects of health care. Indeed, the memberships of both the National Osteoporosis Foundation and the Society for Clinical Densitometry reflect this unique diversity. Primary care, family practice, internal medicine, geriatrics, endocrinology, rheumatology, gynecology, orthopedic surgery, radiology, gastroenterology, nephrology, and epidemiology are among the fields likely to benefit from this volume. In addition, the book contains information relevant to public health officials, nurses, technologists, physical therapists, and even the general public.

As this book goes to press, rapid improvements are occurring in the ability to diagnose, treat, and monitor osteoporosis, and major public educational efforts are underway to increase therapeutic compliance and minimize the risk of fall-related fractures. An arsenal of new drugs awaits evaluation by the Food and Drug Administration, and efforts to identify sensitive serum markers for osteoporosis are paralleling technological breakthroughs in the noninvasive quantification of bone density, architecture, and strength. It is indeed a renaissance time in our understanding of this disorder, and we hope this volume will be successful in both educating and stimulating its readers.

David J. Sartoris

Contents

Contributors

Reimer Andresen, M.D. Radiologist, Department of Radiology, Behring Municipal Hospital, Free University of Berlin, Berlin, Germany

Earl Brien, M.D. Associate Director, Musculoskeletal Tumor Service, and Assistant Clinical Professor, University of California at Irvine, Orange, and Assistant Clinical Professor, University of Southern California, Los Angeles, California

Kim Brixen, M.D. Department of Endocrinology and Metabolism, Aarhus University Hospital, Aarhus, Denmark

Gary W. Edelson, M.D. Assistant Professor, Department of Medicine, Grace Hospital and Wayne State University School of Medicine, Detroit, Michigan

Eric Fink Eriksen, M.D. D.M.Sc. Department of Endocrinology, Aarhus Amtssygehus, Aarhus, Denmark

Harry K. Genant, M.D. Professor of Radiology, Medicine, and Orthopedic Surgery, Department of Radiology, University of California, San Francisco, San Francisco, California

Claus C. Glüer, Ph.D. Professor of Medical Physics, Department of Diagnostic Radiology, University of Kiel, Kiel, Germany

Stephan Grampp, M.D. Assistant Adjunct Professor, Musculoskeletal Section, Department of Radiology, University of California, San Francisco, San Francisco, California

John H. Healey, M.D. Chief, Orthopedic Surgery, Memorial Sloan-Kettering Cancer Center, and Associate Professor of Surgery (Orthopedic), Cornell University Medical College, New York, New York

Michael Jergas, M.D. Assistant Adjunct Professor, Department of Radiology, University of California, San Francisco, San Francisco, California

Michael Kleerekoper, M.D., F.A.C.P. Professor and Associate Chairman, Department of Internal Medicine, Wayne State University School of Medicine, Detroit, Michigan

Joseph M. Lane, M.D. Professor and Chairman, Department of Orthopedic Surgery, University of California at Los Angeles Medical Center, Los Angeles, California

Philipp Lang, M.D. Resident, Diagnostic Radiology, Department of Radiology, University of California, San Francisco, San Francisco, California

L. Joseph Melton, III, M.D. Eisenberg Professor of Epidemiology, Mayo Medical School, and Consultant, Section of Clinical Epidemiology, Department of Health Sciences Research, Mayo Clinic and Foundation, Rochester, Minnesota

Elizabeth R. Myers, Ph.D. Assistant Professor, Orthopedic Biomechanics Laboratory, Department of Orthopedic Surgery, Charles A. Dana Research Institute, and Harvard Thorndike Laboratory, Beth Israel Hospital and Harvard Medical School, Boston, Massachusetts

Donald L. Resnick, M.D. Professor of Radiology, University of California, San Diego, School of Medicine, and Department of Radiology, Veterans Affairs Medical Center, San Diego, California

David J. Sartoris, M.D. Professor of Radiology, Musculoskeletal Imaging Section, University of California, San Diego, School of Medicine, and Chief, Quantitative Bone Densitometry, University of California, San Diego, Medical Center, San Diego, California

Jill E. Spadia, M.D. Research Associate, Department of Radiology, University of California, San Diego, School of Medicine, and University of California, San Diego, Medical Center, San Diego, California

Torben Steiniche, M.D., Ph.D. Pathologist, Department of Pathology, Aarhus Kommunehospital, Aarhus University Hospital, Aarhus, Denmark

John A. M. Taylor, D.C., D.A.C.B.R.* Research Associate, Department of Radiology, University of California, San Diego, Medical Center, San Diego, California

Heinz W. Wahner, M.D., F.A.C.P. Section of Nuclear Medicine, Department of Radiology, Mayo Clinic, Rochester, Minnesota

Bruce Wollman, M.D. Research Associate, Department of Radiology, University of California, San Diego, School of Medicine, San Diego, California

Dexter M. Wong Research Associate, Department of Radiology, University of California, San Diego, Medical Center, San Diego, California

---

**Present affiliation*: Western States Chiropractic College, Portland, Oregon.

OSTEOPOROSIS

1

Pathophysiology of Osteoporosis

GARY W. EDELSON

*Grace Hospital and Wayne State University School of Medicine
Detroit, Michigan*

MICHAEL KLEEREKOPER

*Wayne State University School of Medicine
Detroit, Michigan*

I. NORMAL BONE PHYSIOLOGY

While many factors contribute to the strength of the skeleton and its ability to withstand trauma without fracture, the major determinant accounting for at least 70% of bone strength is bone mineral density (mass per volume). Approximately 80% of the total skeletal mass is cortical (compact) bone with a low surface: volume ratio, while the remaining 20% is cancellous (spongy) bone with a much higher surface:volume ratio. However, the microarchitecture of cancellous bone appears to develop along patterns governed by mechanical loading of the skeleton, and presumably makes a contribution to bone strength greater than can be accounted for by mass alone. Alterations in this interrelationship among mass, volume, surface, and architecture must all be considered in the pathogenesis and pathophysiology of the loss of bone strength with an increased risk of fracture that is hallmark of osteoporosis. In this chapter, we will review the several factors (known and postulated) that contribute to the development of peak bone mass and strength and which, under pathologic conditions, result in loss of this mass and strength. The major focus of our discussion will be on the factors governing the balance between bone resorption and formation, and the impact of normal aging and many diseases on this balance.

The skeleton is a complex organ system that is under a constant state of flux. It serves mechanical, metabolic, and protective functions. There are two general types of bone, cortical and cancellous. Cortical bone is found primarily in the shafts of the long bones of the appendicular skeleton. It is also found as the outer layer of virtually all bones. Cancellous bone is found primarily in the bones of the axial skeleton and in the ends of the long bones. The cellular process of bone activity by which both cortical and cancellous bone are maintained is referred to as bone remodeling. This remodeling process takes place on bone surfaces in discrete packets known as basic multicellular units (1). Initially, a cell from the hematopoietic granulocyte-macrophage colony-forming unit lineage along a bone surface is activated and proliferates or transforms into an osteoclast (2). An osteoclast creates a bone cavity. Subsequently, osteoblasts, derived from pluripotent mesenchymal stem cells of the bone marrow, fill in the area of resorption with type I collagen (3). Type I collagen ultimately becomes mineralized, probably as a function of the osteoblasts, thereby completing the process of new bone formation. There is an interdependency of the osteoclastic and osteoblastic activities whereby osteoclasts are initially recruited to a particular site on the bone surface, and when their task is completed, they signal the osteoblasts to attend to that same site. This interrelationship is known as coupling and is a crucial link in the chain of bone-remodeling events (4). Any situation that interferes with the coupling process or causes imbalance between the bone-forming and bone-resorbing relationship can lead to significant loss of bone mass over time.

Regulation of the bone-remodeling process is complex. Undoubtedly, there are numerous systemic hormones, such as parathyroid hormone, 1,25-dihydroxyvitamin D (calcitriol), calcitonin, estrogens, and androgens which serve in part to regulate the process. Vitamin D is recognized as a stimulator of osteoclastic formation and a promoter of osteoblast differentiation (5). There are also numerous local factors that play an important role in the physiology of bone remodeling—interleukins (IL-1 and IL-6), transforming growth factors, prostaglandins, tumor necrosis factor, lymphotoxin, colony stimulating factors, and gamma interferons to name a few (6–9). Interleukin 1 is a potent osteoclast stimulator whose action can be locally partially inhibited by the prostaglandin inhibitor indomethacin, suggesting a prostaglandin-mediated mode of action (8). In vivo, it has been demonstrated that IL-1 has an effect on bone formation as well (10). The effect is suppression of bone formation. For these reasons, IL-1 has been implicated by some as a prime mediator of osteoporosis. IL-6 may play a role in the regulation of osteoclast transformation and/or maturation (7). Certain transforming growth factors appear to play a role in the stimulation of bone formation while prostaglandins stimulate bone resorption. Tumor necrosis factor, lymphotoxin, colony stimulating factors, and gamma interferons all appear to have some influence on osteoclast development.

We know that, in both men and women, skeletal mass gradually increases during growth and development and reaches some maximum point between the ages of 18 and 35. We further know that both men and women gradually lose bone after that point in time as part of the aging process. It appears that the cancellous bone mass begins to be lost earlier on than the cortical bone mass, perhaps by as much as a 20-year differential (11). This difference can be accounted for by the greater surface: volume ratio of cancellous bone that makes it more susceptible to any deleterious effects of bone remodeling, which only takes place on skeletal surfaces. The exact factors that cause age-related bone loss have not been well defined, but most experts would agree that it is probably related to some endocrinologic or hormonal alteration seen as part of the normal physiologic aging process. A major etiologic component is estrogen deficiency, an inevitable result of menopausal ovarian senescence which has been shown to increase osteoclastic resorbing capacity (12–14). Furthermore, estrogen deficiency both directly and indirectly decreases the efficiency of intestinal and renal calcium absorption and reabsorption, respectively (Fig. 1).

Testosterone deficiency in men, which is the major identifiable cause of male osteoporosis, has analogous mineral metabolism effects. Evidence in support of

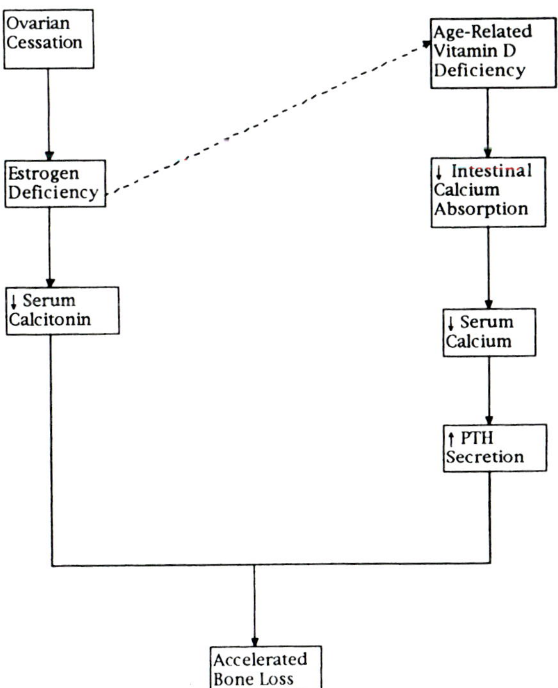

Figure 1 Pathophysiology of age-related bone loss. Ovarian cessation and age-related vitamin D deficiency ultimately result in accelerated bone loss.

gonadal hormone deficiency as the cause of increasing bone resorption is that specific receptors for estrogen and testosterone have been identified on the surface of bone cells (15). Much harder to explain than the obvious reduction in ovarian hormone production at the menopause are the effects of aging on the kidney and the gut as they affect the skeleton. The kidney is the sole site of production of calcitriol, and for unknown reasons, renal production of this hormone decreases with age to a greater extent than can be explained by age-related decrements in glomerular filtration rate. Synthesis of calcitriol from its precursor 25-hydroxy-vitamin D via the enzyme 1-alpha hydroxylase is catalyzed by parathyroid hormone. Thus the age-related fall in renal production of calcitriol is associated with secondary hyperparathyroidism and increased bone resorption. Even as this secondary hyperparathyroidism maintains normal production of calcitriol to the maximum extent possible, the situation is aggravated by the aging gut with impaired absorptive capacity for many nutrients including calcium. Thus, with aging, more vitamin D may be required to maintain adequate absorption of calcium, further aggravating any tendency toward secondary hyperparathyroidism and accelerated bone loss. Of course this explanation begs the question since it provides an acceptable explanation for parathyroid hormone (PTH)-mediated bone loss but not for the age-related changes in the kidney and the gut.

Also, cellular and immune changes that occur with aging also undoubtedly contribute to the regulation and alteration of bone remodeling. The prime candidates for these effects include interleukins, tumor necrosis factor, and transforming growth factor (TGF beta). It has been fairly well demonstrated that these cellular changes are a result of estrogen deficiency, whereby estrogen in sufficient concentration suppresses the osteoblastic biosynthesis of these factors. It has also been shown that at least a couple of these cytokines are able to sensitize bone to the resorptive effects of parathyroid hormone and thereby have an indirect effect on bone remodeling.

Finally, there are the effects of declining physical activity with aging. Just as peak bone mass during growth and development is influenced by load-bearing exercise and other mechanical factors, bone loss during aging and in disease, is so influenced. The biochemical, hormonal, and local factors that regulate the interaction between the neuromuscular system and the skeleton have not been elucidated. What is known, particularly from extreme circumstances such as immobilization following acute spinal cord injury or the weightlessness of space travel, is that there is no more rapid acceleration of bone loss than the removal of mechanical and neuronal influences on bone remodeling. Since muscle mass and function decline with age, as do physical fitness and the amount of time devoted to physical activity, it is tempting to suggest that this contributes to age-related bone loss. However, it has proven quite difficult to document this in either cross-sectional or prospective studies, suggesting that in normal aging the effect is quite small. Nonetheless, in susceptible persons it might be the one factor that makes the ultimate difference between sustaining an osteoporotic fracture or not. Aside from any direct influence on bone remodeling, bone mass, and bone strength, there is a significant interaction between muscle strength, neurologic function, and the likelihood of falling, as well as the ability to sustain a fall without injury.

II. CONCEPT OF PEAK ADULT BONE MASS

There are two factors that determine the level of bone mass at any particular age in both males and females. These are peak adult bone mass and the duration and rate of bone loss. Peak adult bone mass represents the maximal result of growth and consolidation and is reached between the ages of 18 and 35. Peak adult bone mass is about 25–30% higher in males than it is in females and about 10% higher in blacks than in whites (22). Bone mass accounts for 75–80% of bone strength and, as such, is the most important determinant of bone strength (23). Genetic factors account for 70% or more of the variance in bone mass in healthy young women (24). Adequate production of sex hormones is crucial to the development of optimal/genetically predetermined peak adult bone mass. However, there are many environmental factors that may modify peak bone mass, resulting in a suboptimal peak. The recognition of such nongenetic factors impacting bone mass has occurred mainly as a result of retrospective analyses. It has been determined that low calcium and protein intake, deficient intake of other nutrients, endocrine dysfunction, chronic illness, malnutrition, and immobilization may all result in a suboptimal peak adult bone mass and thereby increase the risk of developing osteoporosis later in life (20,23). The role of physical activity on achievement of peak bone mass is somewhat unclear, based on available data to date. Most investigators agree that weight-bearing exercise is generally an enhancer of bone formation and bone mass as well as a contributor to general skeletal strength. Furthermore, we well know that relative inactivity, immobilization being the extreme of inactivity, causes an abrupt halt in bone formation and apparently even causes an increase in the rate of bone resorption (25). It is clear that exercise is site-specific with respect to bone mass benefits. In other words, those involved with weight-bearing exercises that place a great deal of stress on the femoral neck, such as running or ice skating, are more effective in sustaining and achieving a higher bone mass in the femoral neck area than they are for the spine or the forearm (26).

There are some interesting data that suggest a possible association between the vitamin D receptor gene and bone density, although this work is preliminary and not yet well established (27). We should mention that any of the causes of secondary osteoporosis, which we will delineate later in this chapter, certainly will impair the attainment of peak bone mass should they develop prior to the age of completion of bone growth maturation. Primary hyperparathyroidism, Cushing's syndrome, rheumatoid arthritis, and neoplasms such as lymphoma or leukemia are but a few examples.

III. FACTORS AFFECTING RATE OF BONE LOSS

Once peak bone mass has been attained, men without secondary causes of osteoporosis, and women prior to the age of menopause lose approximately 0.25% to 1% of bone yearly. In the perimenopausal and immediate postmenopausal period, women may lose 2–5% of bone yearly. Over an entire life span, men may experience 20–30% skeletal mineral loss whereas women experience approximately 15% loss every 10 years after the menopause (28,29). Without doubt, the single greatest contributor to bone loss is loss of gonadal function. Relatively rapid loss of bone mass is seen after ovarian failure of any cause, but the most common is after spontaneous menopause. Other reported causes include Turner's syndrome (30) hypogonadotropic hypogonadism due to hyperprolactinemia (31), anorexia nervosa (32), and extreme physical activity (33). Likewise, irrespective of the cause, men experience significantly increased rates of bone loss when hypogonadism develops. It has been reported in hyperprolactinemic syndromes (34), idiopathic hypogonadotropic hypogonadism (35), surgical and medical castration (36), Klinefelter's syndrome (37), hemochromatosis (38), and even in delayed puberty (39). Hypogonadism, however, is clearly not the only factor accounting for osteoporosis in men since nearly two-thirds of osteoporotic men have normal gonadal function (40). Often such men will have other identifiable secondary causes for osteoporosis.

A classification system of type I, or postmenopausal-type, osteoporosis and type II, or senile-type, osteoporosis has been adapted and become increasingly popular since its introduction approximately 15 years ago (41). Type I osteoporosis tends to occur at younger ages and is characterized best by vertebral and wrist fractures. Type II osteoporosis is thought etiologically to be due to age-related bone loss, thus occurring at an older age, and is best characterized by hip fractures. Since bone resorption accelerates significantly in the perimenopausal period as a result of the fairly abrupt cessation of estrogen production by the ovaries, it is believed that this is the most likely etiology for type I osteoporosis, but again, this has not been proven beyond doubt. It is during this period in a woman's life that cancellous bone loss is greatest. In type II osteoporosis, there is relative universal bone loss. The extent of bone loss appears to be well correlated with the degree of estrogen deficiency, which is another fact supporting the importance of the relationship between estrogen adequacy and bone mass maintenance (14). Whether estrogen deficiency directly stimulates bone resorption or there is an indirect effect via immune system cytokines, remains a question to be answered. Nevertheless, estrogen deficiency is the single most important cause of bone loss in women, and replacement of estrogen is the single best preventive therapy for osteoporosis.

At the same time, however, it is clear that there are factors involved other than estrogen deficiency, because despite the fact that all postmenopausal women have endogenous estrogen deficiency, osteoporosis only develops in 10–20% of them (6). Since bone remodeling represents a balance between bone formation and bone resorption, it is understandable that any condition that increases the rate of bone resorption and/or interferes with the process of bone formation would increase the risk of developing osteoporosis. Primary factors associated (to varying degrees) with an increased risk of osteoporosis are advancing age, Caucasian or Asian race, early or premature menopause, thin/petite body habitus, relative physical inactivity, calcium-poor diets, and long-term use of antiepileptics of corticosteroids (42). There are also some fairly convincing data to suggest that a family history of osteoporosis in a first-degree relative (43), cigarette smoking (44), and excessive consumption of alcohol (45) also increase the risk of developing osteoporosis.

Dietary calcium deficiency and vitamin D deficiency is associated with an increased risk of premenopausal loss of bone as well as an increased risk of osteoporosis postmenopausally. Calcium is best thought of as a threshold nutrient, having its greatest effect on retarding bone loss in the immediate postmenopausal period in those who start out with the lowest daily intakes of calcium. Factors contributing to vitamin D deficiency in the elderly population are decreased dietary intake of vitamin D, decreased conversion of 25-hydroxyvitamin D to calcitriol due to the decrease in alpha-1-hydroxylase activity normally seen with aging, and decreased skin synthesis of vitamin D primarily due to a lack of sunlight exposure in the elderly who are more prone to remain indoors (46).

Physical activity has effects on bone loss similar to the effects it has on attainment of peak adult bone mass. That is to say that a lack of physical activity will increase the rate of bone loss whereas regular weight-bearing activities will decrease the rate of bone loss in a site-specific fashion. Young tennis players have significantly higher forearm bone densities in their racquet holding or dominant arm than in their nondominant arm (47). Ballet dancers have higher bone densities in the hip regions than do nondancers when matched for osteoporosis risk factors (48).

No matter which of the aforementioned causes is operative in a particular patient, the basic mechanism of bone loss is consistently an uncoupling of bone formation and bone resorption in such a manner that there is an absolute greater amount of bone resorbed than there is bone formed. This may occur as a result of a relatively greater increase in bone resorption (or osteoclastic activity) than bone formation (or osteoblastic activity) or relative deficiency of osteoblastic bone formation with a normal rate of bone resorption. This latter mechanism is more typical of senile, or age-related, type II osteoporosis and of that seen in men who develop osteoporosis. The former mechanism is the typical type of bone remodeling seen in a postmenopausal or estrogen-deficient woman and is often referred to as high-turnover-type osteoporosis. The term "high turnover" signifies the fact that the rates of bone resorption and bone formation are occurring rapidly in a coupled fashion.

IV. PATHOPHYSIOLOGY OF MALE OSTEOPOROSIS

The pathophysiology of osteoporosis in men is quite analogous to that seen and described thus far in women. Certainly, osteoporosis is a much less frequent affliction of males, with an incidence ratio of approximately 2 to 1, females to males (49). Of all hip fractures experienced by the elderly population, only about 30% occurred in men (50). Healthy boys and young men develop a higher peak bone mass than their female counterparts, which must account for the lower incidence and prevalence of osteoporosis in men later in life. However, whenever factors are present during the years of bone maturation which prohibit the attainment of this preprogrammed genetic peak bone mass, then the risk of osteoporosis is significantly increased in that individual. In addition to the peak adult bone mass benefit that men enjoy, there are also sex-related differences in the rates of age-related bone loss. In general, women lose more bone mass with aging than men do, and men do not experience a dramatic decrease in gonadal hormone synthesis such as women do at the time of menopause. Just as in women, though, age-related increases in bone resorption rates in men may be related to various hormonal factors. Serum parathyroid hormone levels increase with age, while at the same time calcitonin levels do not fall, and in fact remain at higher levels than those seen in women (40) (Fig. 2). The decreased synthesis of calcitriol described previously in aged females is also seen in men and may result in a negative

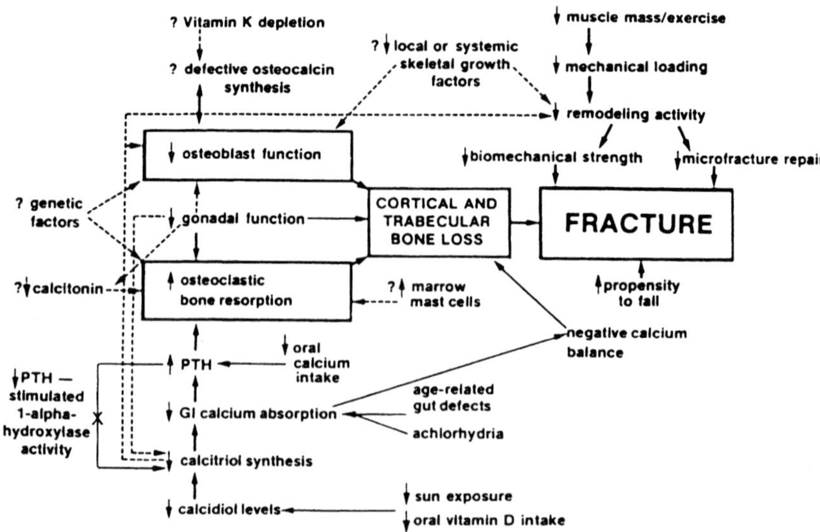

Figure 2 Multifactorial pathophysiology of involutional bone loss in men.

calcium balance via decreasing the ability of the intestine to absorb calcium. Whether or not an age-related decline in gonadal function that does not frankly reach the hypogonadal range contributes to some extent to the age-related bone loss phenomenon in men has not been established. However, Leydig cell number and thus testosterone levels decrease with age; there are discrete hypothalamic-pituitary function changes with aging; there is an increased incidence of coexistent illness and pharmaceutical use, and similar decreases in muscle mass, weight-bearing activities, and the ability to avoid or withstand falls as seen in women (50).

Any of the so-called secondary causes of osteoporosis broadly categorized as endocrinopathies, neoplasms, hereditary disorders, drug-induced osteoporoses, osteomalacia, and other disorders can induce osteoporosis in men just as they do in women. The mechanisms of these will be described in the next section.

V. PATHOPHYSIOLOGY OF DISEASE-SPECIFIC OSTEOPOROSES

There are numerous medical disorders and drugs that have been identified as causing osteoporosis. These are listed in Table 1 and generally include endocrine

Table 1 Secondary Causes of Osteoporosis

Endocrine/metabolic	Beta-thalassemia	*Pharmacologic agents*
Diabetes mellitus type I	PTHrP-secreting solid tumors (esp. squamous, renal, bladder, ovarian)	Aluminum-containing antacids
Cushing's syndrome	*Gastrointestinal*	Anticonvulsants
Hypogonadism—primary and secondary	Inflammatory bowel disease	Cisplatin
Hyperparathyroidism—primary and secondary	Gluten enteropathy	Cyclosporine
Hyperthyroidism	Postgastrectomy	Glucocorticoids
Homocystinuria	Primary biliary cirrhosis	Heparin
Acromegaly	Hepatic insufficiency	Methotrexate
Hypovitaminosis D	Hemochromatosis	Plicamycin
Scurvy	Wilson's disease	Thyroid hormone excess
Hematologic/oncologic	Malnutrition	Diuretics except thiazides
Leukemia	*Chronic inflammatory diseases*	Alcohol
Lymphoma	Rheumatoid arthritis	*Other*
Multiple myeloma	*Renal*	Immobilization
Waldenstrom's macroglobulinemia	Idiopathic hypercalciuria	Osteogenesis imperfecta
Systemic mastocytosis	Renal failure	Disuse/paralysis
Hemolytic anemias	Renal tubular acidosis	Ehlers-Danlos syndrome
Sickle cell disease		Marfans syndrome
		Post organ transplantation
		Pregnancy
		Gaucher's disease

and metabolic diseases, hematologic/oncologic diseases, gastrointestinal disorders, chronic inflammatory disorders, renal diseases, and a good number of pharmacologic agents. Among the endocrine-mediated osteoporoses is hypogonadism, which has already been discussed at length, but the point should be made that the causes of hypogonadism are fairly extensive. The more common ones include central causes of hypogonadism, such as hypothalamic and pituitary diseases. For example, anorexia nervosa causes an alteration of hypothalamic gonadotropic releasing hormone secretion resulting in low estradiol levels, and in addition, patients with anorexia nervosa tend to have low dietary calcium intake associated with their overall low dietary caloric intake, further contributing to the increasing bone resorption and state of negative calcium balance (32). This is also fairly commonly seen in female athletes, especially competitive athletes in whom bone density is severely reduced in association with prolonged amenorrhea.

Both primary and secondary hyperparathyroidism increase rates of bone resorption, although patients with these conditions are not typically diagnosed by their presentation with osteoporosis. Rather, those with primary hyperparathyroidism are diagnosed when they have a notably high calcium on serum screening profiles, and those with secondary hyperparathyroidism are diagnosed when they present with symptoms of osteodystrophy. The exact mechanism by which parathyroid hormone induces osteoporosis is by a direct stimulatory effect on osteoblasts which, through the coupling mechanism, stimulates osteoclast activity and accelerates bone resorption (51). The type of bone loss that is seen is a generalized loss of bone density, however, with a more dramatic cortical than cancellous bone loss (52). It is not unusual to detect this differential bone loss through bone density testing wherein forearm bone density, representing a more cortically rich site of bone, will demonstrate a greater deficit than will vertebral bone density, which is richer in cancellous bone. Although correction of the hyperparathyroidism through parathyroidectomy will cause a cessation of the accelerated bone loss, it does not allow for reestablishment of bone density which had previously been lost (53). In the majority of patients with primary hyperparathyroidism, however, the condition is fairly mild, and significant bone disturbances are not typically seen.

Secondary hyperparathyroidism in the United States is most commonly caused by renal failure and worldwide by vitamin D deficiency or malnutrition. It is more commonly associated with osteomalacia than with osteoporosis per se. In this condition, the high levels of parathyroid hormone stimulate bone resorption by the same mechanisms as they do in primary hyperparathyroidism by directly affecting osteoblasts and, secondarily, stimulating osteoclasts. When this is superimposed on the already preexisting calcium deficiency, the end result may be simultaneously occurring osteomalacia and osteoporosis. Interestingly, hypovitaminosis D itself is associated with osteoporosis as well (53).

Cushing's syndrome, whether from a pituitary adenoma, adrenal overproduction of glucocorticoids, an ectopic ACTH syndrome, or exogenous steroid use, results in significant loss of bone mass. The exact mechanism of this pathophysiology is multifactorial (see Fig. 3) and includes a decrease in the activity of osteoblasts with decreased bone formation, increased osteoclastic activity with resultant increased rates of bone resorption, decreased intestinal calcium absorption, and increased renal calcium excretion, and is an independent effect on the hypothalamic pituitary axis impairing the action of gonadotropin releasing hormone and resulting in a hypogonadotropic hypogonadism (54–56). The type of bone deficit typically seen with Cushing's syndrome is greater degrees of cancellous bone loss than cortical bone loss, but with increased fragility of both types (55).

Accelerated bone loss may also be seen in thyrotoxicosis and in patients treated with supraphysiologic doses of thyroid hormone. The mechanism of bone loss acceleration is likely a direct action of thyroid hormone on osteoclasts whereby

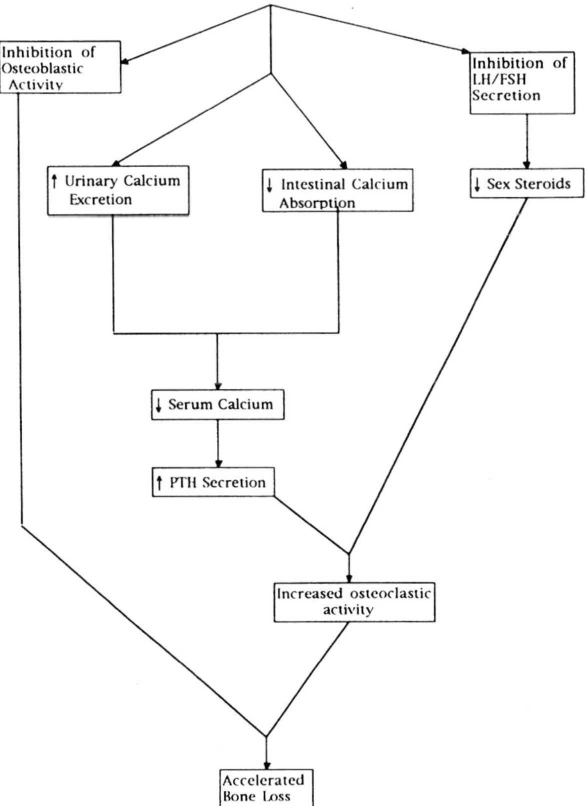

Figure 3 Pathophysiology of glucocorticoid-induced accelerated bone loss.

osteoclastic activity and the rate of bone resorption are increased (57). It has been demonstrated that hyperthyroidism causes increases in serum calcium levels with simultaneous decreases in parathyroid hormone levels and calcitriol levels (58). Markers of bone formation, such as osteocalcin and alkaline phosphatase, have been found to be elevated consistent with the direct effects of thyroid hormone on bone cells and consistent with the fact that T_3 receptors have been identified on osteoblastlike cell lines (57). Further, consistent findings in thyrotoxicosis are the blunting of intestinal calcium absorption and hypercalciuria (59).

The exact mechanisms by which type I diabetes mellitus causes osteoporosis remains somewhat controversial, but the general consensus is that it is related to an alteration of growth factors, perhaps increased levels of insulinlike growth factor 1 (60). The data on bone density in patients with type II diabetes mellitus is even less clear, with some studies showing increased and others decreased bone density (61). The suggestion is that insulin either directly or indirectly stimulates bone formation and that this effect is even more pronounced when insulin resistance and its resultant hyperinsulinemia are present.

Neoplastic diseases such as multiple myeloma (62), Waldenstrom's macroglobulinemia (61), and systemic mastocytosis (63) appear to be causes of osteoporosis through various immune mechanisms. Substances such as osteoclast activating factor (OAF), interleukins, and tumor necrosis factors are local stimulators of osteoclastic activity and thereby induce an increased rate of bone resorption.

Connective tissue disorders causing osteoporosis are fairly rare occurrences. Gaucher's disease (61), osteogenesis imperfecta (64), Ehlers-Danlos syndrome (65), Marfans syndrome (66), homocystinuria (67), and scurvy (61) are all recognized causes. In osteogenesis imperfecta, generalized osteoporosis is seen as a result of defective osteoid formation whereas in homocystinuria the exact mechanism is as yet unknown; however, there is probably a disorder of collagen metabolism involved.

Since local hormones may play a very important role in the initiation of physiologic bone resorption and have a crucial role in the maintenance of osteoblast and osteoclast coupling, it is quite reasonable to comprehend that rheumatoid arthritis causes localized bone loss around affected joints. A more generalized type of osteoporosis may also be seen with rheumatoid arthritis (68), but is usually seen in the most severe disease cases and in the more chronic cases.

Both Crohn's disease and ulcerative colitis are associated with osteoporosis, although much less frequently than rheumatoid arthritis (69). The pathophysiologic mechanism of osteoporosis in inflammatory bowel disease is multifactorial and includes the stimulation of local inflammatory cells as described in rheumatoid arthritis, the frequent coexistence of hypogonadotropic hypogonadism, an increased propensity to immobilization, in some cases calcium and vitamin D malabsorption, and corticosteroid therapy.

Hepatic insufficiency is also associated with lower mean bone mineral densities, and the mechanisms are varied depending on the exact cause of the hepatic insufficiency. Most typically, there are a decreased rate of bone formation and a low turnover type of osteoporosis as indicated by markers of bone remodeling (70). Often there are identifiable toxins which may have mutually caused the hepatic disease and the bone disease. When this is not the case, malnutrition, calcium malabsorption, and hypogonadism associated with this condition may be the prime etiologic factors. Surprisingly, vitamin D Deficiency does not seem to play a major pathophysiologic role (70). The exact mechanism of posttransplantation osteoporosis is not clear; however, multiple mechanisms and possible contributing factors have been proposed. The most likely factors are prolonged postsurgical immobilization and concomitant relatively high-dose corticosteroid use (71, 72). The immunosuppressant cyclosporine unfortunately also has deleterious effects on bone remodeling, but in a dose-dependent fashion (73). The end result is a greater than threefold increase in fracture rates in posttransplant patients.

Immobilization or disuse of bone is a prominent cause of both focal and generalized bone mass loss (25). It may occur very quickly in the setting of complete immobilization. An analogous but more readily apparent situation is that of a patient who has had a limb casted due to a fracture who after 6 weeks of muscular immobilization in that limb has significant muscular atrophy noted upon removal of the cast. If we could see bone as easily as we can see muscle, a similar profound atrophy would be noted.

Finally, there are multiple diet-related osteoporoses, such as chronic deficiency in calcium, protein, and vitamin C (74). Both tobacco use and excessive alcohol consumption decrease osteoblastic function, contributing to increased rates of bone loss in men and women (75). Additionally, alcohol diminishes calcium absorption by interfering with hepatic 25-hydroxyvitamin D metabolism.

The last category of secondary osteoporoses is the drug-induced osteoporoses. As discussed previously, thyroid hormones act directly on a cellular level to stimulate bone resorption (57), but the precise mode of this interaction has yet to be identified. Glucocorticoids directly inhibit osteoblastic bone formation and indirectly stimulate osteoclastic bone resorption (54–56,76). The increased bone resorption seen with glucocorticoid administration is likely an indirect effect due to the increased parathyroid hormone levels resulting from glucocorticoid inhibition of calcium absorption from the gut and increased urinary calcium excretion. These secondary elevations in parathyroid hormone lead to a generalized increase in osteoclastic bone resorption although cancellous bone loss predominates. Gonadal hormone production is also affected in that glucocorticoids blunt gonadotropin secretion and decrease gonadal testosterone and estrogen production. The deleterious effects of steroids on bone and mineral metabolism appear to be both dose- and duration-dependent. Anticonvulsant drugs, such as phenytoin and barbiturates, cause increased inactivation of 25-hydroxyvitamin D, which is the precursor to the more biologically active form of vitamin D, calcitriol (76). This impairs the gastrointestinal mechanism for calcium absorption. Interestingly, high doses of heparin produce osteoporosis apparently through stimulation of osteoclast formation and osteoclastic activity and decreased osteoblastic activity leading to increased bone resorption (30).

The chemotherapeutic agent methotrexate has a fairly profound calciuric effect and may also be toxic to osteoblasts, resulting in a negative calcium balance and an uncoupling of osteoclastic and osteoblastic activity with resultant rapid bone mass loss (77). Cyclosporin A is an immunosuppressant drug which either directly or indirectly down-regulates osteoblastic activity to a relatively greater degree than osteoclastic activity, and results in a significant bone-remodeling imbalance (78). As mentioned, this becomes quite important given the fact that accelerated bone loss is known to occur in association with organ transplantation independent of any drug effect. Aluminum-containing phosphate binders are directly toxic to bone and can cause osteoporosis as well as osteomalacia (79). Ethanol, when imbibed in large quantities over long periods of time, through a multifactorial mechanism also is a common culprit for causing osteoporosis.

VI. CONCLUSION

The pathophysiology of osteoporosis, while seemingly complex on the surface, is really not so complex when there is first a basic understanding of normal bone physiology. Primary genetic determinants of peak adult bone mass play a major role in predicting the ultimate risk of osteoporosis in patients; however, as delineated in this chapter, there are numerous environmental and lifestyle factors which may modify this peak outcome. On the cellular level, toxins to osteoblasts, osteoclasts, or the interference with mineralization can and will induce profound osteoporosis. Ultimately, the most dramatic determinant and contributor to osteoporosis is the rate of bone loss. This is clearly affected by hormonal factors as well as local cytokines, and there are multiple primary and secondary causes of increased rates of bone loss, impairment of bone formation, and alterations in vitamin D metabolism. An understanding of the pathophysiology of osteoporosis provides a framework for comprehending biochemical and histologic approaches to evaluating osteoporosis, provides a framework for assessing quantitative osteoporosis assessment methods, and drives the interest of industry in the direction of developing new treatment strategies and treatment-specific pharmacologic agents for the prevention and treatment of osteoporosis.

REFERENCES

1. Parfitt AM. Bone remodeling and bone loss: understanding the pathophysiology of osteoporosis. Clin Obstet Gynecol 1987; 30(4):789–811.

2. Christiansen C. Skeletal osteoporosis. J Bone Miner Res 1993; 8(2):S475–S480.
3. Puzas JE. The osteoblast. In: Favus MJ, ed. Primer on the Metabolic Bone Diseases and Disorders of Mineral Metabolism, 2nd ed. New York: Raven Press; 1993:15–21.
4. Parfitt AM. Morphologic basis of bone mineral measurements: transient and steady state effects of treatment in osteoporosis. Min Electr Metab 1980; 14:273–287.
5. DeLuca HF. Vitamin D revisited. Clin Endocrinol Metab 1980; 9:1–26.
6. Vaananen HK. Pathogenesis of osteoporosis. Calcif Tissue Int 1991 (suppl); 49: S11–S14.
7. Epstein FH. Bone marrow, cytokines, and bone remodeling: emerging insights into the pathophysiology of osteoporosis. N Engl J Med 1995; 332(5):305–311.
8. Mundy GR. Cytokines and growth factors in the regulation of bone remodeling. J Bone Miner Res 1993; 8(2):S505–S510.
9. Arnaud CD. An integrated view of the role of the endocrine system in the genesis of the osteoporosis associated with aging. Osteoporos Int 1993 (suppl); 1:S37–S39.
10. Gowen M, Wood DD, Russell RGG. Stimulation of the proliferation of human bone cells in vitro by human monocyte products with interleukin 1 activity. J Clin Invest 1985; 75:1223–1229.
11. Simon L. Pathogenesis of osteoporosis. Bull Rheum Dis 1993; 42(5):1–3.
12. Heaney RP, Recker RR, Saville PD. Menopausal changes in bone remodeling. J Lab Clin Med 1978; 92:964–970.
13. Marcus R. Understanding osteoporosis. West J Med 1991; 155:53–60.
14. Mazzuoli GF, D'Erasmo E, Minisola S, et al. Pathogenetic aspects of involutional osteoporosis. Clin Rheumatol 1989; 8(2):22–29.
15. Eriksen EF, Berg NJ, Graham ML, et al. Multiple sex steroid receptors in cultured human osteoblast-like cells. In: Jensen J et al, eds. Abstracts of the International Symposium on Osteoporosis, Denmark, 1987:N.67.
16. Fleming LA. Osteoporosis: clinical features, prevention, and treatment. J Gen Int Med 1992; 7:554–562.
17. Marcus R, Madvig P, Young G. Age-related changes in parathyroid hormone and parathyroid hormone action in normal humans. J Clin Endocrinol Metab 1984; 58: 223–230.
18. Girasole G, Jilka RL, Passeri G, et al. 17-Beta-estradiol inhibits interleukin-6 production by bone marrow–derived stromal cells and osteoblasts in vitro—a potential mechanism for the antiosteoporotic effect of estrogens. J Clin Invest 1992; 89: 883–891.
19. Mack PB, LaChance PA, Vose GP, et al. Bone demineralization of foot and hand of Gemini-Titan IV, V, and VII astronauts during orbital flight. AJR 1967; 100:503–511.
20. Cormier C. Physiopathology and etiology of osteoporosis. Curr Opin Rheumatol 1991; 3:457–462.
21. Lohman T, Going S, Pamenter R, et al. Effects of resistance training on regional and total bone mineral density in premenopausal women: a randomized prospective study. J Bone Miner Res 1995; 10(7):1015–1024.
22. Pollitzer WS, Anderson JJB. Ethnic and genetic differences in bone mass: a review with a hereditary vs. environmental perspective. Am J Clin Nutr 1989; 40:1244–1259.

23. Edelson GW, Kleerekoper M. Bone mass, bone loss, and fractures. Physical Med Rehab Clinics N Amer 1995; 6(3):455–464.
24. Krall EA, Dawson-Hughes B. Heritable and lifestyle determinants of bone mineral density. J Bone Miner Res 1993; 8:1–9.
25. Elias AN, Gwinup G. Immobilization osteoporosis in paraplegia. J Am Paraplegia Soc 1992; 15(3):163–170.
26. Slemenda CW, Johnston CC. High intensity activities in young women: site specific bone mass effects among female figure skaters. Bone Miner 1993; 20(2):125–132.
27. Morrison NA, Qi JC, Tokita A, et al. Prediction of bone density from vitamin D receptor alleles. Nature 1994; 367:284–287.
28. Nilas L. Assessment of the physiological bone loss in women, with special emphasis on the menopausal changes. Danish Med Bull 1991; 38(4):317–327.
29. Thomsen K, Gotfredsen A, Christiansen C. Is post-menopausal bone loss an age-related phenomenon? Calcif Tissue Int 1986; 39:123–127.
30. Odell WD, Heath H III. Osteoporosis: pathophysiology, prevention, diagnosis, and treatment. DM 1993; XXXIX(11):789–868.
31. Koppelman MCS, Kurtz DW, Morrish KA, et al. Vertebral body bone mineral content in hyperprolactinemic women. J Clin Endocrinol Metab 1984; 59:1050–1053.
32. Seeman E, Szmukler GI. Formica C, et al. Osteoporosis in anorexia nervosa: the influence of peak bone density, bone loss, oral contraceptive use, and exercise. J Bone Miner Res 1992; 7(12):1467–1474.
33. Drinkwater BL, Nilson K, Chestnut CH III, et al. Bone mineral content of amenorrheic and eumenorrheic athletes. N Engl J Med 1984; 311:277–281.
34. Jackson JA, Kleerekoper M, Parfitt AM. Symptomatic osteoporosis in a man with hyperprolactinemic hypogonadism. Ann Intern Med 1986; 105:543–545.
35. Finkelstein JS, Klibanski A, Neer RM, et al. Osteoporosis in men with idiopathic hypogonadotropic hypogonadism. Ann Intern Med 1987; 106:354–361.
36. Stepan JJ, Lachman M, Zverina J, et al. Castrated men with bone loss: effect of calcitonin treatment on biochemical indices of bone remodeling. J Clin Endocrinol Metab 1989; 69:523–527.
37. Jackson JA, Kleerekoper M, Parfitt AM, et al. Bone histomorphometry in hypogonadal and eugonadal men with spinal osteoporosis. J Clin Endocrinol Metab 1987; 65:53–58.
38. Diamond T, Stiel D, Posen S. Osteoporosis in hemochromatosis: iron excess, gonadal deficiency, or other factors. Ann Intern Med 1989; 110:430–436.
39. Gilchrist N, Espiner EA, Cook HB. Familial short stature and coeliac disease: a family case report. N Z Med J 1983; 96(736):563–565.
40. Jackson JA, Kleerekoper M. Osteoporosis in men: diagnosis, pathophysiology, and prevention. Medicine 1990; 69(3):137–152.
41. Riggs BL, Melton LJ III. Evidence for two distinct syndromes of involutional osteoporosis. Am J Med 1983; 75:899–901.
42. Lindsay R. Osteoporosis: A Guide to Diagnosis, Prevention, and Treatment. New York: Raven Press; 1992.
43. Anderson JJ, Pollitzer WS. Ethnic and genetic differences in susceptibility to osteoporotic fractures. Adv Nutr Res 1994; 9:129–149.

44. Hopper JL, Seeman E. The bone density of female twins discordant for tobacco use. N Engl J Med 1994; 330:387–392.
45. Diamond T, Stiehl O, Lunzer M, et al. Ethanol reduces bone formation and may cause osteoporosis. Am J Med 1989; 86:282–288.
46. Gallagher JC. Pathophysiology of osteoporosis. Semin Nephrol 1992; 12(2):109–115.
47. Kannus P, Haapasalo H, Sievanen H, et al. The site-specific effects of long-term unilateral activity on bone mineral density and content. Bone 1994; 15(3):279–284.
48. Nilsson BE, Andersson SM, Havdrup T, Westlin NE. Ballet-dancing and weight-lifting—effects on BMC. AJR 1978; 131:541–542.
49. Orwoll ES, Bliziotes M. Heterogeneity in osteoporosis: men versus women. Rheum Dis Clin North Am 1994; 20(3):671–689.
50. Seeman E. The dilemma of osteoporosis in men. Am J Med 1995; 98(suppl 2A): 765–885.
51. McSheehy PMJ, Chambers TJ. Osteoblastic cells mediate osteoclastic responsiveness to parathyroid hormone. Endocrinology 1986; 118(2):824.
52. Seeman E, Wahner HW, Offord KP, et al. Differential effects of endocrine dysfunction on the axial and appendicular skeleton. J Clin Invest 1982; 69:1302–1309.
53. Bone HG III. The dynamics of osteoporosis. In: Kelley WN, Harris ED Jr, Ruddy S, Sledge, CB, eds. Textbook of Rheumatology. Philadelphia: WB Saunders; 1994:2–14.
54. Lukert BP, Raisz LG. Glucocorticoid-induced osteoporosis: pathogenesis and management. Ann Intern Med 1990; 112:352–364.
55. Sambrook PN, Jones G. Corticosteroid osteoporosis. Br J Rheumatol 1995; 34:8–12.
56. Joseph JC. Corticosteroid-induced osteoporosis. Am J Hosp Pharm 1994; 52:188–197.
57. Baran DT, Braverman LE. Editorial: Thyroid hormones and bone mass. J Clin Endocrinol Metab 1991; 72(6):1182–1183.
58. Krolner B, Jorgensen JV, Nielsen SP. Spinal bone mineral content in myxoedema and thyrotoxicosis. Effects of thyroid hormone(s) and antithyroid treatment. Clin Endocrinol (Oxf) 1983; 18:439–446.
59. Peerenboom H, Keck E, Kruskemper HL, Strohmeyer G. The defect of intestinal calcium transport in hyperthyroidism and its response to therapy. J Clin Endocrinol Metab 1984; 59:936–940.
60. Selby PL. Osteopenia and diabetes. Diabet Med 1988; 5:423–428.
61. McKenna MJ. Miscellaneous causes of osteoporosis. In: Favus MJ, ed. Primer on the Metabolic Bone Diseases and Disorders of Mineral Metabolism, 2nd ed. New York: Raven Press; 1993:258–262.
62. Kaplan FS. Osteoporosis. Pathophysiology and prevention. Clin Symp 1993; 39(1): 2–32.
63. Chines A, Pacifici R, Avioli LV, et al. Systemic mastocytosis presenting in osteoporosis: a clinical and histomorphometric study. J Clin Endocrinol Metab 1991; 72: 140–144.
64. Baron R, Gertner JM, Lang R, Vighery A. Increased bone turnover with decreased bone formation by osteoblasts in children with osteogenesis imperfecta tarda. Pediatr Res 1983; 17:204–207.
65. Kivirikko KI. Collagens and their abnormalities in a wide spectrum of diseases. Ann Med 1993; 25(2):113–126.

66. Gray JR, Bridges AB, Mole PA, et al. Osteoporosis and the Marfan syndrome. Postgrad Med J 1993; 69(811):373–375.
67. Piper BA, Galsworthy TD, Bockman RS. Clinical insights from the etiopathology of osteoporosis. Contemp Int Med 1995; 7(5):58–68.
68. Cooper C, Coupland C, Mitchell M. Rheumatoid arthritis, corticosteroid therapy, and hip fracture. Ann Rheum Dis 1995; 54:49–52.
69. Greenstein AJ, Janowitz HD, Sacher DB. The extra-intestinal complications of Crohn's disease and ulcerative colitis in a study of 700 patients. Medicine 1976; 55:401–412.
70. McCaughan GW, Feller RB. Osteoporosis in chronic liver disease: pathogenesis, risk factors, and management. Dig Dis 1994; 12:223–231.
71. Meys E, Fontanges E, Fourcade N, et al. Bone loss after orthotopic liver transplantation. Am J Med 1994; 97:445–450.
72. Nisbeth V, Lindh F, Ljunghall S, et al. Fracture frequency after kidney transplantation. Transplant Proc 1994; 26:1764.
73. Massari PU, Garay G, Ulla MR. Bone mineral content in cyclosporine-treated renal transplant patients. Transplant Proc 1994; 26:2646–2648.
74. Heaney RP. Nutritional factors in osteoporosis. Annu Rev Nutr 1993; 13:287–316.
75. De Vernejoul MC, Bielakoff J, Herve M, et al. Evidence for defective osteoblastic function. A role for alcohol and tobacco consumption in osteoporosis in middle aged men. Clin Orthop 1983; 179:107–115.
76. Hahn HJ. Steroid and drug-induced osteopenia. In: Favus MJ, ed. Primer on the Metabolic Bone Diseases and Disorders of Mineral Metabolism, 2nd ed. New York: Raven Press; 1993:250–255.
77. Mazanec DJ, Grisanti JM. Drug-induced osteoporosis. Clev Clin J Med 1989; 56(3): 297–303.
78. Rich GM, Mudge GH, Laffel GL, Leboff MS. Cyclosporine A and prednisone-associated osteoporosis in heart transplant recipients. J Heart Lung Transpl 1992; 11(5):950–958.
79. Spencer H, Kramer L. Osteoporosis: calcium, fluoride, and aluminum interactions. J Am Coll Nutr 1986; 4(1):121–128.

2

Biochemistry and Histology of Osteoporosis

ERIK FINK ERIKSEN

Aarhus Amtssygehus
Aarhus, Denmark

TORBEN STEINICHE and KIM BRIXEN

Aarhus University Hospital
Aarhus, Denmark

I. INTRODUCTION

This chapter deals with two different approaches to the analysis of bone remodeling: assessment by biochemical markers in serum or urine, and histological analysis of bone biopsies. Both approaches have undergone tremendous technical developments in recent years and have contributed immensely to our understanding of the skeleton and its most prevalent disease—osteoporosis.

Bone remodeling constitutes the lifelong renewal process of bone whereby the mechanical integrity of the skeleton is preserved. It implies the continuous removal of bone (bone resorption) followed by synthesis of new bone matrix and subsequent mineralization (bone formation). Moreover, bone remodeling is an integral part of the calcium homeostatic system together with the kidneys and the gut. The ongoing removal of old bone by osteoclastic resorption and subsequent coupled osteoblastic formation of new bone leads to liberation of calcium and matrix constituents to serum. The liberation of calcium to the serum pool creates the basis for calcium kinetic methods for estimation of whole skeletal metabolism. The matrix constituents liberated to blood during bone resorption can be used as markers of bone resorption in serum or urine, and components liberated during osteoblastic matrix synthesis are putative markers of bone formation.

Disturbances in bone remodeling lead to alterations in bone architecture—removal of structural elements followed by loss of mechanical competence and fractures. Restoration of bone structure and mechanical competence can only be achieved if these processes are reversed by treatment regimens creating a positive balance between resorption and formation. Thorough understanding of bone remodeling is therefore very important, not only in relation to clinical decision making, interpretation of bone marker levels in serum, and bone mass assessment or calcium kinetic indices, but also for the design of more effective treatments of metabolic bone diseases.

On the following pages we will describe the biochemistry of the most important biochemical markers and relate them to the histological changes observed in normal and osteoporotic bone.

II. BIOCHEMICAL MARKERS OF BONE TURNOVER

In recent years, several specific and sensitive biochemical assays facilitating noninvasive and repeated measurement of bone turnover have been developed (Table 1). In addition to technical demands on precision, accuracy, and specificity, such markers should be validated by comparison with independent measurement of bone formation and resorption at organ level (i.e., combined calcium kinetics and balance studies) or at least tissue level (i.e., histomorphometric analyses of bone biopsies) and not merely by clinical experience. Although some of the markers are highly specific for bone formation or resorption, these two processes tend to vary in the same direction in almost all clinical situations due to the tight coupling between formation and resorption discussed above. The markers, however, relate to different aspects of the remodeling process, have different metabolic pathways and different sensitivity and sources of error, and thus offer additive information.

Table 1 Validated Biochemical Markers of Bone Turnover

Osteoblastic activity	Osteoclastic activity
S-alkaline phosphatase	U-Hydroxyproline (U-OHPr)
Total alkaline phosphatase (S-tAP)	U-collagen crosslinks
Bone alkaline phosphatase (S-bAP)	Pyridinoline (U-Pyr)
S-osteocalcin (S-BGP)	Deoxypyridinoline (U-D-Pyr)
S-carboxyterminal propeptide of human type I collagen (S-PICP)	S-C-terminal pyridinium crosslinked telopeptide domain of type I collagen (S-ICTP)
	S-Tartrate-resistant acid phosphatase (S-TRAP)

S, assessment in serum; U, assessment in urine.

A. Biochemical Markers of Bone Formation

The ideal marker of bone formation should be a structural protein released to the blood in a rate proportional to its incorporation into bone, and the fraction of release should be unchanged by disease. It should have a well-characterized function and should not be released unaltered during bone resorption. Furthermore, its metabolic pathway and serum half-life should be known.

Osteoblasts produce collagen, a number of noncollagenous matrix protein, and enzymes participating in the regulation of bone mineralization. Although none of these meet all the ideal demands, several can be measured in serum as fairly reliable indicators of osteoblastic activity.

1. Alkaline Phosphatase

Total alkaline phosphatase (tAP) is still the most widely used bone marker in clinical work. Three isoenzymes encoded by separate genes are found in blood: liver-bone-kidney AP, intestinal AP, and placental AP (1). Thus, liver and bone isoforms are only distinguished by subtle differences in posttranslational glycosylation. The functional enzyme is bound as tetrameres to cell membranes and cytoplasmatic vesicles (2) while serum tAP seems to represent spillover.

AP may have several physiological substrates. It splits inorganic phosphate from organic phosphate, increasing the calcium-phosphate product and enabling mineralization, but also splits inorganic pyrophosphate, which is a potent inhibitor of mineralization. Furthermore, it splits phosphoetanolamine and pyridoxal-5′-phosphate. Mutations in the functional region of the enzyme as seen in *hypophosphatasia* are characterized by varying degrees of osteomalacia and rickets, indicating that AP is essential for normal mineralization of bone (3). Serum tAP is markedly increased in osteomalacia, induced by vitamin D deficiency. This is probably explained by the focal nature of this disease and due to the often secondary hyperparathyroidism seen in this condition. Even in this condition, however, serum tAP activity is closely correlated with mineralization rate as measured by calcium kinetics (3).

Bone AP (bAP) constitutes approximately 50% of serum AP (4,5) and has a serum half-life of 24–48 hours. Despite this relatively long half-life, it varies in a circadian rhythm, with peak levels in the afternoon and at night (6). The exact metabolic pathway is unknown, but clearance is independent of renal function.

AP activity in serum is measured spectrophotometrically using p-nitrophenyl phosphate as substrate (7). Bone and liver AP may be separated by electrophoresis (4,8), but this method yields only semiquantitative results and is time-consuming. bAP may be determined by precipitation with wheat germ lectin which preferentially binds to the glycosylated bAP (9–11) or by inactivation with heat or urea

(12). Finally, bAP concentration may be measured using two antibodies with small differences in affinity toward the isoforms (13). All the above methods, however, have their shortcomings, and there is some evidence suggesting that the metabolism of bAP is altered in certain liver diseases such as primary biliary cirrhosis (14).

a. Total Alkaline Phosphatase (tAP) in Osteoporosis. The majority of osteoporotic patients exhibit normal tAP levels. Thus, when increased AP levels are encountered in osteoporosis, either a new recent fracture or osteomalacia should be suspected first. The latter condition will lead to much higher levels as recent fracture. Hulth et al. (15) reported tAP levels of 6.7 ± 2.0 U in osteoporotics (normals range 2–8 U). Twelve patients revealed high levels, of 10–14 U, without histological evidence of osteomalacia. Delmas et al. (16) studied 62 postmenopausal women with at least one low-energy fracture and normal routine serum biochemistries. When compared to 142 matched controls the osteoporotic women exhibited a significant 27% increase in tAP and 23% had levels > SD (16). Charles et al. (3) reported mean levels of tAP in a group of 52 osteoporotics to be significantly increased when compared to 22 controls, but the controls were somewhat younger (Table 2).

In osteoporosis tAP correlates poorly to bone mass (15,16), but significant correlations to calcium accretion have been reported by Lauffenburger et al. ($r = 0.69$; $P < .01$) (17) and Charles et al. ($r = 0.48$; $P > .001$) (3) (Table 3). In the material of Lauffenburger et al. (17), poor correlations between tAP and bone histomorphometric indices of bone formation (osteoid and osteoblastic surfaces) were found. Based on histomorphometric evaluation of bone biopsies, Brown et al. (18) subdivided an osteoporotic material into three groups: low-turnover, normal-turnover, and high-turnover. Serum tAP levels were not different among the three groups.

Table 2 Serum Levels of Carboxyterminal Propeptide of Human Procollagen Type I (S-PICP), Osteocalcin (S-BGP), Alkaline Phosphatase (S-AP), and Serum Crosslinked Carboxyterminal Telopeptide of Human Collagen Type I (S-ICTP) (mean ± SD) in Normals and Patients With Osteoporosis

	N	S-PICP μg/L	S-BGP μg/L	S-AP U/L	S-ICTP μg/L
Normals	22	114 ± 22	14.7 ± 5.9	127 ± 30	2.3 ± 0.6
Osteoporosis	52	112 ± 47	18.2 ± 5.9**	200 ± 52***	4.0 ± 5.3***

*$P < .05$.
**$P < .01$.
***$P < .001$.

Table 3 Linear Regression Analysis of Serum Markers of Bone Formation: Serum Carboxyterminal Propeptide of Human Procollagen Type I (S-PICP), S-alkaline Phosphatase (S-AP), S-Osteocalcin (S-BGP), and One Marker of Bone Resorption Serum Crosslinked Carboxyterminal Telopeptide of Human Collagen Type I (S-ICTP) on the Calcium Kinetic Index of Bone Formation (mineralization rate (m)) in Normal Subjects, Metabolic Bone Disease, and Osteoporosis

Marker	*r*	*P*	SEE	SEE/Y	Marker	*r*	*P*	SEE	SEE/Y
Normals (n = 22)					Osteoporosis (n = 52)				
S-PICP	0.53	<.05	2.0	0.44	S-PICP	0.49	<.001	1.8	0.50
S-BGP	0.20	NS	—	—	S-BGP	0.45	<.001	1.9	0.53
S-AP	0.15	NS	—	—	S-AP	0.48	<.001	2.2	0.61

r: regression coefficient.
P: level of significance; NS: not significant.
SEE: standard of error of estimate.
SEE/Y: Standard error of estimate divided by mean value of dependent variable.

The osteoblastic production of alkaline phosphatase has been found to be increased in osteoporosis (3) (Fig. 1). After correction for turnover by division with the calcium kinetic mineralization rate, S-tAP was found to be increased (45 U/L/mmol/day vs. 25 U/L/mmol/day in controls). The reason for this difference is unknown.

b. Bone Alkaline Phosphatase (bAP) in Osteoporosis. Stepan et al. (19) reported bAP to be significantly increased in osteoporosis (16.4 U/L (range 11.1–24.4) vs. 9.2 U/L (7.1–12.0 in controls). Bone alkaline phosphatase was increased in 60% of osteoporotics, but tAP was only increased in 22%. Farley et al. (20) also reported increased levels in 43 patients with osteoporosis (10.4 ± 7.2 U/L vs. 7.1 ± 3.6 U/L in controls). The serum levels of bAP did not correlate to tAP in this study.

In conclusion, tAP is not a good marker of osteoporosis. Bone alkaline phosphatase reveals more pronounced increases in osteoporosis, but the overlap to normals precludes a specific diagnosis based on this enzyme alone.

2. *Osteocalcin*

Osteocalcin, also called bone γ-carboxy glutamic acid-containing protein (BGP), is the most abundant noncollagenous matrix protein of bone, comprising 1–2% of total bone protein (21,22). It is solely produced by osteoblasts (23) and odontoblasts (24), and remains the most specific marker of osteoblastic activity. It consists of 49 amino acids (molecular weight (MW) 5800) and is unique due to its content of three glutamic acid residues which in varying degrees are carboxylated by a vitamin K–dependent process to γ-carboxy glutamic acid, providing the molecule with a strong affinity toward hydroxyapatite (Fig. 2) (25). The physio-

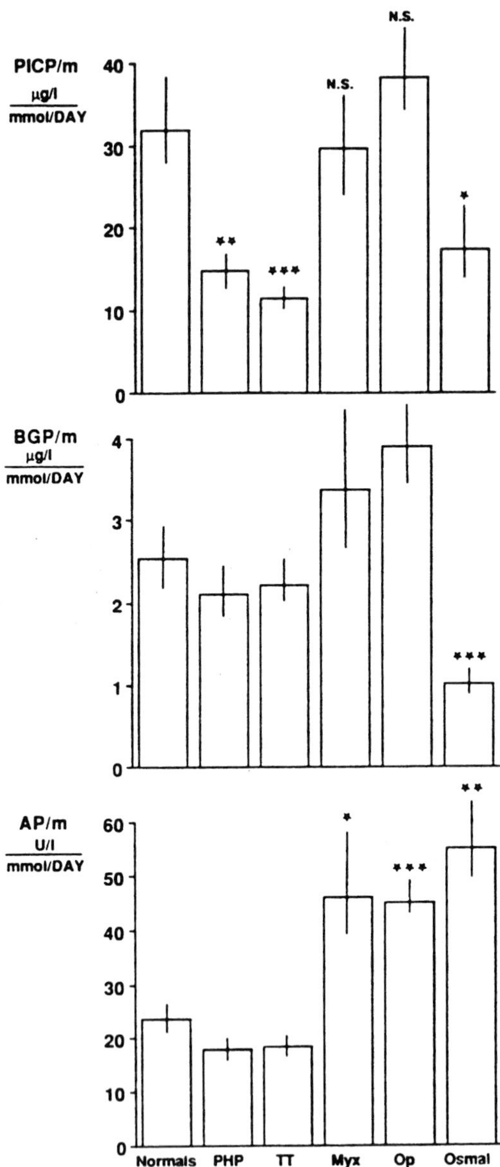

Figure 1 Synthesis of carboxyterminal propeptide of human procollagen type I (S-PICP), osteocalcin (S-BGP), alkaline phosphatase (S-AP) at the osteoblastic level (S-PICP/m, S-BGP/m, S-AP/m, respectively) in osteoporosis (Op) compared to other metabolic bone diseases (primary hyperparathyroidism (PHP), thyrotoxicosis (TT), myxedema (Myx), and osteomalacia (Osmal). Serum levels of the different bone markers are expressed as percent of values obtained in normals. Error bars denote 95% confidence intervals for the mean. (Reproduced with permission from Charles et al. (3).)

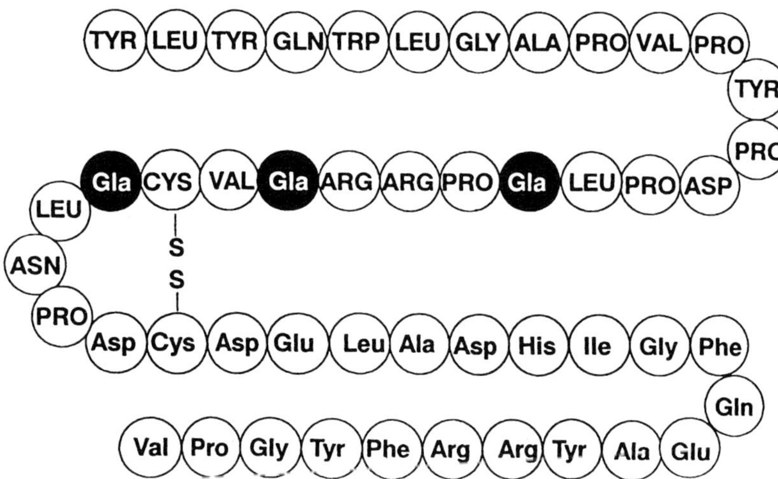

Figure 2 Structure of osteocalcin. Note the 3 GLA residues.

logical significance of osteocalcin is still unknown, but its structure is highly conserved through evolution (26). The secretion of osteocalcin is highly dependent on $1,25(OH)_2D_3$, which increases the transcription of the osteocalcin gene (27,28). Osteocalcin inhibits precipitation of hydroxyapatite and may be involved in the regulation of matrix mineralization. Furthermore, it attracts osteoclast precursors chemotactically (29), and resorption of osteocalcin-deprived bone is retarded (29-31), suggesting that it may be involved in the regulation of bone resorption. Osteocalcin found in serum results from de novo synthesis, and no intact osteocalcin seems to be released during bone resorption (23,32). Osteocalcin is cleared by the kidneys, and serum levels thus depend on renal function (33). Moreover, serum half-life is short (25–70 minutes) (34), and consequently serum osteocalcin varies in a circadian rhythm (35).

Serum osteocalcin can be measured by radioimmunoassay (RIA), enzyme-linked adsorbent assay (ELISA) methods (36–38), and several assays are commercially available. Recently, dual-antibody assays measuring only intact osteocalcin have been presented (39). Serum level of osteocalcin is greatly influenced by several endocrine (vitamin D status (40), menstruation cycle (41), circadian rhythm (35), alcohol (42), and season (43)). Strictly controlled sampling conditions are therefore needed to secure proper evaluation of osteocalcin levels.

a. Osteocalcin in Osteoporosis. In patients with postmenopausal osteoporosis, osteocalcin levels have been reported as being normal (44,45) or slightly elevated (16,46). In one study bone mass was found to be negatively correlated to bone mass ($r = 0.36$; $P < .001$) (16). Osteocalcin also reflects bone formation as assessed by histomorphometry. Brown et al. (44) found significant correlations between osteoid and tetracycline-based parameters measured in bone biopsies obtained from 22 patients with untreated postmenopausal osteoporosis. In the same study, patients with low turnover exhibited mean osteocalcin levels of 2.9 ± 0.9 ng/mL, while the mean level in high turnover osteoporosis was 9.7 ± 0.8 ng/mL.

In a study on 52 osteoporotics Charles et al. (3) found mean BGP levels of 18.2 ± 5.9 ng/mL vs. 14.7 ± 5.9 ng/mL ($P < .01$) (Table 2). A significant correlation between S-BGP and bone mineralization rate assessed by calcium kinetics was also demonstrable ($r = 0.45$; $P < .001$). Osteocalcin production at the osteoblastic level is similar to that of normal individuals. In another study osteoporotic patients were found to display reduced osteocalcin levels, while tAp was similar to levels found in nonosteoporotic women (47). The differences may be explained by differences in bone mass between the two populations.

During corticosteroid treatment or in vitamin D deficiency states osteoblastic synthesis of BGP is reduced due to direct inhibition at the cellular level (Fig. 1). In other conditions BGP synthesis at the osteoblastic level is also relatively constant (Fig. 1), making this serum marker the most accurate marker of osteoblastic activity and bone turnover so far (3).

3. *Type I Procollagen Propeptide (PICP)*

Collagen comprises more than 90% of the organic bone matrix (48) of which 97% is type I collagen and only minute amounts are of types III, V, and IX (3%), mostly localized in blood vessels within bone (49). Collagen is synthesized as procollagen-containing peptide extensions in both the C- and N-terminal ends which are cleaved from the rest of the molecule before its incorporation into collagen fibrils (Fig. 3). These propeptides are produced in equimolar ratios to collagen production similar to the C-peptide of insulin (50). PICP is cleared from the blood by the liver (51). It has a very short serum half-life (in rats 6–8 minutes) and shows a pronounced circadian variation (52,53). Despite structural similarities, procollagen peptides from different collagen types differ immunologically, and type I procollagen propeptide can be measured by commercially available RIA (54). Though several connective tissues apart from bone (especially skin) also contain type I collagen, their contribution to serum PICP seems to be small in most situations. This view is supported by experimental evidence from pigs demonstrating that the concentration of PICP in lymph and serum are similar (55). In women, PICP increases by 34% between the ages 50 and 83 (56).

a. PICP in Osteoporosis. Due to the novelty of PICP, the clinical data pertaining to osteoporosis are sparse. Charles et al. (3) could not demonstrate any difference in PICP levels in osteoporosis and normal controls (112 ± 47 μg/L vs. 114 ± 22 μg/L) (Table 2). A significant correlation to bone mineralization at the organ level as assessed by calcium kinetics ($r = 0.49$; $P < .001$) (Table 3) was, however, demonstrable. In osteoporosis the osteoblastic synthesis of PICP seems similar to that of controls (3) (Fig. 1).

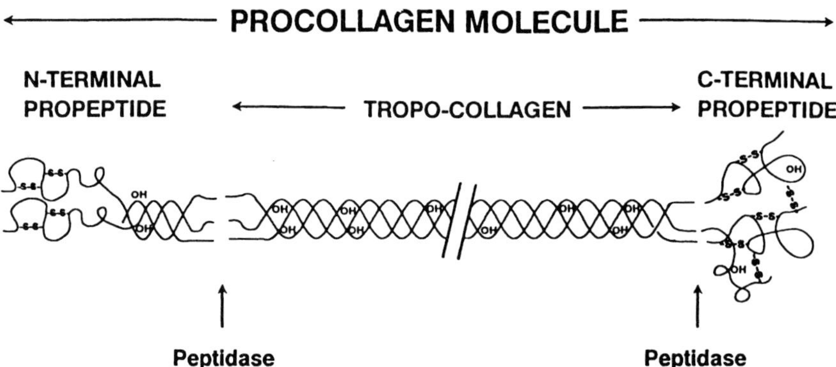

Figure 3 Structure of type I collagen. The peptide is synthesized as a propeptide with two propeptides (C- and N-terminal). After synthesis the two propeptides are split off by peptidases.

B. Biochemical Markers of Bone Resorption

The ideal marker of bone resorption should be a degradation product of a matrix component not found in any other tissue. Its serum level should not be under separate endocrine control, and it should not be reutilized in new bone formation. During the degradation of collagen, several metabolites are released into circulation and excreted in the urine, some of which are specific for bone or predominantly originate from bone. Furthermore, osteoclasts produce several enzymes, among which tartrate-resistant acid phosphatase, with some reservations, may be used as a marker of bone resorption. The close metabolic control of both calcium absorption, excretion, and nonresorptive release from bone, as well as reutilization during bone formation, however, precludes the use of serum levels or urinary calcium excretion as a measure of bone resorption.

1. Hydroxyproline

Collagen is unique by its high content of hydroxyproline (approximately 13%) (57). Hydroxyproline is formed by the vitamin C–dependent hydroxylation of the nonessential amino acid proline and contributes by formation of hydrogen bonds significantly to the stability of collagen fibrils (50) as illustrated by the inferior quality of collagen in scurvy. During collagen breakdown hydroxyproline is released into circulation in free, oligopeptide- and polypeptide-bound forms. Free hydroxyproline is excreted in the urine but completely reabsorbed and degraded in the liver while the peptide-bound fractions are excreted in the urine (57). A significant proportion of urinary hydroxyproline, however, originates from the breakdown of nonbone collagen, degradation of procollagen propeptides, and intracellular breakdown of collagen chains (i.e., collagen formation) (58). Finally, a gelatine-restricted diet is necessary during urine collection since dietary hydroxyproline is readily absorbed (57). Alternatively, spot urine collected after an overnight fast may be used if hydroxyproline concentration is expressed in relation to creatinine concentration (59). Hydroxyproline is measured by colorimetry (57,60) or high-pressure liquid chromatography (HPLC) (61).

a. Hydroxyproline in Osteoporosis. Similar to most other biochemical markers in osteoporosis, urinary hydroxyproline excretion has been found to be normal in most studies on osteoporotic populations (44,62,63). If the distributions are studied, however, 30% of osteoporotics exhibit levels above the normal range (62).

In a group of 34 untreated women with postmenopausal osteoporosis Gallagher et al. (62) reported a linear correlation between urinary hydroxyproline excretion and organ level bone resorption rate as assessed by calcium kinetics ($r = 0.59$; $P < .001$). Lauffenburger (17) found the same correlation in a group of 15 osteoporotics ($r = 0.77$), but surprisingly enough, urinary hydroxyproline correlated inversely to cancellous bone erosion surface in the same material ($r = -0.53$; $P < .05$). A similar inverse correlation to osteoclastic erosion surface was also reported by Whyte et al. (63). The reason for the negative correlations to erosion surface are probably explained by the fact that erosion surface is a bad measure of bone resorption. Further studies employing newer methods for the histomorphometric assessment of bone resorption (64) are clearly needed to resolve this apparent discrepancy.

2. *Collagen Crosslinks*

The individual collagen molecules are held together by hydrogen bonds and covalent crosslinks (50). The structure of the latter varies among the different types of collagen, and in collagen types I, II, III, and IX, crosslinks of pyridinoline (Pyr) and deoxypyridinoline (D-Pyr) structure are found (Fig. 4) (65). Crosslink formation is initiated enzymatically within the matrix following the aggregation of collagen molecules into fibers (66,67). The $\alpha 1$ and $\alpha 2$ chains of type I collagen has four and three potential crosslinking sites, respectively (Fig 4). There is one locus in each of the nonhelical C- and N-terminal regions (telopeptide regions) and two or one sites, respectively, approximately 90 residues from each terminus within the helical part of the molecules (66). Pyridinolines are not degraded during bone resorption but circulate in serum as part of peptide fragments and are excreted in the urine as free (30%) and peptide-bound (70%) pyridinolines (66). Pyr is found in bone and cartilage and in small quantities in other types of collagen (68). D-Pyr is found almost exclusively in bone and dentin and only in minute amounts in aorta and ligaments (68–70). Since neither of the pyridinolines is found in the skin and collagen turnover in the aforementioned tissues is slow in comparison with bone, it may be assumed that most of the pyridinoline (and in

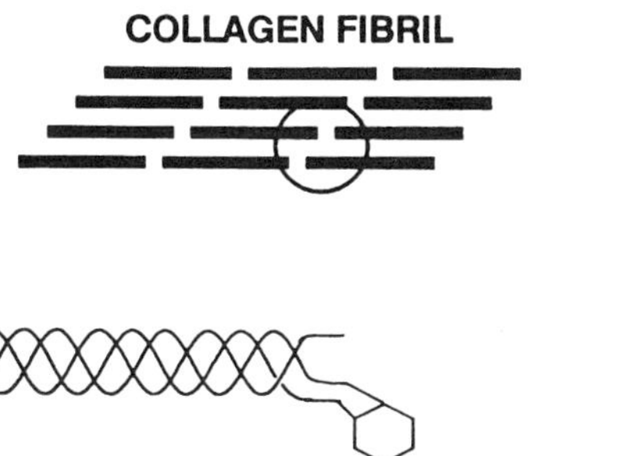

Figure 4 During deposition in bone matrix, type I collagen chains are linked together with crosslinks, creating an ordered staggered array (upper panel). The crosslink consists of a 6-C carbon ring connecting two collagen molecules. The α1 and α2 chains of type-I collagen have four and three potential crosslinking sites, respectively. There is one locus in each of the nonhelical C- and N-terminal regions (telopeptide regions) and two or one sites, respectively, approximately 90 residues from each terminus within the helical part of the molecules. Following degradation of type I collagen during bone resorption, the crosslink circulates in serum as part of the C-terminal crosslinked telopeptide domain of type I collagen (ICTP), which can be assessed using RIA. After further metabolism a smaller fragment containing the crosslink portion is excreted in urine and can be estimated by HPLC.

particular D-Pyr) in urine originates from bone. This is supported by excellent correlation between pyridinoline excretion and bone resorption rate as measured by tracer kinetics (71).

Thus, pyridinolines have the following advantages over hydroxyproline: non-bone collagen contributes much less to crosslinks, thus obviating dietary restraints during urine collection; and only bone collagen that has matured contributes. Finally, Pyr and D-Pyr in the diet do not appear to be absorbed (72). Both urinary pyridinoline excretion (73) and the serum levels of the C-terminal pyridinoline-crosslinked telopeptide of type I collagen (ICTP) vary in a circadian rhythm (53).

Total urinary Pyr and D-Pyr can be measured by HPLC using fluorescence detection after hydrolysis of the sample (74). A commercial ELISA for measurement of free Pyr is, furthermore, available. Recently, an RIA detecting ICTP in serum has been described and validated (75). Finally, an ELISA measuring ICTP has been described (76). Pyridinoline excretions are excellent markers of bone turnover around menopause. In a recent study, deoxypyridinoline was found to increase 82% after cessation of ovarian estrogen secretion (77). A less pronounced increase of 34% was described by Eastell et al. (56).

a. Collagen Crosslinks in Osteoporosis. Pyridinolines correlate significantly to erosion surface in osteoporotics ($r = 0.35–0.45$) (78). In a recent study of 12 osteoporotics Eastell et al. (71) reported a very high correlation between crosslink excretion in urine and bone resorption ($r = 0.92$; $P < .001$). This result makes urinary collagen crosslinks one of the best markers of bone resorption currently available.

We have found the correlation between the serum marker of bone resorption (pyridinoline crosslinked telopeptide regions of collagen type I (S-ICTP) and resorption assessed by calcium kinetics to be poor, though significant ($r = 0.40$; $P < .01$) (Table 3).

3. *Tartrate-Resistant Acid Phosphatase (TRAP)*

Acid phosphatases are a group of lysosomal enzymes capable of hydrolyzing phosphomonoesters under acid conditions. They are found in bone, prostate, thrombocytes, erythrocytes, and the spleen. TRAP is measured by spectrophometric methods (79).

There are at least six isoenzymes (types 0–5), which can be separated electrophoretically (80). Type 5, which is resistant to tartrate inhibition, is found in the spleen, placenta, lung macrophages, epidermis, and bone, but these subtypes differ slightly in respect to substrate specificity and kinetics. In bone, osteoclasts produce TRAP as, adhering to the bone surface by their ruffled border, they release several lysozomal enzymes dissolving the bone (81). TRAP varies with bone turnover—e.g., in relation to treatment with sex steroids (82). In practice, however, it has been difficult to measure bone TRAP without contamination from other sources. Furthermore, the release of TRAP does not necessarily reflect the work performed by the osteoclasts, as exemplified by patients with type II autosomal-dominant osteopetrosis who have high levels of TRAP but severely decreased bone resorption.

4. *Potential New Bone Markers*

Several other noncollagenous bone proteins found in serum or urine may prove useful as bone markers in the future but have not been fully evaluated. *Matrix GLA protein* is, like osteocalcin, a vitamin K–dependent protein produced by osteoblasts (83). It appears before osteocalcin in developing bone; however, it is also produced by cartilage and other connective tissues. There is some evidence that MGP and osteocalcin are produced by osteoblasts of different phenotype. *Osteonectin* is a glycoprotein found in bone, but it is also produced by thrombocytes and released during the coagulation process (49). It binds to collagen and has several calcium binding sites and may play a role in mineralization. *Osteopontin* (bone sialoprotein) is a sialic acid–rich protein probably involved in cell-matrix adhesion, but it is produced by several other tissues apart from bone (49).

C. Variation with Age and Sex

Both markers of formation and resorption are high during childhood and decreases after puberty (84,85). In later life, serum osteocalcin (86), bone AP (87), and urinary pyridinoline and hydroxyproline excretion (86,88) tend to increase slowly with age, especially in women, while no increase is seen in PICP (89). In accordance with the increase in turnover observed by histomorphometry, bone markers increase in women around the menopause, whether spontaneous or surgical (Fig. 5) (90,91).

D. Role of Biochemical Markers in Diagnostic Workup

Assessment of bone turnover is important for the interpretation of bone mass measurements made by DEXA-scans (dual energy x-ray absorptiometry), which

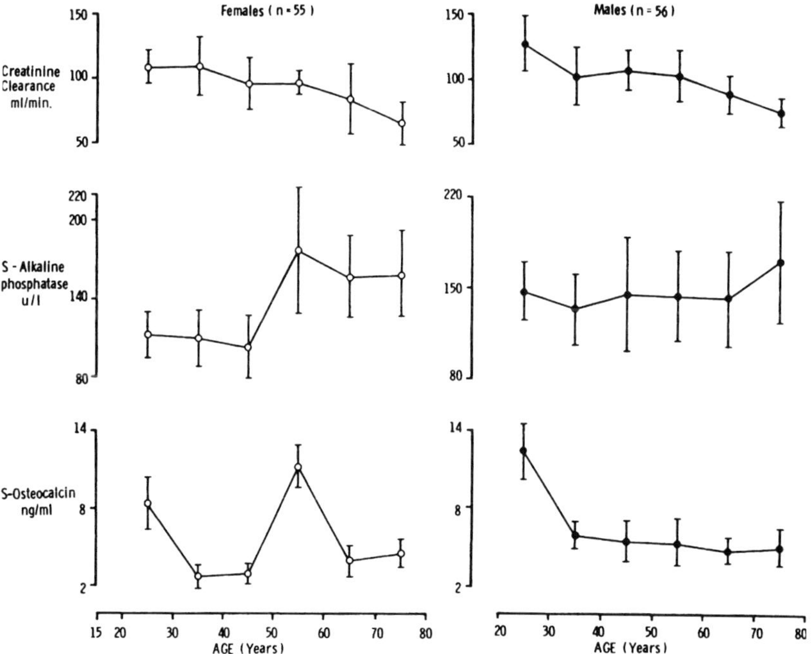

Figure 5 Age-dependent changes in formative bone markers (alkaline phosphatase and osteocalcin). Note the marked increase for both markers around menopause in women. Changes in creatinine clearance are shown in both sexes to demonstrate that it is changes in bone turnover and not reduced renal function that is responsible for the increase in osteocalcin. (Reproduced with permission from Eriksen EF, Osteoporosis, NOVO-Nordisk A/S (1991).)

have become widely available in recent years. Significant changes in "bone mass" may be accounted for merely by changes in bone turnover due to two mechanisms. First, increased turnover leads to an increase in the remodeling space (see section B). Second, it decreases the mean age of the bone, and since newly formed bone is less mineralized than old bone, the mineral content will decrease, leading to apparent osteopenia. Patients with high turnover due to thyrotoxicosis, for instance, may prove to have normal bone mass, when the high-turnover state is cured by antithyroid treatment. In theory, apparent bone mass may change 4–8% as a result of turnover changes alone (83), and this corresponds to the changes seen in many treatments; indeed, there is experimental evidence that the increase in "bone mass" seen following estrogen-progesterone treatment is mainly due to these mechanisms (92).

E. Evaluation of Bone Turnover in Relation to Decisions on Treatment

There is some histomorphometric evidence suggesting a bimodal distribution of bone turnover in patients with postmenopausal osteoporosis. In the study of Arlot et al. (93), patients with high turnover (30%) had lower bone mass, fewer trabeculae, but also increased serum osteocalcin compared with those with normal turnover (70%), and it was suggested that the former group had decreased formative capacity at the level of the individual osteoblasts. The distribution of turnover rates probably varies with general calcium intake of the population studied and the resulting degree of secondary hyperparathyroidism. Thus, treatment trials employing calcium supplements should always be evaluated against this background.

Antiresorptive treatment regimens like estrogen/progestogen, bisphosphonates, and calcitonin act mainly by reducing bone turnover. They have not been shown to significantly change bone balance in humans. Thus they act mainly by protecting against irreversible bone loss due to trabecular perforations (92,94,95). These widespread regimens will therefore theoretically be most effective in high-turnover states. Indeed, in a recent study on the effects of calcitonin, high-turnover osteoporotics were found to respond most favorably (96).

Around menopause most women will be in a high-turnover state (Fig. 5). Thus, all the antiresorptive regimens will probably be effective. In the later postmenopause, however, some osteoporotics will exhibit normal and low turnover, and antiresorptive regimens will have a limited effect. The decision whether to employ an antiresorptive regimen or an anabolic treatment (fluoride or PTH) should therefore probably rely on prior assessment of bone turnover. In this setting bone markers are prime candidates for the evaluation of bone turnover, and with the knowledge summarized above, serum osteocalcin or collagen crosslinks seem to be the most sensitive markers.

F. Monitoring Treatment

It has been shown in several studies that estrogen and estrogen-progesterone treatment decreases bone turnover (97). This reduction is reflected in lower levels of serum osteocalcin, AP, PICP, urinary hydroxyproline, and pyridinoline excretion (98–100). Bisphosphonates also efficiently slow down turnover as measured both histomorphometrically (101) and biochemically (102). Similarly, salmon calcitonin decreases bone turnover as measured biochemically. In contrast, serum osteocalcin and AP increase during treatment with fluoride (103), which stimulates bone formation. Not all patients respond favorably to this treatment, and it has been proposed that biochemical markers of bone turnover could be used to identify responders. Data on this, however, are contradictory (103–106).

G. Evaluation of Bone Balance With Biochemical Markers

It is tempting to propose that bone balance could be evaluated noninvasively by means of two or more biochemical markers of bone turnover. Bone balance is, however, the small difference between two large numbers (i.e., volume of bone formed − volume of bone resorbed). With most biochemical markers carrying errors of 10–15% in assay error, it is obvious that evaluation in single individuals is impossible. Whether reasonable estimates in large grouped materials can be achieved remains to be established.

H. Prediction of Bone Loss

Bone turnover increases around the menopause. The decrease in bone mineral content in the period 2–4 years thereafter as measured by photon absorptiometry can be predicted by a combination of biochemical bone markers. This has been proposed as a screening procedure to identify women at high risk of developing osteoporosis (107). Several questions, however, remain unanswered. First, there is evidence that a substantial proportion of women change their rate of bone loss in both directions during long-term follow-up (108). Second, there are no long-term studies linking women with high bone turnover immediately after the menopause with increased fracture incidence at the age when osteoporosis usually becomes evident, i.e., 15–20 years later. Finally, most subjects above the age of 40 or 50 *are* in negative bone balance at BMU level, and high turnover in these subjects *will* lead to increased bone loss, but some subjects—certainly those at a younger age—have positive balance at BRU level and do not suffer bone loss in relation with high turnover. Thus, the above generalization, which may well be applied on groups of patients, cannot be applied on individual patients. In our opinion, therefore, it is premature to implement a screening strategy based on biochemical markers of bone turnover.

III. BONE MATRIX IN OSTEOPOROSIS

Mutations in the α1(I) and α2(I) chains of type I collagen have been demonstrated to cause osteogenesis imperfecta, and a few cases with such mutations phenotypically overlapping with osteoporosis (109) have been reported, but there are no definite biochemical disturbances in the vast majority of patients with osteoporosis and thus no diagnostic biochemical tests.

Shapiro et al. described a family with osteopenia and abnormal collagen chains (110), and other cases were found to exhibit abnormal levels of type III and type II collagen in their bone matrix (111). In a recent study Diebold et al. (111) extracted collagen from bone obtained from individuals over an age range of 22–93 years. They were able to demonstrate that the degree of hydroxylation of the α2(I) collagen chain correlated inversely with trabecular bone volume. They also found a higher degree of hydroxylation in postmenopausal women when compared to premenopausal levels. The abnormalities described above are, however, diverse and have only been described in a very limited number of osteoporotics. Thus, whether a generalized defect of osteoblastic collagen synthesis can be characterized in osteoporotic patients is still an open question.

For osteocalcin, disturbances in γ-carboxylation (112) or glycation (113) have been implicated in the development of osteoporosis. Reduced γ-carboxylation of osteocaclin might theoretically interfere with binding to hydroxypatite. Indeed, vitamin K supplementation has been shown to normalize bone turnover in osteoporotics and increase hydrozyapatite binding of serum osteocalcin (112). However, no clear separation between osteoporotics and normal controls has been demonstrated so far.

IV. BONE HISTOMORPHOMETRY AND OSTEOPOROSIS

Throughout life, bone is renewed through internal reorganization, by which bone is turned over by localized osteoclastic resorption followed by osteoblastic formation (remodeling) (114) (Fig. 6). In adults, bone remodeling accounts for more than 90% of normal bone turnover. Cancellous bone is continuously renewed by these processes in order to adjust architecture to changes in prevailing mechanical forces, to preserve the viability of the embedded osteocytes, and to avoid stress fractures. The remodeling process may further be essential for the microfracture repair. Remodeling is regulated by a number of systemic hormones and local cytokines.

A unique feature of bone is that remodeling leaves traces behind, traces that can be quantitated using microscopical and stereologic analysis. Moreover, bone lends itself to incorporation of a time marker (115). This feature creates the basis for the calculation of rates of activity for the different cell types (95,115). Quantitative bone histology is the only method by which alterations in cellular activity can be separated from changes in cell number. Other techniques of calcium metabolic research (e.g., bone densitometry, assays for biochemical markers in serum, calcium kinetics) only yield data on tissue or organ activity. Consequently these indices are the products of individual cell activity and number of cells.

Recently, advanced stereological methods have further facilitated accurate measurements of all elements in cancellous and cortical bone remodeling and allowed a three-dimensional reconstruction of the remodeling sequence in normals and in various bone diseases (95,116). By the use of these methods on iliac crest bone biopsies from normals, and from osteoporotic patients before and after various treatment regimens and in diseases related to osteoporosis, new knowledge is added to the growing understanding of the pathophysiology of osteopenia and how to prevent and/or treat it.

Age-related bone loss is an inescapable condition, affecting all groups that have been studied, whether defined on the basis of sex, race, economic status, geographic location, or historical epoch (117). In normal individuals, peak bone mass is reached at age 25–35 years, and thereafter a decrease with age occurs in both sexes (118). All women are furthermore subject to an accelerated bone loss after menopause (119,120). Furthermore, the loss of trabecular volume with age seems to be accompanied by structural changes which may reduce the strength of the bone to a greater extent than the reduction in the amount of bone itself would suggest (121–125). Because of either a low peak bone mass (126) or a more pronounced bone loss and/or more pronounced changes in bone structure with age or during menopause, a significant proportion of women and men over 50 reach the fracture threshold for bone mass and suffer spontaneous fractures (symptomatic osteoporosis).

A. Bone-Remodeling Sequence

Remodeling occurs as a distinct sequence of events in both cancellous and cortical bone (Fig. 6). After activation, osteoclasts start to erode and form a resorption cavity. When a certain resorption depth is reached, the osteoclasts are replaced by mononuclear cells, which complete the resorption. The resorption period lasts for about 4–6 weeks, and the end result of the resorptive process is a resorption lacuna with a certain final resorption depth. After completion of resorption, preosteoblasts invade the resorption cavity, differentiate to osteoblasts, and start bone matrix formation. After a certain period of time, the initial mineralization lag time, the bone matrix is subsequently mineralized to lamellar bone. Osteoblasts will now continue to form bone matrix, which subsequently will mineralize (mineralization lag time) and thereby refill the lacunae with lamellar bone and thus in essence repair the resorption-mediated defect. Some of the osteoblasts are incorporated during this process in the matrix and later mineralized bone as osteocytes. These osteocytes are interconnected by canaliculi and connected to surface lining

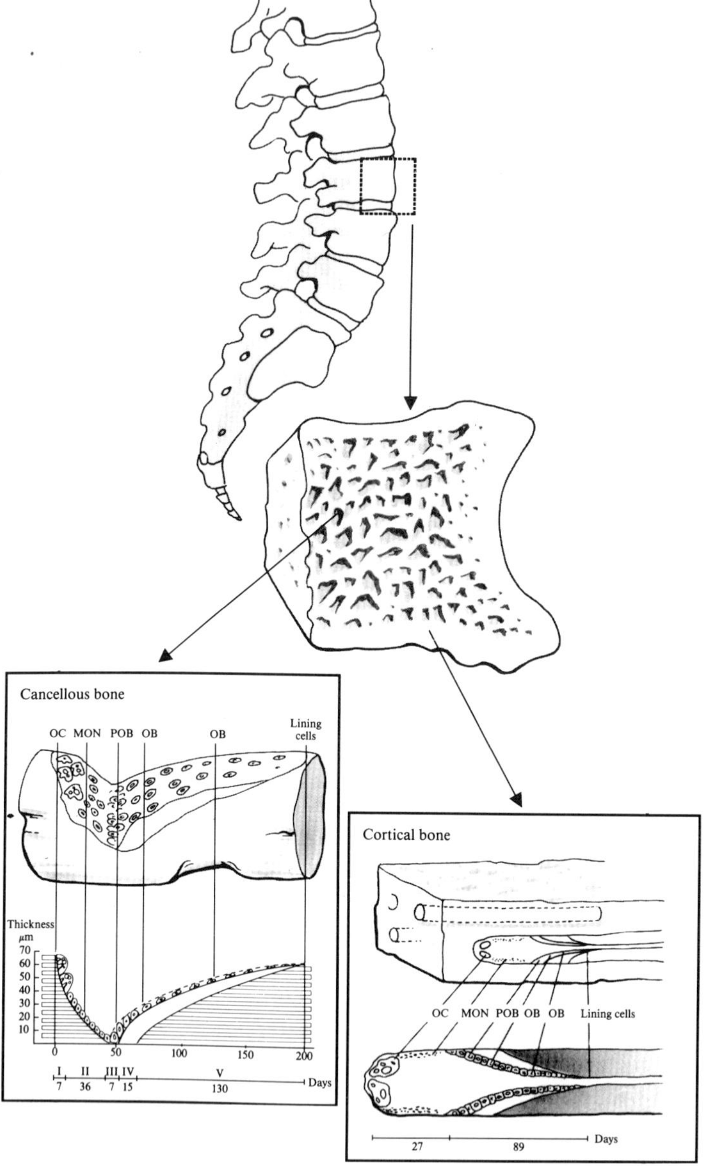

Figure 6 Remodeling in cancellous and cortical bone. In cortical bone the bone multicellular unit (BMU) consists of a tunnel (cutting cone) drilled out by advancing osteoclasts (OC) followed by mononuclear (MON) cells. In younger normal individuals the resorption period lasts around 30 days. Bone formation is initiated by the emergence of preosteoblasts (POB) in the BRU. Later on, preosteoblasts differentiate into osteoblasts (OB) that form a

cells, which occur after the end of formation. The duration of the bone formation period is 2–3 months, and the end result is a new bone structural unit (BSU), characterized by a certain thickness (mean wall thickness).

As described above, resorption and formation are closely associated with each other both temporally and spatially (64,114,115,127). In the normal remodeling process, resorption will always be followed by formation, and formation will always be preceded by resorption. The frequency by which a given place on the trabecular bone surfaces undergoes remodeling is termed the activation frequency.

B. Bone Remodeling and Bone Loss

As described previously bone mass significantly decreases with age in both men and women (118), and in osteoporotic patients a further reduction is observed (128). Therefore it is not surprising that age is a main risk factor for both types of primary osteoporosis. Bone may be gained or lost by the remodeling process by three different mechanisms.

1. Reversible Bone Loss/Gain

The remodeling space is the amount of bone that has been removed by osteoclasts and is not yet reformed by the osteoblasts during the remodeling sequence (129). The total remodeling space within the skeleton depends on the number of ongoing remodeling cycles, the duration of the resorptive and formative periods, and the depths of the resorption lacunae. In normal individuals the remodeling space is around 6–8% of the skeletal volume (131). An increase in activation frequency leads to an increase in the number of ongoing remodeling cycles. This will increase the remodeling space and thereby proportionally decrease the amount of bone (Fig. 7). Obviously the opposite effect is seen if the activation frequency is decreased. The process is reversible because the remodeling space and thus the bone volume return to normal when the metabolic challenge to the bone is removed.

---

matrix, which subsequently becomes mineralized and fills out the tunnel except for a central Haversian canal (closing cone). The formative period lasts 90 days. The finished new Haversian system constitutes a new cortical bone structural unit (BSU).
In cancellous bone the sequence of events is identical, except that the process takes place on trabecular surfaces. The resorption period lasts about 50 days in younger individuals, and can be subdivided into an osteoclastic period (I), a mononuclear period (II), and a preosteoblastic period (III). Matrix formation lasts 15 days (IV), followed by mineralization for another 130 days (V). Thus after a total of around 150 days a new cancellous BSU is formed. (Reproduced with permission from Eriksen EF, Osteoporosis, NOVO-Nordisk A/S (1991).)

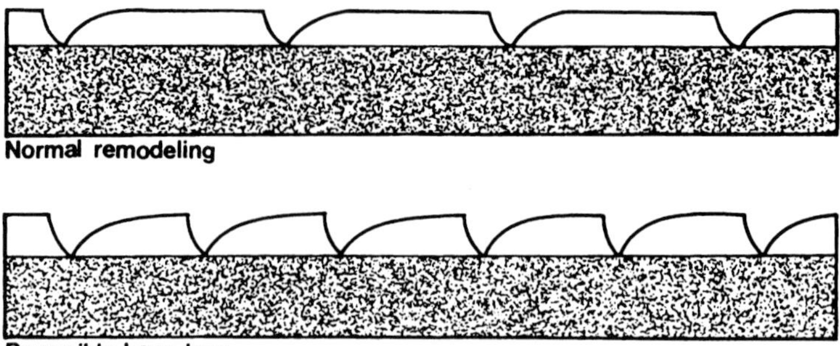

Figure 7 High-turnover states may lead to a transient deficit of bone due to resorption preceding formation (reversible bone loss). The remodeling space is the amount of bone temporarily missing due to ongoing remodeling. If bone turnover is increasing, this space will increase and an apparent decrease in bone mass will be detectable. If, however, bone turnover goes down again, the remodeling space will be reduced and an apparent increase in bone mass will be detectable. Such changes are primarily responsible for the changes in bone mass observed after treatment with antiresorptive drugs such as estrogen, bisphosphonates, and calcitonin.

2. *Irreversible Bone Loss/Gain by Changes in Bone Balance*

In normal young adults, the amount of bone formed by the osteoblasts at the modeling site is equal to the amount of bone previously resorbed. An imbalance may occur leading to a thinning of the trabeculae and osteopenia (Fig. 8). Obviously, an increase in trabecular thickness will occur if the bone balance per remodeling site is positive.

3. *Irreversible Loss of Whole Trabecular Elements*

A very deep resorption lacuna may perforate a trabecular plate, removing the basis for the subsequent bone formation, and thereby cause a loss of a structural element and a disintegration of the trabecular network (122) (Fig. 8). The risk of trabecular plate perforations depends on the activation frequency, resorption depth, and trabecular thickness. Antiresorptive regimens mainly protect bone mass by lowering bone turnover, thus reducing the risk for perforations. Although the loss of bone volume by this mechanism may be limited, the effect on the biomechanical competence (strength) may be very pronounced (123). Recent studies have demonstrated that women exhibit a more pronounced degree of perforative resorption (130) (Fig. 9).

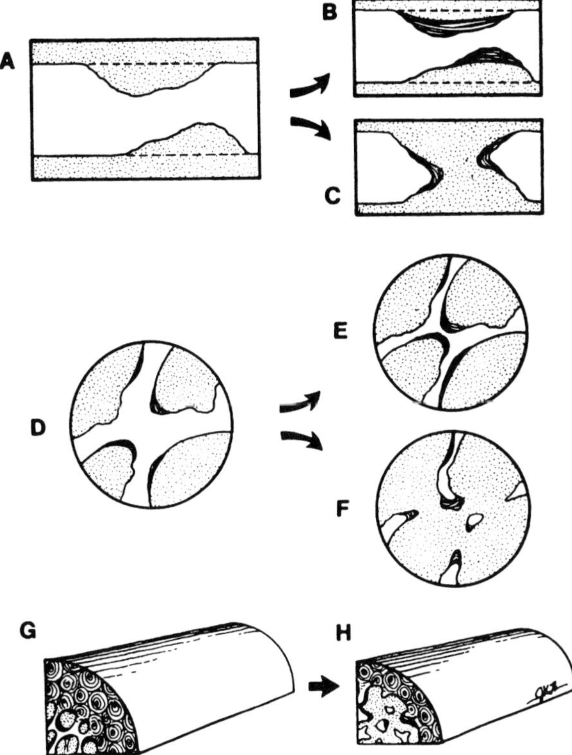

Figure 8 Irreversible bone loss may occur either through thinning of trabeculae (A → B and D → E), perforation of trabeculae (A → C and D → F), or thinning of cortical bone (G → H). (Reproduced with permission from Eriksen et al. New Developments in Medicine, Matthew Bender and Co. Inc., New York 1987; 2:11–23.)

4. *Implications for Bone Mass Measurements*

Due to the differences in architecture and bone remodeling, cortical and cancellous bone have different mechanisms of bone loss, which may lead to different alterations in bone densitometry in different areas of the skeleton dependent on the proportion of cancellous bone to cortical. Changes in turnover not only lead to changes in porosity and absolute bone mass, but also affect the mean bone age. As older bone is more heavily mineralized than younger bone, changes in mean bone age introduce an extra variable (131–133). Mathematical modeling based on the histomorphometry data available suggests that bone mass measurements may be off by 40% from "true" bone mass in extreme cases; more commonly, however,

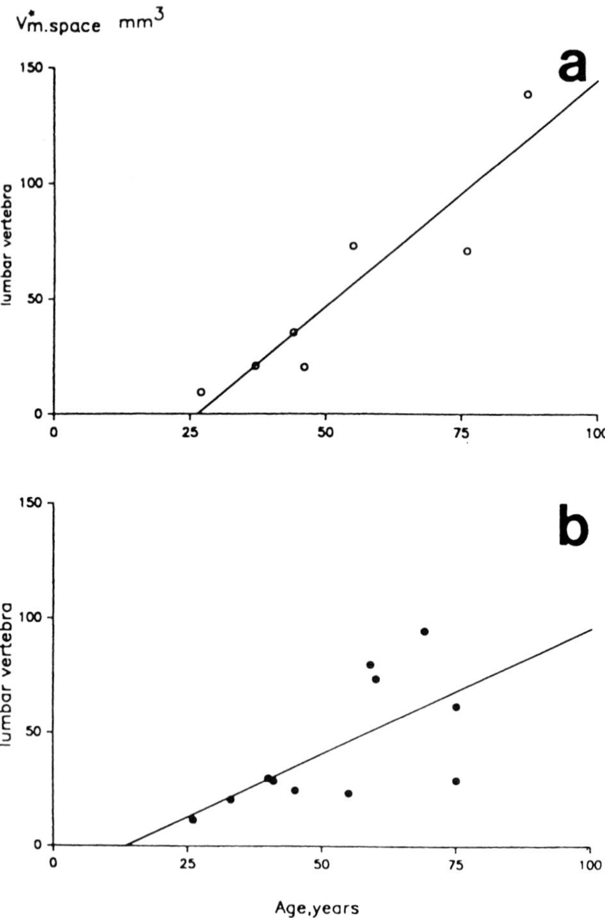

Figure 9 Age-dependent changes in marrow star volume in women (a) and men (b). The marrow star volume is a measure of the degree of perforative resorption in bone. Note the pronounced increase with increasing age. (Redrawn with permission from Vesterby A, et al. Bone 1990; 11:46–59.)

the deviation amounts to 5–10% (131,132). It is important to take these processes into consideration if one is dealing with bone density measurements; otherwise, false conclusions may be reached.

When analyzing the changes in bone mass obtained using different treatment regimens, three different patterns stand out (Fig. 10). One variant shows a 5–10% increase in bone mass after 1 year; then bone mass levels off and ultimately starts

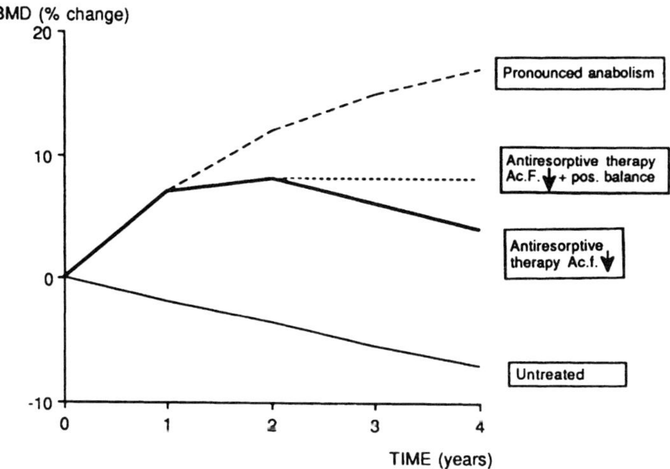

Figure 10 Characteristic patterns for changes in bone mineral density (BMD). Untreated subjects will undergo age-dependent or accelerated bone loss (lower curve). Curves describing changes in bone mass associated with antiresorptive treatment regimens like estrogen, bisphosphonates, or calcitonin mostly exhibit a plateau after 2–3 years (two curves in the middle). Later on, either complete stabilization of bone mass or a slower decline, probably attributable to age-dependent bone loss, has been described. In the former case a certain degree of positive bone balance has to be present to offset the inevitable age-dependent bone loss. A pure anabolic regimen (e.g., fluoride or parathyroid hormone) will result in a steady increase during treatment, as shown in the upper curve. (Reproduced with permission from Eriksen et al. Handbook of Experimental Pharmacology (Mundy GR, Martin TJ eds.). Springer Verlag 1993; 107:67–109.)

to decrease. This initial increase is explained by a lowering of bone turnover, leading to an apparent increase in bone mass. Ultimately, after 2–3 years, however, the age-dependent bone loss offsets the initial gain, and bone mass goes down again. This pattern is seen in some reports on bone mass changes after antiresorptive therapy (estrogen/progestogen (134–136), bisphosphonates (94), and calcitonin (137). Other papers dealing with effects of antiresorptive therapy describe the same initial gain in bone mass, around 5–10%, but then bone mass stays constant (136). Provided no change of radiation source in the BMD apparatus or mean bone age occurs, this pattern can only be explained by a certain anabolic effect offsetting the age-dependent bone loss. The third pattern shows a gradual increase in bone mass over the treatment period. This development is explained by a pronounced anabolic effect leading to pronounced changes in bone balance, and has only been reported after fluoride (138) or parathyroid hormone (139) treatment so far.

C. Bone Loss in Osteoporosis

Bone mass at any age is the result of two variables—the amount of bone achieved during growth and maturation, and the subsequent rate of age-related bone loss. A stochastic model of bone loss published by Horsman et al. (*Lunar News* 1989) suggested that about two-thirds of all hip fractures are found in women who at skeletal maturity were in the lowest quartile of BMD (bone mineral density). Thus, peak BMD at maturity, and not the rate of postmenopausal bone loss, is in the above-mentioned investigation considered of greatest importance in determining lifetime fracture risk.

Peak bone mass depends on bone growth and bone modeling. The growth and modeling of the skeleton results from its genetic makeup, nutritional and hormonal factors, and mechanical demands (126).

The reduction in estrogen production after menopause increases bone turnover for an unknown period of time. The mechanism behind the perimenopausal high-turnover state is still subject to discussion, but reduced circulating estrogen levels may enhance the stimulating effect of circulating parathyroid hormone on bone remodeling (140). The increased bone turnover induces a reversible as well as an accelerated irreversible bone loss. Such changes in bone remodeling taking place around menopause cannot be expected to be present in bone biopsies obtained 10–15 years later. In order to gain information of the pathophysiology of osteoporosis, longitudinal studies are necessary to investigate further not only bone dynamics in osteoporotic patients but also the dynamics taking place during the normal menopause.

In epidemiological studies, obesity has been shown to be protective against bone loss after menopause (141,142). An inverse relation between body weight and hip fracture rate has been reported in several studies (143,144). Obesity may protect the skeleton in several ways. An increased conversion of adrenal androgens to estrogen in the fat tissue may protect against the abrupt decrease in estrogen level after the menopause and thus the accelerated bone loss during this period (145). Obese individuals may be less likely to fall because of inactivity, and when a fall does occur, the extensive body fat may act as a buffer absorbing the fall energy and thereby protecting against fractures (144). Obesity during childhood may also induce changes in bone modeling, which may increase peak bone mass and alter the bone architecture in a more favorable direction. During growth and modeling obese individuals develop a greater skeleton with larger cortical areas and larger marrow spaces (146). Thus, the absolute amount of trabecular bone is normal, but distributed over a larger space. This hypothesis is supported by the fact that the largest biopsy lengths were found in subjects who had been suffering from obesity since childhood.

Trabecular bone volume is reduced by 20–30% in osteoporotic patients compared with age- and sex-matched normal controls, but a substantial overlap exists.

Several studies have shown that beside the slight reduction in trabecular bone volume, significant differences in microstructure exist between osteoporotic patients and normal controls. Parfitt et al. (128) found that the reduction in trabecular bone volume observed in patients with osteoporotic vertebral fracture was mainly due to a reduction in plate density and not in thickness. Only in patients with hip fracture did trabecular thinning contribute substantially to the additional loss of trabecular bone. Kimmel et al. (147) and Arlot et al. (93) both found a highly significant reduction in trabecular number (around 30%) and a significant increase in trabecular separation (around 40%) in patients with postmenopausal osteoporosis compared with normal controls. Unlike Parfitt et al. (128), trabecular thickness was found slightly reduced in both studies in the osteoporotic patients (11% and 22%, respectively). The data suggest that besides a moderate loss of trabecular bone mass, osteoporotic patients have significant structural changes with a discontinuity of the trabecular lattice due to perforations.

The mechanical properties of trabecular bone depend on structural continuity as well as on the amount of bone present. Discontinuity of the trabecular lattice due to perforations may produce greater loss of strength than the same extent of bone loss due to thinning of the trabecular plate alone. Mosekilde (148,149) has shown that the vertebral bone mass expressed as the ash density from the age of 20 years to the age of 80 decreased to 50%, whereas the vertical compressive stress decreased to 25% and the horizontal compressive stress to only 5% of the value at the age of 20. That changes in the trabecular structure may be a key factor in the development of osteoporosis is supported by a recent study by Recker et al. (150). In this study transiliac bone biopsies were obtained from 23 patients with postmenopausal osteoporosis with manifest vertebral compression fractures and matched by trabecular bone volume with 23 normal controls. Although the patients and controls had the same trabecular volume, histomorphometric measurements of trabecular microstructure showed significant differences between the two groups, suggesting a loss of trabecular connectivity in the patients. Osteoporotic patients exhibited reduced bone surface density, increased trabecular thickness, reduced trabecular number, and greater trabecular separation.

D. Bone Remodeling in Osteoporosis

Are there any changes in the ongoing remodeling process in the osteoporotic patients that can explain the observed changes in bone volume and especially in bone structure? Various and conflicting answers to this question have been reported in the literature (63,147,151,152).

In 50 untreated postmenopausal osteoporotic patients Arlot et al. (151) found a wide spectrum of bone turnover as compared with normal controls. Based on a bimodal distribution of cancellous osteoid perimeter, patients were subdivided into two groups: one with normal turnover, and one with high turnover, representing 30% of the cases. In our own studies on osteoporotic patients, the data for bone turnover did not deviate from a log-normal distribution (no bimodality), and no subsets of osteoporotic patients could be identified. Likewise, Kimmel et al. (149) were unable to identify subgroups of osteoporotic patients in a large study. In the study by Recker et al. (150) the change in microstructure was not accompanied by changes in bone remodeling dynamics.

In a study from the Mayo Clinic comprising 89 osteoporotic women, Eriksen et al. (152) found a significant negative bone balance (Fig. 11). This imbalance was mainly due to a significant reduction in wall thickness. Age-matched women without spinal fractures did not show any significant imbalance. Darby and Meunier (153) and Cohen-Solal et al. (154) also reported a significant reduction in wall thickness in osteoporotic patients. In a Danish study of osteoporotic women, however, the negative balance between resorption and formation in osteoporotic patients did not deviate from the balance in age-matched controls.

Steiniche et al. (147) studied 66 patients with postmenopausal spinal osteoporosis and 25 normal controls from our center. No significant difference in the extent of resorptive or formative (osteoid covered) surfaces was observed. For the

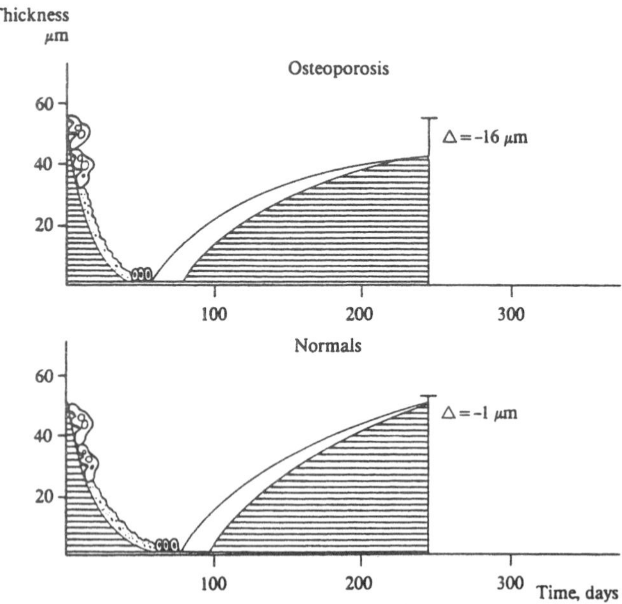

Figure 11 Bone remodeling sequences in osteoporotic women and age-matched controls. Note the more pronounced negative balance in osteoporotics. (Reconstruction based on data from Eriksen EF et al. (1990). J Bone and Mineral Res 5:311–319.)

tetracycline-based data the control group (n = 13) was considerably younger, and this probably explains the observed reduction in bone formation rate and adjusted appositional rate in the patients. In a study of 90 women with postmenopausal osteoporosis compared with 34 healthy postmenopausal normal controls, Kimmel et al. (147) found no major differences in the dynamic indices of bone remodeling. Thus it seems that osteoporotic patients comprise a very heterogeneous group with patients having low, normal, or even increased bone turnover. A similar conclusion was drawn by Whyte et al. (63).

V. CONCLUSION

Although the results concerning static and dynamic remodeling parameters and bone balance in clinically manifest osteoporosis are not completely concordant, the persisting negative bone balance in adult life and hormonal changes around menopause with increased risk of perforations seem to be of primary importance. Most studies point toward an osteoblastic defect as the main factor behind this negative balance in osteoporosis. Whether osteoporotic women exhibit excessive imbalance around menopause is still unsettled. However, if this is the case, the high turnover in the postmenopausal period would tend to exacerbate bone loss in this group of individuals. Although minor changes in matrix biochemistry have been described in osteoporotic subjects, bone loss due to excessive remodeling imbalance still seems to be the most plausible explanation for the low bone mass in osteoporosis.

The longitudinal data available so far suggest that it is peak bone mass more than bone turnover that is the main determinant for later osteopenia and fracture. Thus, securing attainment of peak bone mass seems to be a major task in the long-term prophylaxis against osteoporosis. For the current large population of women with low peak bone mass at risk for osteoporotic fracture, the main task will be to protect against excessive bone loss in individuals by antiresorptive treatment with estrogens or bisphosphonates.

The biochemical bone markers currently available cannot be used for the diagnosis of osteoporosis, and they are too imprecise for the noninvasive evaluation of bone balance. They are well suited for monitoring changes in bone turnover in longitudinal studies, and in the future they will probably enable clinicians to separate a high-risk group of women. Recent data obtained by Wand et al. (155) suggest that osteoporotic women exhibit a prolonged high-turnover state after menopause. If this observation holds up to further study, bone markers may play an increasing role in the diagnostic workup of individuals at risk.

The best markers currently available for clinical use seem to be osteocalcin for evaluation osteoblastic activity, and pyridinium crosslinks for assessment of bone resorption. It has to be kept in mind, however, that all women exhibit high turnover after menopause, and it is still an open question, which cutoff level to choose for a given marker in order to get maximal separation between the population at risk and normal women.

REFERENCES

1. Weiss MJ, Henthorn PS, Lafferty MA, Slaughter C, Raducha M, Harris H. Isolation and characterization of a cDNA encoding a human liver/bone/kidney-type alkaline phosphatase. Biochemistry 1986; 83:7182–7186.
2. Hamilton BA, Mcphee JL, Hawrylak K, Stinson RA. Alkaline phosphatase releasing activity in human tissues. Clin Chim Acta 1990; 186:249–254.
3. Charles P, Hasling C, Risteli L, Risteli J, Mosekilde L, Eriksen EF. Assessment of bone formation by biochemical markers in metabolic bone disease: separation between osteoblastic activity at the cell and tissue level. Calcif Tissue Int 1992; 51: 406–411.
4. Hoof VO, Haylaerts MF, Geryl H, Mullem M, Leputre LG, Broe ME. Age and sex distribution of alkaline phosphatase isoenzymes by agarose electrophoresis. Clin Chem 1990; 36:875–878.
5. Brixen K, Nielsen HK, Eriksen EF, Charles P, Mosekilde L. Efficacy of wheat germ lectin-precipitated alkaline phosphatase in serum as an estimator of bone mineralization rate: comparison to serum total alkaline phosphatase and serum bone Gla-protein. Calcif Tissue Int 1989; 44:93–98.
6. Nielsen HK, Brixen K, Mosekilde L. Diurnal rhythm in serum activity of wheat-germ lectin-precipitable alkaline phosphatase: temporal relationships with the diurnal variation of serum osteocalcin. Scand J Clin Lab Invest 1990; 50:851–856.
7. Keiding R, Hörder M, Gerhardt W, et al. Recommended methods for the determination of four enzymes in the blood. Scand J Clin Lab Invest 1974; 33:291–306.
8. Onica D, Sundblad L, Waldenlind L, Shanwell A. Characterization of serum alkaline phosphatase isoenzymes by affinity electrophoresis in agarose gel containing lectin combined with agar gel electrophoresis. Scand J Clin Lab Invest 1987; 47:239–245.
9. Brixen K, Nielsen HK, Eriksen EF, Charles P, Mosekilde L. Efficacy of wheat germ lectin-precipitated alkaline phosphatase in serum as an estimator of bone mineralization rate: comparison to serum total alkaline phosphatase and serum bone gla-protein. Calcif Tissue Int 1989; 44:93–98.
10. Rosalki SB, Foo AY. Two new methods for separating and quantifying bone and liver alkaline phosphatase isoenzymes in plasma. Clin Chem 1984; 30:1182–1186.
11. Behr W, Barnert J. Quantification of bone alkaline phosphatase in serum by precipitation with wheat-germ lectin: a simplified method and its clinical plausibility. Clin Chem 1986; 32:1960–1966.
12. Moss DW. Alkaline phosphatase isoenzymes. Clin Chem 1982; 28:2007–2016.
13. Bailyes EM, Seabrook RN, Calvin J, et al. The preparation of monoclonal antibodies to human bone and liver alkaline phosphatase and their use in immunoaffinity purification and in studying these enzymes when present in serum. Biochem J 1987; 244:725–733.
14. Puche RC, Caferra DA, Rosillo I. Bone isoenzyme of serum alkaline phosphatase measured with wheat-germ agglutinin. Clin Chem 1988; 34:1372–1375.

15. Hulth AG, Nilsson BE, Westlin NE. Alkaline phosphatase in women with osteoporosis. Acta Med Scand 1979; 22:201–206.
16. Delmas PD, Wahner HW, Mann KG, Riggs BL. Assessment of bone turnover in postmenopausal osteoporosis by measurement of serum bone gla-protein. J Clin Med 1983; 102:470–476.
17. Lauffenburger T, Olah AJ, Dambacher MA, Guncaga J, Lentner C, Haas HG. Bone remodeling and calcium metabolism: a correlated histomorphometric, calcium kinetic and biochemical study in patients with osteoporosis and Paget's disease. Metabolism 1977; 26:589–606.
18. Brown JP, Delmas PD, Arlot M, Meunier PJ. Active bone turnover of the cortico-endosteal envelope in postmenopausal osteoporosis. J Clin Endocrinol Metab 1987; 64:954–959.
19. Stepan J, Pacovsky V, Horn V, et al. Relationship of the activity of the bone isoenzyme of serum alkaline phosphatase to urinary hydrozyproline excretion in metabolic and neoplastic bone diseases. Eur J Clin Invest 1978; 8:373–377.
20. Farley JR, Chesnut CH, Baylink DJ. Improved method for quantitative determination in serum of alkaline phosphatase of skeletal origin. Clin Chem 1981; 27:2002–2007.
21. Hauschka PV, Lian JB, Gallop PM. Direct identification of the calcium-binding amino acid, γ-carboxyglutamate, in mineralized tissue. Proc Natl Acad Sci USA 1975; 72:3925–3417.
22. Price PA, Otsuka AS, Poser JW, Kristaponis J, Raman N. Characterization of a γ-carboxyglutamic acid-containing protein from bone. Proc Natl Acad Sci USA 1976; 73:1447–1451.
23. Price PA, Williamson MK, Lothringer JW. Origin of the vitamin K–dependent bone protein found in plasma and its clearance by kidney and bone. J Biol Chem 1981; 256:12760–12766.
24. Butler WT, D'Souza RN, Bronckers AL, Happonen RP, Somerman MJ. Recent investigations on dentin specific proteins. Proc Finn Dent Soc 1992; 88(suppl 1):369–376.
25. Poser JW, Esch FS, Ling NC, Prince PA. Isolation and sequence of the vitamin K–dependent protein from human bone. J Biol Chem 1980; 225:5685–8691.
26. Nishimoto SK, Price PA. The vitamin K–dependent bone protein is accumulated within cultured osteosarcoma cells in the presence of the vitamin K antagonist warfarin. J Biol Chem 1985; 260:2832–2836.
27. Beresford JN, Gallagher JA, Poser JW, Russell RGG. Production of osteocalcin by human bone cells in vitro. Effects of 1,25(OH)2D3, 24,25(OH)2D3, parathyroid hormone, and glucocorticoids. Metab Bone Dis Rel Res 1984; 5:229–234.
28. Morrison N, Shine J, Eisman J. 1,25-Dihydroxyvitamin D responsive element and glucocorticoid repression of the osteocalcin gene. Science 1990; 246:1158–1161.
29. Lian JB, Tassinari M, Glowacki J. Resorption of implanted bone prepared from normal and warfarin-treated rats. J Clin Invest 1984; 73:1223–1226.
30. Defranco DJ, Glowacki J, Cox KA, Lian JB. Normal bone particles are preferentially resorbed in the presence of osteocalcin-deficient bone particles in vivo. Calcif Tissue Int 1991; 49:43–50.

31. Glowacki J, Rey C, Glimcher MJ, Cox KA, Lian J. A role for osteocalcin in osteoclast differentiation. J Cell Biochem 1991; 45:292–302.
32. Riggs BL, Tsai KS, Mann KG. Effect of acute increases in bone matrix degradation on circulating levels of bone-gla protein. J Bone Min Res 1986; 1:539–541.
33. Delmas PD, Wilson DM, Mann KG, Riggs BL. Effect of renal function on plasma levels of bone Gla-protein. J Clin Endocrinol Metab 1983; 57:1028–1030.
34. Melick RA, Farrugia W, Carolyn CL, Quelch KJ, Scoggins BA, Wark JD. The metabolic clearance rate of osteocalcin in sheep. Calcif Tissue Int 1988; 42: 736–739.
35. Gundberg CM, Markowitz ME, Mizruchi M, Rosen JF. Osteocalcin in human serum: a circadian rhythm. J Clin Endocrinol Metab 1985; 60:736–739.
36. Price PA, Nishimoto SK. Radioimmunoassay for the vitamin K–dependent protein of bone and its discovery in plasma. Proc Natl Acad Sci USA 1980; 77:2234–2238.
37. Egsmose C, Daugaard H, Lund B. Determination of bone Gla protein (osteocalcin) by enzyme-linked immunosorbent assay. Clin Chim Acta 1989; 184:279–288.
38. Garnero P, Grimaux M, Demiaux B, Preaudat C, Seguin P, Delms P. Measurement of serum osteocalcin with a human specific two-site immunoradiometric method. J Bone Min Res 1992; 7:1389–1398.
39. Shiraki M, Hosoda K, Seino Y. The region specific sandwich enzyme immunoassays for intact and N-fragment osteocalcin. J Bone Min Res 1991; 6(suppl 1):S245.
40. Nielsen HK, Brixen K, Kassem M, Mosekilde L. Acute effects of 1,25-dihydroxy-vitamin D_3, prednisone, and 1,25-dihydroxyvitamin D_3 plus prednisone on serum osteocalcin in normal individuals. J Bone Min Res 1991; 6:435–441.
41. Nielsen HK, Brixen K, Bouillon R, Mosekilde L. Changes in biochemical markers of osteoblastic activity during the menstrual cycle. J Clin Endocrinol Metab 1990; 70:1431–1437.
42. Laitinen K, Valimaki M. Alcohol and bone. Calcif Tissue Int 1991; 49(suppl): S70–S73.
43. Thomsen K, Eriksen EF, Jørgensen JCR, Charles P, Mosekilde L. Seasonal variation of serum bone GLA-protein. Scand J Clin Lab Invest 1989; 49:605–611.
44. Brown JP, Malaval L, Chapuy MC, Delmas PD, Edouard C, Maunier PJ. Serum bone Gla-protein: a specific marker for bone formation in postmenopausal osteoporosis. Lancet 1984; 1091–1993.
45. Gundberg CM, Cole DEC, Lian JB, Reade TM, Gallop PM. Serum osteocalcin in the treatment of inherited rickets with 1,25-dihydroxyvitamin D3. J Clin Endocrinol Metab 1983; 56:1063–1067.
46. Price PA, Parthemore JG, Deftos LJ. New biochemical marker for bone metabolism. J Clin Invest 1980; 66:878–883.
47. Pietschmann P, Resch H, Krexner E, Woloszczuk W, Willvonseder R. Decreased serum osteocalcin levels in patients with postmenopausal osteoporosis. Acta Med Austriaca 1991; 18:114–116.
48. Herring GM. The organic matrix of bone. In: Bourne GH, ed. The Biochemistry and Physiology of Bone, Vol 1. New York: Academic Press; 1972:127–189.
49. Robey PG, Bianco P, Termine JD. The cellular biology and molecular biochemistry

of bone formation. In: Coe FL, Favus MJ, eds. Disorders of Bone and Mineral Metabolism. New York: Raven Press; 1992:241–263.

50. Prockop DJ, Kivirikko KI, Tuderman L, Guzman NA. The biosynthesis of collagen and its disorders. N Engl J Med 1979; 301:13–23.
51. Smedsrød B, Melkko J, Risteli L, Risteli J. Circulating C-terminal propeptide of type I procollagen is cleared mainly via the mannose receptor in liver endothelial cells. Biochem J 1990; 271:345–350.
52. Hassager C, Risteli J, Risteli L, Jensen SB, Christiansen C. Diurnal variation in serum markers of type I collagen synthesis and degradation in healthy premenopausal women. J Bone Min Res 1992; 7:1307–1311.
53. Nielsen HK, Risteli J, Brixen K, Risteli L, Charles P, Eriksen EF. Circadian variation in new biochemical markers in normals. Bone Miner 1992; 7:1307–1311.
54. Melkko J, Niemi S, Risteli L, Risteli J. Radioimmunoassay of the carboxyterminal propeptide of human type I procollagen. Clin Chem 1990; 36:1328–1332.
55. Jensen LT, Olesen HP, Risteli J, Lorentzen I. External thoragic duct–venous shunt in pigs for long term studies of connective tissue metabolites in lymph. Lab Anim Sci 1990; 40:620–624.
56. Eastell R, Peel NFA, Hannon RA, et al. The effect of age on bone turnover as assessed by pyridinium crosslinks and procollagen I C-terminal peptide. Osteoporosis Int 1993; suppl 1:S100–S101.
57. Kivirikko KI, Laitinen O, Prockop DJ. Modifications of a specific assay for hydroxyproline in urine. Anal Bio 1967; 19:249–255.
58. Bienkowski RS, Cowan MJ, Mcdonald JA, Crystal RG. Degradation of newly synthesized collagen. J Biol Chem 1978; 253:4356–4363.
59. Pødenphant J, Larsen NE, Christiansen C. An easy and reliable method for determination of urinary hydroxyproline. Clin Chim Acta 1984; 142:145–148.
60. Goverde BC, Veenkamp FJN. Routine assay of total urinary hydroxyproline based on resin-catalyzed hydrolysis. Clin Chim Acta 1993; 41:29–40.
61. Macek J, Adam M. Method for rapid determination of hydroxyproline by high-performance liquid chromatography and its exploitation for the study of collagen formation. J Chromat 1986; 374:125–128.
62. Gallagher JC, Aaron J, Horsman A, Marshall DH, Wilkinson R, Nordin BEC. The crush fracture syndrome in postmenopausal women. J Clin Endocrinol Metab 1973; 2:293–305.
63. Whyte MP, Bergfeld MA, Murphy WA, Avioli LV, Teitelbaum SL. Postmenopausal osteoporosis: a heterogeneous disorder as assessed by histomorphometric analysis of iliac crest bone from untreated patients. Am J Med 1982; 72:193–202.
64. Eriksen EF, Melsen F, Mosekilde L. Reconstruction of the resorptive site in iliac trabecular bone: a kinetic model for bone resorption in 20 normal individuals. Metab Bone Dis Rel Res 1984; 5:235–242.
65. Eyre DR. Collagen cross-linking amino acids. In: Cunningham LW, ed. Method in Enzymonology. Orlando: Academic Press; 1987:115–139.
66. Eyre D. New biomarkers of bone resorption. (Editorial.) J Clin Endocrinol Metab 1992; 74:470A–470C.

67. Forsman RW, Obrien JF. Quantifying bone and liver alkaline phosphatase by the resolution of two-component inactivation data obtained with a centrifugal analyzer. Clin Chem 1991; 37:347–350.
68. Eyre DR, Koob TJ, Van Ness KP. Quantitation of hydroxypyridinium crosslinks in collagen by high-performance liquid chromatography. Anal Biochem 1984; 137: 380–388.
69. Robins SP, Duncan A. Pyridinium crosslinks of bone collagen and their location in peptides isolated from rat femur. Biochim Biophys Acta 1987; 914:233–239.
70. Linde A, Robins SP. Quantitative assessment of collagen crosslinks in dissected predentine and dentine. Collagen Rel Res 1988; 8:443–450.
71. Eastell R, Hampton L, Colwell A. Urinary collagen crosslinks are highly correlated with radioisotopic measurements of bone resorption. In: Christiansen C, Overgaard K, eds. Osteoporosis. Copenhagen: Osteopress; 1990:469–470.
72. Colwell A, Eastell R, Assiri AMA, Russell RGG. Effect of diet on deoxypridinoline excretion. In: Christiansen C, Overgaard K, eds. Osteoporosis. Copenhagen: Osteopress; 1990:590–591.
73. Schlemmer A, Hassager C, Jensen SB, Christiansen C. Marked diurnal variation in urinary excretion of pyridinium cross-links in premenopausal women. J Clin Endocrinol Metab 1992; 74:476–480.
74. Robins SP, Black D, Paterson CR, Reid DM, Duncan A, Seibel MJ. Evaluation of urinary hydroxypyridinium crosslink measurements as resorption markers in metabolic bone diseases. Eur J Clin Invest 1991; 21:310–315.
75. Risteli J, Niemi S, Elomaa I, Risetli L. Bone resorption assay based on a peptide liberated during type I collagen degradation. J Bone Min Res 1991; 6(suppl 1):A670.
76. Hanson DA, Eyre DR. A specific immunoassay for bone resorption based on cross-linked collagen peptides in urine. J Bone Min Res 1991; 6(suppl 1):A669.
77. Uebelhart D, Schlemmer A, Johansen JS, Gineyts E, Christiansen C, Delmas PD. Effect of menopause and hormone replacement therapy on the urinary excretion of pyridinium cross-links. J Clin Endocrinol Metab 1991; 72:367–373.
78. Delmas PD, Schlemmer A, Gineyts E, Riis B, Christiansen C. Urinary excretion of pyridinoline crosslinks correlates with bone turnover measured on iliac crest biopsy in patients with vertebral osteoporosis. J Bone Min Res 1991; 6:639–644.
79. Bollerslev J. Autosomal dominant osteopetrosis: bone metabolism and epidemiological, clinical, and hormonal aspects. Endocrinol Rev 1989; 10:45–67.
80. Yam LT. Clinical significance of the human acid phosphatases. Am J Med 1974; 56:604–617.
81. Minkin C. Bone acid phosphatase as a marker of osteoclast function. Calcif Tissue Int 1982; 34:285–290.
82. Stepan JJ, Pospichal J, Schreiber V, et al. The application of plasma tartrate-resistant acid phosphatase to assess changes in bone resorption in response to artificial menopause and its treatment with estrogen or norethisterone. Calcif Tissue Int 1989; 45:273–280.
83. Fraser JD, Otawara Y, Price PA. 1,25-Dihydroxyvitamin D3 stimulates the synthesis of matrix alpha-carboxyglutamine acid protein by osteosarcoma cells: mutually

exclusive expression of vitamin K–dependent bone proteins by clonal osteoblastic cell lines. J Biol Chem 1988; 263:911–916.
84. Johansen JS, Giwercman A, Hartwell D, et al. Serum bone Gla-protein as a marker of bone growth in children and adolescents: correlation with age, height, serum insulin-like growth factor I, and serum testosterone. J Clin Endocrinol Metab 1988; 67:273–278.
85. Gundberg CM, Lian JB, Gallop PM. Measurements of gamma-glutamate and circulating osteocalcin in normal children and adults. Clin Chim Acta 1983; 1218:1–8.
86. Delmas PD, Stenner D, Wahner HW, Mann KG, Riggs BL. Serum bone gla protein increases with aging in normal women: implications for the mechanism of age related bone loss. J Clin Invest 1983; 71:1316–1321.
87. Gonchoroff DG, Branum EL, Cedel SL, Riggs BL, Obrien JF. Clinical Evaluation of high-performance affinity chromatography for the separation of bone and liver alkaline phosphatase isoenzymes. Clin Chim Acta 1991; 199:43–50.
88. Fujimoto D, Suzuki M, Uchiyama A, Miyamoto S, Inoue T. Analysis of pyridinoline, a cross-linking compound of collagen fibers in human urine. J Biochem 1983; 94:1133–1136.
89. Melkko J, Niemi S, Risteli L, Risteli J. Radioimmunoassay of the carboxyterminal propeptide of human type-I procollagen. Clin Chem 1990; 36:1328–1332.
90. Uebelhart D, Schlemmer A, Johansen JS, Gineyts E, Christiansen C, Delmas PD. Effect of menopause and hormone replacement therapy on the urinary excretion of pyridinium cross-links. J Clin Endocrinol Metab 1991; 72:367–373.
91. Fogelman I, Poser JW, Smith ML, Hart DM, Bevan JA. Alterations in skeletal metabolism following oophorectomy. In: Christiansen C, Arnaud CC, Nordin BEC, Parfitt AM, Peck WA, Riggs BL, eds. Osteoporosis. Aalborg: Aalborg Stiftsbogtrykkeri; 1984:519–522.
92. Steiniche T, Hasling C, Charles P, Eriksen EF, Mosekilde L, Melsen F. A randomized study on the effects of estrogen/gestangen or high dose oral calcium on trabecular bone remodeling in postmenopausal osteoporosis. Bone 1989; 10:313–320.
93. Arlot ME, Delmas PD, Chappard D, Meunier PJ. Trabecular and endocortical bone remodeling in postmenopausal osteoporosis: comparison with normal postmenopausal women. Osteoporos Int 1990; 1:41–49.
94. Storm T, Thamsborg G, Steiniche T, Genant HK, Sørensen OH. Effect of intermittent cyclical etidronate therapy on bone mass and fracture rate in women with postmenopausal osteoporosis. N Engl J Med 1990; 322:1265–1271.
95. Eriksen EF. Normal and pathological remodeling of human trabecular bone: three dimensional reconstruction of the remodeling sequence in normal and in metabolic bone disease. Endocrinol Rev 1986; 7:379–408.
96. Civitelli R, Gonnelli S, Zacchei F, et al. Bone turnover in postmenopausal osteoporosis effect of calcitonin treatment. J Clin Invest 1988; 82:1268–1274.
97. Steiniche T, Hasling C, Charles P, Eriksen EF, Mosekilde L, Melsen F. A randomized study on the effects of estrogen gestation or high dose oral calcium on trabecular bone remodeling in postmenopausal osteoporosis. Bone 1989; 10:313–320.
98. Johansen JS, Riis BJ, Delmas PD, Christiansen C. Plasma BGP: an indicator of

spontaneous bone loss and of the effect of oestrogen treatment in postmenopausal women. Eur J Clin Invest 1988; 18:191–195.

99. Lufkin EG, Wahner HW, Ofallon WM, et al. Treatment of postmenopausal osteoporosis with transdermal estrogen. Ann Intern Med 1992; 117:1–9.
100. Hasling C, Eriksen EF, Melkko J, et al. Effects of a combined estrogen-gestagen regimen on serum levels of the carboxy-terminal propeptide of human type-I procollagen in osteoporosis. J Bone Miner Res 1991; 6:1295–1300.
101. Steiniche T, Hasling C, Charles P, Eriksen EF, Melsen F, Mosekilde L. The effect of etidronate on trabecular bone remodeling in postmenopausal spinal osteoporosis—a randomized study comparing intermittent treatment and an ADFR regime. Bone 1991; 12:155–163.
102. Mallmin H, Ljunghall S, Larsson K, Lindh E. Short-term effects of pamidronate on biochemical markers on bone metabolism of osteoporosis—a placebo-controlled dose-finding study. Upsal J Med Sci 1991; 96:205–212.
103. Pouilles JM, Tremollieres F, Causse E, Louvet JP, Ribot C. Fluoride therapy in postmenopausal osteopenic women: effect on vertebral and femoral bone density and prediction of bone response. Osteoporos Int 1991; 1:103–109.
104. Tremollieres F, Pouilles JM, Louvet JP, Ribot C. Transitory bone loss during substitution treatment for hypothyroidism. Results of a two year prospective study. Rev Rhum Mal Osteoartic 1991; 58:869–875.
105. Hasling C, Nielsen HE, Melsen F, Mosekilde L. The safety of osteoporosis treatment with sodium fluoride, calcium phosphate and vitamin D. Miner Electrolyte Metab 1987;
106. Baylink DJ, Duane PB, Farley SM, Farley JR. Monofluorophosphate physiology: the effects of fluoride on bone. Caries Res 1983; 17(suppl 1):56–76.
107. Christiansen C, Riis BJ, Rødbro P. Prediction of rapid bone loss in postmenopausal women. Lancet 1987; 1105–1108.
108. Hui SL, Slemenda CW, Johnston CC. The contribution of bone loss to postmenopausal osteoporosis. Osteoporos Int 1990; 1:30–34.
109. Spotila LD, Constantinou CD, Sereda L, Ganguly A, Riggs BL, Prockop DJ. Mutation in a gene for type-I procollagen (COL1A2) in a woman with postmenopausal osteoporosis—evidence for phenotypic and genotypic overlap with mild osteogenesis imperfecta. Proc Natl Acad Sci USA 1991; 88:5423–5427.
110. Shapiro JR, Stover ML, Burn VE, et al. An osteopenic nonfracture syndrome with features of mild osteogenesis imperfecta associated with the substitution of a cysteine for glycine at triple helix position 43 in the pro alpha 1(I) chain of type I collagen. J Clin Invest 1992; 89:567–573.
111. Diebold J, Batge B, Stein H, Muller PK, Lohrs U. Vertebral trabecular bone in various age groups and in osteoporosis—morphometry and bone matrix biochemistry. Verh Dtsch Ges Pathol 1990; 74:243–247.
112. Knapen MH, Hamulyak K, Vermeer C. The effect of vitamin K supplementation on circulating osteocalcin (bone Gla protein) and urinary calcium excretion. Ann Intern Med 1989; 111:1001–1005.
113. Gundberg CM, Anderson M, Dickson I, Gallop PM. "Glycated" osteocalcin in human and bovine bone. The effect of age. J Biol Chem 1986; 261:14557–14561.

114. Parfitt AM. The actions of parathyroid hormone on bone: relation to bone remodeling and turnover, calcium homeostasis, and metabolic bone diseases. Part II of IV, parts. PTH and bone cells: bone turnover and plasma calcium regulation. Metabolism 1976; 25:909–955.
115. Frost HM. Tetracycline-based histological analysis of bone remodeling. Calcif Tissue Int 1969; 3:211–237.
116. Eriksen EF, Steiniche T, Mosekilde L, Melsen F. Histomorphometric analysis of bone in metabolic bone disease. Endocrinol Metab Clin North Am 1989; 18:919–954.
117. Milhaud G, Christiansen C, Gallagher C, Reeve J, Seeman E, Chestnut C. Pathogenesis and treatment of postmenopausal osteoporosis. Calcif Tissue Int 1983; 35: 708–711.
118. Melsen B, Melsen F, Mosekilde L, Bergmann S. Histomorphometric analysis of normal bone from the iliac crest. Acta Path Micr Scand Sect A 1978; 86:70–81.
119. Krølner B, Nielsen SP. Bone mineral content of the lumbar spine in normal and osteoporotic women: cross-sectional and longitudinal studies. Clin Sci 1982; 62: 329–332.
120. Garn SM, Rohmann CG, Wagner B. Bone loss as a general phenomenon in man. Fed Proc 1967; 26:1729–1736.
121. Kleerekoper M, Villanueva AR, Stanciu J, Rao DS, Parfitt AM. The role of three-dimensional trabecular microstructure in the pathogenesis of vertebral compression fractures. Calcif Tissue Int 1985; 37:594–597.
122. Parfitt AM. Age-related structural changes in trabecular and cortical. Calcif Tissue Int 1984; 36(suppl 1):S123–S128.
123. Parfitt AM. Trabecular bone architecture in the pathogenesis and prevention of fracture. Am J Med 1987; 82:68–72.
124. Vesterby A, Gundersen HJG, Melsen F. Star volume of marrow space and trabeculae of the first lumbar vertebra: sampling efficiency and biological variation. Bone 1989; 10:7–13.
125. Vesterby A, Mosekilde L, Gundersen HJG, Melsen F, Holme K, Sorensen S. Biologically meaningful determinants of the in vitro strength of lumbar vertebrae. Bone 1991; 12:219–224.
126. Burckhardt P, Michel C. The peak bone mass concept. Clin Rheumatol 1989; 8(suppl 2):16–21.
127. Eriksen EF, Gundersen HJG, Melsen F, Mosekilde L. Reconstruction of the formative site in iliac trabecular bone in 20 normal individuals employing a kinetic model for matrix and mineral apposition. Metab Bone Dis Rel Res 1984; 5:243–252.
128. Parfitt AM, Mathews CHE, Villanueva AR, Kleerekoper M, Frame B, Rao DS. Relationships between surface, volume, and thickness of iliac trabecular bone in aging and in osteoporosis. J Clin Invest 1983; 72:1396–1407.
129. Parfitt AM. The physiologic and clinical significance of bone histomorphometric data. In: Recker RR, ed. Bone Histomorphometry: Techniques and Interpretation. Boca Raton: CRC Press; 1983:143–224.
130. Vesterby A, Gundersen HJG, Melsen F, Mosekilde L. Marrow space star volume in the iliac crest decreases in osteoporotic patients after continuous treatment with fluoride, calcium, and vitamin-D2 for five years. Bone 1991; 12:33–37.

131. Parfitt AM. Morphologic basis of bone mineral measurements: transient and steady state effects of treatment in osteoporosis. Min Elect Metab 1980; 4:273–287.
132. Frost HM. Some effects of basic multicellular unit-based remodelling on photon absorptiometry of trabecular bone. Bone Miner 1989; 7:47–65.
133. Jerome CP, Gubler HP. Experimental determination of the law of bone remodeling and effect of rat parathyroid hormone (1–34) infusion on derived parameters. Calcif Tissue Int 1991; 49:398–402.
134. Munk-Jensen N, Nielsen SP, Obel EB, Eriksen PB. Reversal of postmenopausal vertebral bone loss by oestrogen and progestogen: a double blind placebo controlled study. Br Med J 1988; 296:1150–1152.
135. Horsman A, Gallagher JC, Simpson M, Nordin BEC. Prospective trial of oestrogen and calcium in postmenopausal women. Br Med J 1977; 2:789–792.
136. Lindsay R, Hart DM, Forrest C, Baird C. Prevention of spinal osteoporosis in oophorectomized women. Lancet 1980; 2:1151–1154.
137. Marie PJ, Rasmussen H, Kuntz D, Gueris J, Caulin F. Treatment of postmenopausal osteoporosis with phosphate and intermittent calcitonin. In: Christiansen C, Arnaud CD, Nordin BEC, Parfitt AM, Peck WA, Riggs BL, eds. Osteoporosis. Ålborg: Ålborg Stiftsbogtrkkeri; 1985:575–579.
138. Riggs BL, Hodgson SF, Ofallon WM, et al. Effect of fluoride treatment on the fracture rate in postmenopausal women with osteoporosis. N Engl J Med 1990; 322: 802–809.
139. Reeve J, Davis UM, Hesp R, McNally E, Katz D. Treatment of osteoporosis with human parathyroid peptide and observations on effect of sodium fluoride. Br Med J 1990; 301:314–318.
140. Orimo H, Fujita T, Yoshikawa M. Increased sensitivity of bone to parathyroid hormone in ovariectomized rats. Endocrinology 1972; 90:760–765.
141. Seeman E, Melton LJ III, O'Fallon WM, Riggs BL. Risk factors for spinal osteoporosis in men. Am J Med 1983; 75:977–983.
142. Daniell HW. Osteoporosis of the slender smoker. Vertebral compression fractures and loss of metacarpal cortex in relation to postmenopausal cigarette smoking and lack of obesity. Arch Intern Med 1976; 136:298–304.
143. Alderman BW, Weiss NS, Daling JR, Ure CL, Ballard JH. Reproductive history and postmenopausal risk of hip and forearm fracture. Am J Epidemiol 1986; 124: 262–267.
144. Kiel DP, Felson DT, Anderson JJ, Wilson PWF, Moskowitz MA. Hip fracture and the use of estrogens in postmenopausal women. N Engl J Med 1987; 317:1169–1174.
145. Siiteri PK. Postmenopausal estrogen production. Front Hormone Res 1973; 3:40–44.
146. Steiniche T, Vesterby A, Eriksen EF, Mosekilde L, Melsen F. A histomorphometric determination of iliac bone structure and remodeling in obese subjects. Bone 1986; 7:77–82.
147. Kimmel DB, Recker RR, Gallagher JC, Vaswani AS, Aloia JF. A comparison of iliac bone histomorphometric data in postmenopausal osteoporotic and normal subjects. Bone Miner 1990; 11:217–222.
148. Mosekilde L. Sex differences in age-related loss of vertebral trabecular bone mass and structure—biomechanical consequences. Bone 1989; 10:425–432.

149. Mosekilde L. Normal vertebral body size and compressive strength: relations to age and to vertebral and iliac trabecular bone compressive strength. Bone 1986; 7: 207–212.
150. Recker RR, Smith RT, Kimmel DB. Loss of trabecular connectivity in osteoporosis demonstrated with independent methods. Bone 1993; xx:A28 (abstract).
151. Arlot M, Edouard C, Meunier PJ, Neer RM, Reeve J. Impaired osteoblast function in osteoporosis: comparison between calcium balance and dynamic histomorphometry. Br Med J 1984; 289:417–520.
152. Eriksen EF, Hodgson SF, Eastell R, Cedel SL, O'Fallon WM, Riggs BL. Cancellous bone remodeling in type I (postmenopausal) osteoporosis: quantitative assessment of rates of formation, resorption, and bone loss at tissue and cellular levels. J Bone Miner Res 1990; 5:311–319.
153. Darby AJ, Meunier PJ. Mean wall thickness and formation periods of trabecular bone packets in idiopathic osteoporosis. Calcif Tissue Int 1981; 33:199–204.
154. Cohen-Solal ME, Shih MS, Parfitt AM. Erosion depth and bone balance in overt osteoporosis. J Bone Miner Res 1991; 6:S225.
155. Wand JS, Green JR, Hesp R, et al. Bone remodelling does not decline after menopause in vertebral fracture osteoporosis. Bone Miner 1992; 17:361–375.

3

Epidemiology of Osteoporosis and Fractures

L. JOSEPH MELTON, III

Mayo Medical School and Mayo Clinic and Foundation
Rochester, Minnesota

I. INTRODUCTION

Osteoporosis is a disease characterized by abnormalities in the amount and architectural arrangement of bone tissue, which lead to impaired skeletal strength and an increased susceptibility to fractures (1). In contrast to a disease like cancer, there is no unequivocal dividing line between osteoporosis and "normal" histology. Instead, it is recognized that increasingly severe skeletal derangement is associated with an increased risk of fracture. However, there is no biomechanical threshold below which fractures are inevitable and, because they have other causes, fractures may occur in the absence of skeletal abnormalities. These observations have led to the understanding that osteoporosis is a disease, like hypertension or diabetes mellitus, that must be defined on the basis of a gradient of risk associated with a physiologic abnormality. Thus, osteoporosis can be said to exist at some arbitrarily selected level of skeletal disruption as detected by bone biopsy (Chapter 7) or, more often, as surmised from noninvasive measures of bone density (Chapters 1 and 2). The epidemiology of the condition therefore relates to the determinants of low bone density in the population and to the determinants of fractures, which may involve factors besides bone density. Both aspects of the epidemiology of osteoporosis are reviewed below with a focus on the following questions: How many people have osteoporosis and how does it develop? What is the relationship between low bone mass and fractures? What are the risk factors for fracture? How frequent are fractures and what is their social impact? These insights provide a necessary background for a clear understanding of the various alternatives for evaluating and treating individual patients.

II. EPIDEMIOLOGY OF OSTEOPOROSIS

A. Magnitude of the Problem

The number of people considered to have osteoporosis depends entirely on the way the condition is defined in practice. As in hypertension and diabetes, it has been difficult in osteoporosis to reach consensus on the exact level of bone density that should be considered presumptive evidence of the disease. However, a committee of the World Health Organization recently recommended the definitions shown in Table 1 (2). Under this scheme, it is possible to diagnose and treat osteoporosis (bone density levels more than 2.5 standard deviations (SD) below the young normal mean) prior to the occurrence of fractures (established osteoporosis). This avoids the need to restrict treatment to end-stage disease, where it may be of limited effectiveness. It also circumvents the conceptual confusion that previously existed when a patient was considered normal one day and osteoporotic the next, when a fracture occurred, without any change in underlying bone density (3). This scheme also facilitates prophylaxis by identifying a group of women with bone density levels between 1.0 and 2.5 SD below young normal mean levels as having low bone mass, or osteopenia. Thus, perimenopausal women with bone density that is 1 SD below the young normal mean might not have pathologically low bone mass today but still could be at sufficiently high risk of fracture over their remaining lifetimes that preventive therapy is indicted (4). This is particularly important since currently available treatments can conserve existing bone mass but cannot restore osteoporotic bone to biomechanical normality (5).

Table 1 World Health Organization Definition of Osteoporosis

Normal. A value for bone density higher than 1 SD below the young adult mean value.

Low bone mass ("osteopenia"). A value for bone density more than 1 SD below the young adult mean but less than 2.5 SD below this mean.

Osteoporosis. A value for bone density more than 2.5 SD below the young adult mean.

Severe osteoporosis ("established osteoporosis"). A value for bone density more than 2.5 SD below the young adult mean and one or more fragility fractures.

Source: Ref. 2.

Using the World Health Organization definition of osteoporosis, it has been estimated that 30% of postmenopausal white women could be affected (6). As illustrated in Table 2, the proportion of women ⩾ 50 years of age who have osteoporosis varies from about 16% when bone density is measured in the proximal femur to 17% when measured in the midradius. It is well known that there is only modest correlation in bone density values measured at different skeletal sites (7), and the proportion of women with osteoporosis at any of the three sites is greater, rising from 15% at age 50–59 years to 70% at age 80 years and above, in conjunction with the age-related loss of cortical and cancellous bone (8). These figures are derived from national extrapolations of data from an age-stratified random sample of Rochester, Minnesota, women in whom bone density was assessed in the neck and intertrochanteric regions of the proximal femur and in the lumbar spine by dual-photon absorptiometry and in the midradius by single-photon absorpiometry (6). Comparable data are not yet available for nonwhite women or for men, both because of a lack of population-based data on the distribution of bone density in some of the groups and because of uncertainty about the proper cutoff levels to employ.

The number of affected individuals is likely to increase in the future as the population ages. In the United States, for example, the number of persons aged 65 years and over is expected to rise from 32 million to 69 million between 1990 and 2050, while the number aged 85 years and over will increase from 3 million to 15 million. Because the prevalence of low bone mass rises with age and is quite high in elderly women, these demographic changes alone will eventually result in a

Table 2 Proportion (%) of Rochester, Minnesota, Women With Bone Mineral Measurements More than 2.5 SD Below the Mean for Young Normal Women[a]

Age group	Lumbar spine %	Either hip site %	Midradius %	Spine, hip, or midradius %
50–59	7.6	3.9	3.7	14.8
60–69	11.8	8.0	11.8	21.6
70–79	25.0	24.5	23.1	38.5
⩾80	32.0	47.5	50.0	70.0
Total[b]	16.5	16.2	17.4	30.3

[a]Mean is from 48 subjects under age 40 who were randomly sampled from the Rochester, Minnesota, population. None of them was known to have any disorder that might influence bone metabolism.

[b]Age-adjusted to the population structure of 1990 United States white women 50 years of age and older.

doubling or tripling in the number of affected women. Thus, with these projected increases in the elderly population, the number of postmenopausal white women in the United States with bone mineral more than 2.5 SD below the young normal mean could grow from 9 million now to 23 million by the year 2050. Even today it is probably true that, altogether, 20–25 million Americans are at increased risk of fracture by virtue of low bone mass if one includes nonwhite women and men as well as those with bone density in the osteopenic range (9).

B. Risk Factors for Osteoporosis

Conceptually, at least, the risk factors for osteoporosis are fairly straightforward (Fig. 1). A person's bone mass later in life is determined by the maximal bone mass achieved in young adulthood, as well as by the subsequent rate of bone loss. At age 70 years, these two determinants of bone mass are about equally important (10). The bone loss results from age-related factors that occur universally in the population and account for slow bone loss over life in both sexes; from an accelerated phase of bone loss associated with the menopause in women and hypogonadism in some men; and from medical and surgical conditions that produce "secondary" osteoporosis (8). A person's bone mass is the net result of these factors, the relative importance of which may vary from one individual to another. Thus, race and sex differences in osteoporosis are explained in part by the heritability of skeletal size. Bone mass is greatest in those of African heritage, who have the lowest fracture rates, and is least in Caucasian women of Northern European extraction, who have the highest fracture rates (11). Similarly, the accelerated phase of bone loss in perimenopausal women is superimposed upon

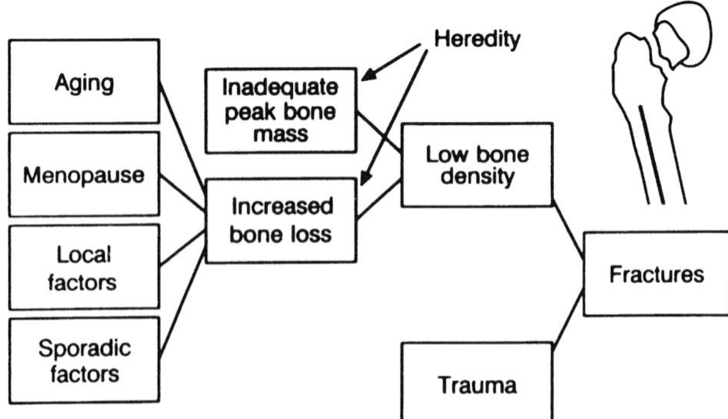

Figure 1 Conceptual model of the pathogenesis of fractures related to osteoporosis. (From Ref. 81.)

the slower, age-related bone loss seen in both sexes and explains in part the twofold higher incidence of fractures among women than men later in life (8). The pathophysiologic basis for these observations is described more fully in Chapter 6.

Attempts to quantify these various risk factors for low bone mass have been less successful. Most studies have been relatively small and have focused on highly selected "normal" women. Only a few population-based investigations have involved postmenopausal women generally, and they have arrived at inconsistent conclusions. This is due in part to the fact that various investigators have emphasized different sets of risk factors or have associated them with different measures of bone mass. For example, age, height, weight, and duration of estrogen replacement therapy accounted for 22–37% of the variability in bone mineral of the calcaneus and forearm among 1,098 Hawaiian women of Japanese ancestry who ranged in age from 43 to 80 years (12). However, height was an important predictor only for bone mineral content (g/cm) of the radius, not for bone mineral density (mg/cm^2), of the calcaneus, where correction for the area scanned partially adjusts for bone width, which is correlated with height. Similarly, age; humeral muscle area; use of estrogen replacement therapy, thiazides, or vitamin D; and calcium intake over 800 mg/day explained 40% of the variance in bone mineral content of the midradius in a population-based study of 324 Iowa women aged 55–80 years (13). While height and weight were also correlated with bone mineral content in the latter study, humeral muscle area appeared to be the better anthropomorphic predictor of bone mass in the multivariate analysis. Humeral muscle area was not evaluated in the study in Hawaii. Moreover, the most recent studies use dual-energy x-ray absorptiometry to assess lean body mass more directly (14), so one must expect continual change in these interrelationships as different combinations of variables are analyzed.

In the most comprehensive study to date, the determinants of appendicular bone density were assessed in 5,430 white or Asian-American women 65 years of age or over in the Study of Osteoporotic Fractures (15). Later age at menopause, estrogen or thiazide use, non-insulin-dependent diabetes, and greater height, weight, strength, and dietary calcium intake were all positively associated with bone mass, while greater age, cigarette smoking, caffeine intake, prior gastric surgery, and maternal history of fracture were negatively associated (Table 3). Despite the large number of potential risk factors that were assessed, models incorporating all of the independent predictors explained only 20–34% of the variance in bone density at the radius or calcaneus. The same is true of clinical studies, where various risk factors together have generally accounted for less than half of the variability in bone mass (4). Moreover, the enormous size of this study permitted identification of risk factors that, while statistically significant, are of marginal importance clinically. Thus, a lifetime caffeine intake equivalent to 10 cups of coffee per day for 30 years was associated with a 1.1% decrease in distal radius bone mineral density (15). Weak effects like that of caffeine, which are

Table 3 Correlates of Distal Radius Bone Mineral Density (BMD)

Variable	Mean or prevalence (%)	Unit change	Percentage change in BMD per unit change (95% C.I.)
Physical characteristics			
Age, years	71.6	5	−2.9 (−3.5 to −2.3)
Weight, kg	67.3	10	3.7 (3.2 to 4.2)
Height, cm	159	10	1.7 (0.7 to 2.8)
Grip strength, kg	20.9	5	3.5 (2.8 to 4.3)
Reproductive and family history			
Age at menopause, years	46.9	54	2.0 (1.4 to 2.5)
Maternal fracture after age 50	30%	yes/no	−2.8 (−4.0 to −1.6)
Medical history			
Non-insulin-dependent diabetes	6%	yes/no	4.8 (2.2 to 7.3)
Gastric surgery	2%	yes/no	−8.2 (−12.9 to −3.5)
Habits			
Current smoker	10%	yes/no	−2.1 (−4.0 to −0.2)
Calcium intake, mg/day	718	400	0.7 (0.1 to 1.3)
Caffeine intake, lifetime, g	4030	2500	−0.2 (−0.3 to −0.1)
Medications			
Estrogen use >2 years	29%	yes/no	7.2 (5.9 to 8.6)
Thiazide use >5 years	24%	yes/no	4.0 (2.6 to 5.3)

Source: Ref. 15.

found in some studies (16) but not others (17), likely reflect the influence of confounding by more important variables which were not assessed.

There have been even fewer population-based studies of risk factors for bone loss in men. In the Hawaiian study mentioned previously, bone mineral content of the forearm in Japanese-American men was negatively correlated with age and positively correlated with height and weight, but these variables accounted for just 11–18% of the variance (12). Age, weight, and amount of strenuous exercise per month accounted for 23% of the variance in bone density of the calcaneus.

Because no consistent set of risk factors has been found in the different studies, it has proven difficult to devise a clinical index to identify patients at high risk of osteoporosis. The difficulties inherent in this approach were demonstrated by Slemenda and colleagues (18), who identified predictors of bone density at various skeletal sites and then compared predicted values at those sites with the results actually observed among 124 perimenopausal women. For femoral neck bone mineral density, the best predictive model was [0.79 + (0.001 × height) + (0.0041 × weight) − (0.00018 × cigarette pack-years) − (0.00023 × urinary calcium/creatinine) + (0.00005 × dietary calcium)]. However, this model accounted for only 17% of the variability in bone mineral measurements at the hip, and correctly classified only 65% of the women whose bone density was in the lowest tertile (Fig. 2). The same risk factors were weighted somewhat differently [0.69 + (0.00099 × height) + (0.0043 × weight) − (0.00046 × pack-years) − (0.0002 × calcium/creatinine) + (0.00002 × dietary calcium)] in a model that correctly identified 61% of the women with low lumbar spine bone density and 45% of those with high values but were different yet [−1.1 + (0.0075 × height) + (0.0022 × weight) − (0.00044 × pack-years) + (0.12 × wrist width) − (0.00016 × calcium/creatinine) + 0.00004 × dietary calcium)] in a model that correctly classified 68% of women with low bone mineral content in the midradius (18). None of these models accounted for more than half the variance in bone mass, and none are adequate for making decisions about interventions in individual patients since bone density can be measured directly with less misclassification error (Chapters 1 and 2).

III. EPIDEMIOLOGY OF FRACTURES

A. Magnitude of the Problem

Except for the possibility of tooth loss (19), the clinical manifestations of osteoporosis relate almost exclusively to fractures. Hip fractures have been recognized

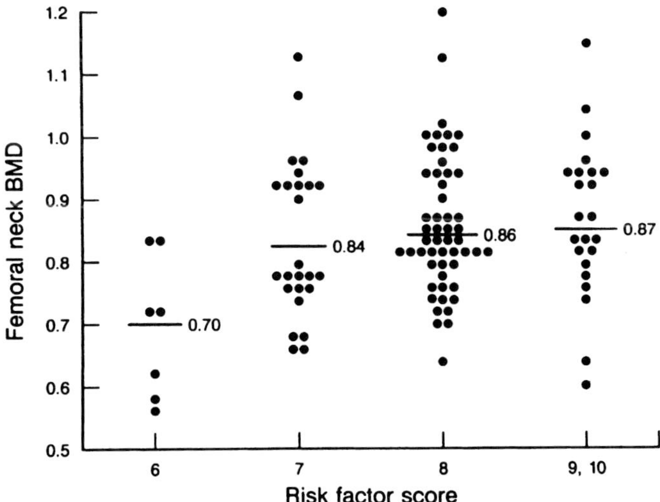

Figure 2 Observed femoral neck bone mineral density (BMD) plotted against risk factor score. (From Ref. 18.)

as a manifestation of osteoporosis for over a century (20), and vertebral fractures have been virtually synonymous with postmenopausal osteoporosis since the time of Albright (21). Only in the past decade, however, has it become obvious that most fractures among the elderly are due in part to low bone mass (22). These fractures are quite common, both individually and in aggregate. Thus, the lifetime risk of a hip fracture has been estimated at about 17% in white women and 6% in white men (Table 4). These figures are approximately equivalent, respectively, to the lifetime risk in women of developing breast, ovarian, or endometrial cancer, and the lifetime risk in men of developing prostate cancer (23). The lifetime risk of a clinically detected vertebral fracture is about 16% in white women and 5% in white men (Table 4). Because a substantial proportion of vertebral fractures are asymptomatic and never diagnosed (24), these are probably low estimates. The lifetime risk of a distal forearm fracture is 16% in white women and a little over 2% in white men (Table 4). The lifetime risk of any one of the three fractures is almost 40% for white women from age 50 years onward and 13% for white men (25). Moreover, as noted above, hip, forearm, and vertebral fractures are not the only ones associated with osteoporosis (22).

The adverse outcomes of these fractures encompass mortality, morbidity, and cost. Hip fractures dominate in each category, leading for example to an overall 5–20% reduction from expected survival (23). The excess deaths occur soon after the fracture and diminish with time so that, after 6 months or so, subsequent survival is comparable to that of similarly aged men and women in the general population (Fig. 3). The deaths can be attributed to interaction of the hip fracture with other medical conditions. Thus, hip fracture patients without serious preexisting diseases have survival no different from controls (26). Mortality increases with the number of comorbid conditions present but, at any level, is greater for hip fracture cases than controls. There is no increased risk of death following distal forearm fractures, nor is there an early excess of vertebral fracture deaths like that seen for hip fractures. Instead, survival appears to worsen with the passage of time

Table 4 Estimated Lifetime Fracture Risk in 50-Year-Old White Women and Men

	Women % (95% C.I.)	Men % (95% C.I.)
Proximal femur fracture	17.5 (16.8–18.2)	6.0 (5.6–6.5)
Vertebral fracture[a]	15.6 (14.8–16.3)	5.0 (4.6–5.4)
Distal forearm fracture	16.0 (15.2–16.7)	2.5 (2.2–3.1)
Any of the three	39.7 (38.7–40.6)	13.1 (12.4–13.7)

[a]Clinically diagnosed fractures only.
Source: Ref. 25.

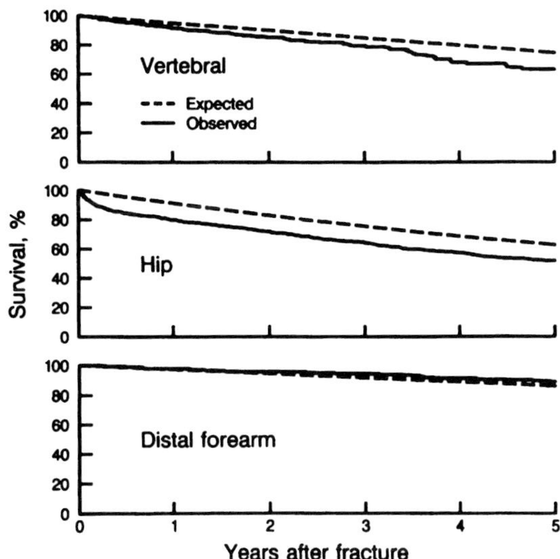

Figure 3 Survival following the diagnosis of vertebral, hip, and distal forearm fracture among Rochester, Minnesota, residents. Figures show observed survival and that expected using death rates of West North Central United States residents in 1980. (From Ref. 27.)

(Fig. 3), probably as the result of underlying diseases that increase the risk of both vertebral fracture and death (27).

From a social perspective, the adverse consequences of osteoporosis relate less to mortality than to long-term disability. Chrischilles and colleagues (28) have estimated that osteoporotic fractures of the hip, spine, and forearm would cause an extra 6.7% of postmenopausal white women to become dependent in the activities of daily living, over and above background levels of dependency in the community, and precipitate admission of an additional 7.8% of these women into nursing homes for long-term care. Again, hip fractures contribute the most to these problems, with up to a third of hip fracture victims becoming totally dependent (29). The majority of vertebral fractures, on the other hand, are not medically attended (24). Nonetheless, vertebral fractures account for 161,000 physician office visits and over 5 million restricted-activity days each year (30). Problems are mostly linked to the minority of elderly women with severe vertebral fractures (31), and only an estimated 4.2% of patients with a vertebral fracture become dependent because of the fracture (28). Similarly, distal forearm fractures lead to over 6 million restricted-activity days annually (30), but they have generally been considered free of long-term disability. While it has been estimated that less than

1% of forearm fracture patients become dependent as a result of the fracture (28), nearly half report only fair or poor functional outcomes at 6 months (32).

The total cost of fractures may be as much as $20 billion per year in the United States (33), and osteoporosis accounts for at least a third of this (30). These costs are likely to rise in the future. Because hip fracture incidence rates rise exponentially with aging (see below), continuation of the demographic trends described earlier could raise the number of hip fractures worldwide from an estimated 1.7 million in 1990 to a projected 6.3 million in 2050 (34). In the United States, the number of hip fractures and their associated costs could triple by 2040 solely on the basis of these demographic changes (35). Any rise in fracture incidence rates, over and above that due to population aging, will increase the number of future fractures still further. Indeed, dramatic increases in incidence have been seen in all areas of the world (Fig. 4), although age-adjusted rates appear to have leveled off in recent years in the United States (36), Sweden (37), and Great Britain (38). No explanation for these changes is known, although speculation has centered on decreases over time in physical activity (36).

B. Risk Factors for Fractures

Incidence rates for proximal femur fractures increase exponentially with aging (Fig. 5), reaching about 3% per year among European-American women aged 85

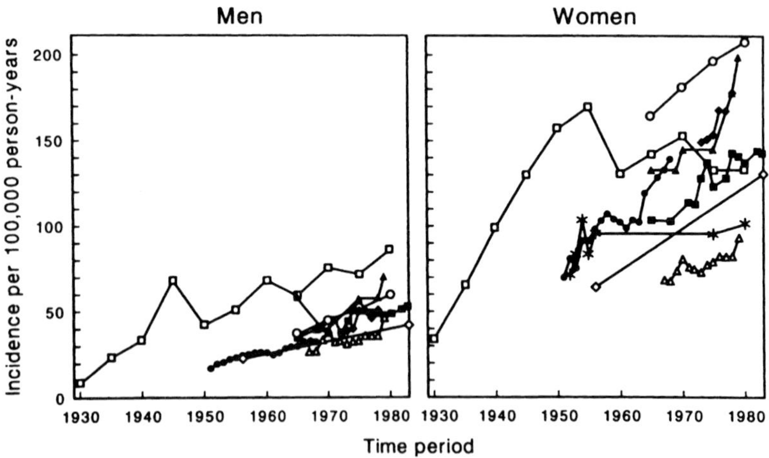

Figure 4 Incidence of hip fractures over time as reported from various studies: ❑–❑ Rochester, Minnesota; ■–■ United States; ◇ – ◇ Oxford, England; ◆ – ◆ Funen County, Denmark; △–△ Holland; ▲–▲ Göteborg, Sweden; ○–○ Uppsala, Sweden; ▪–▪ New Zealand; $*-*$ Dundee, Scotland. (From Ref. 36.)

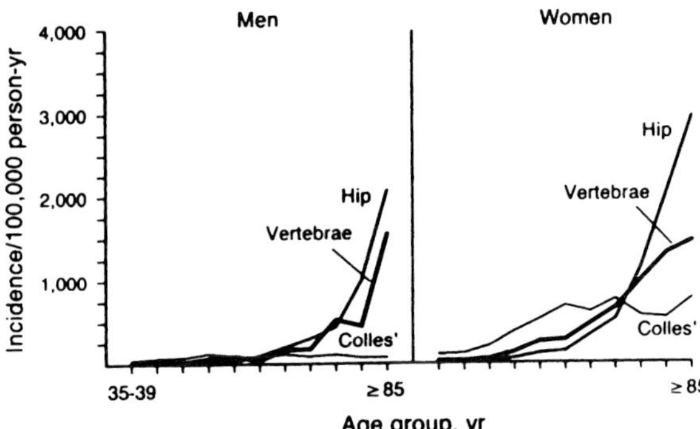

Figure 5 Age-specific incidence rates of hip, vertebral, and Colles' fracture in Rochester, Minnesota, men and women. (From Ref. 82.)

years and over (23). Although this pattern has been seen in virtually every study of white women, incidence rates vary over sevenfold from one European country to another (39) and, within the United States, vary substantially by county nationwide (40). Within counties, hip fracture incidence rates are higher for urban than for rural women (41). These observations indicate a strong role for environmental factors in modulating hip fracture risk among elderly white women. Hip fracture incidence rates for white men at any age are about half those for women in most studies, but, because women live longer, 80% of all hip fractures are in women. This is not true everywhere, however. Among the Maori in New Zealand, men and women have similar hip fracture incidence rates (42), while rates are higher among Bantu men in South Africa (43) and Chinese and Malay men in Singapore (44). Hip fractures are considerably less frequent among African-Americans (45), with less difference in age-adjusted rates between African-American men and women compared to whites. Hip fracture incidence rates among those of Asian ancestry lie between those of whites and blacks, but a sharp increase in hip fracture incidence in some parts of the Far East in recent decades has brought rates closer to those observed in Northern Europe (46). Indeed, when projected population growth is taken into account, it is estimated that about half of the expected 6.3 million hip fractures worldwide in 2050 will occur in Asia (34).

The greater hip fracture incidence in women than men and whites than nonwhites (Fig. 6) has been attributed to differences in bone mass, with African-Americans said to have substantially greater bone mineral density than European-Americans of the same age and sex. However, the African Bantu, who have the lowest hip fracture incidence rates of any population, have values for metacarpal bone density that are lower than those of Johannesburg whites, who display the usual Western pattern of hip fracture incidence (47). The Bantu do have better

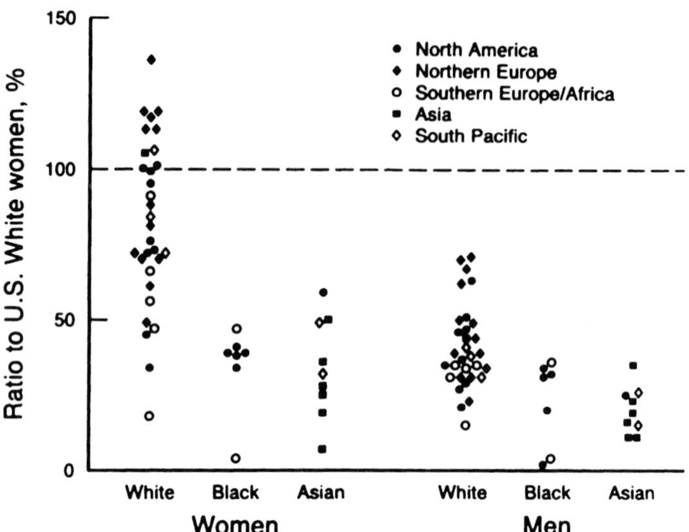

Figure 6 Hip fracture incidence around the world as a ratio of the rates observed to those expected for United States white women of the same age. (From Ref. 11.)

skeletal preservation during midlife, presumably as a result of physically demanding labor. Greater strength and fitness may also account for the lower risk of falling in black than white women (48) and for the lower hip fracture risk that Japanese women enjoy (49). As additional studies reveal differences in bone mass within racial groups (50,51), however, it becomes more difficult to understand how prominent risk factors like age, sex, and race exert their effects.

The incidence of vertebral fractures in white women and men has a similar pattern (Fig. 5), but the number of affected individuals depends on who is counted. A study of clinically diagnosed vertebral fractures in Rochester, Minnesota, found rapidly rising incidence rates with aging in both sexes (24). Rates rose from less than 0.2 per 1,000 per year in men and women under 45 years of age to annual rates of 1.3 per 1,000 men and 1.2 per 1,000 women aged 85 years and over. Since only about a third of all vertebral fractures in Rochester women come to clinical attention, these are underestimates of the true rate (24). Nonetheless, they are greater than those reported in most other incidence studies (52–54). That the true frequency is greater is evidenced by the high prevalence of vertebral fracture found in most studies. A radiographic survey of Rochester women revealed a rapid rise in vertebral fracture prevalence with age, affecting more than half of the women aged 85 years and over (55). Altogether, it is estimated that a fourth of women 50 years of age and over in the general population of Rochester have one or more vertebral fractures, counting crushed, wedged, or ballooned vertebrae. This is consistent with the 21% prevalence reported from a random sample of 70-year-old Danish women (56) and the 24% figure documented among elderly white women from the Study of Osteoporotic Fractures (31). Curiously, the prevalence of vertebral fractures among Asians seems to be as high as that in whites (57), despite their lower hip fracture rates. Few data are available for other ethnic groups.

It has long been held that vertebral fractures are uncommon in men so that the female excess greatly exceeds that seen for other osteoporotic fractures. However, recent population-based studies have documented an unexpectedly high frequency of vertebral fractures in men (58–60). For example, the overall female:male ratio of age-adjusted vertebral fracture incidence rates in Rochester was only 2:1 (24). The sex ratio was 4:1 in the age group 55–64 years, however. The greater discrepancy in rates among middle-aged subjects probably explains the 4:1 ratio reported among women and men with vertebral fractures referred to metabolic bone disease clinics (61). Conversely, prevalence rates were higher in men in two surveys of clinic outpatients in North Dakota, ranging from about 20% in men 45–54 years old to nearly 50% in men 65 years of age and over (62). These inflated figures may reflect occupationally related vertebral fractures insofar as the primary occupation in these rural areas was farming.

There is also a substantial female excess of distal forearm fractures, but the steep rise in incidence begins earlier in life and levels off after about age 60 years (Fig. 5). Consequently, rates in the elderly are only a fraction of those of hip fractures (23). While forearm fractures seem to be less frequent in African-American and Asian populations (63,64), the epidemiologic picture is generally the same. The plateau in forearm fracture incidence may be due to changes in the pattern of bone loss (65), with reversal of the cortical porosity that develops in the distal forearm around the time of menopause or cessation of the bone loss associated with type I osteoporosis (66). Since forearm fracture occurrence is also determined by the risk of falling onto one's hand (67), it has also been suggested that the failure of incidence rates to rise after midlife results from the loss of protective reflexes, with a resulting reduction in the tendency to break falls with an outstretched arm (68). Indeed, the likelihood of falling is great, rising annually from about 1 in 5 women 45–49 years old to nearly half of those aged 85 years and over (69). The risk of falling is generally much less in men.

The pathophysiology of these falls is poorly understood and usually results from a complex interaction of several factors. While environmental factors play a role, half or more of the falls among elderly persons are associated with organic dysfunction such as diminished postural control, gait changes, muscular weakness, decreased reflexes, or poor vision (Table 5). The proportion of persons with

Table 5 Risk Factors for Falling

Reduced visual acuity, dark adaptation and perception
Reduced hearing
Vestibular dysfunction
Proprioceptive dysfunction, cervical degenerative disorders, peripheral neuropathy
Dementia
Musculoskeletal disorders
Foot disorders (calluses, bunions, deformities)
Postural hypotension
Use of medications (benzodiazepines, phenothiazines, antidepressants, antihypertensives, antiarrhythmics, anticonvulsants, diuretics, alcohol, etc.)

Source: Ref. 83.

one of more of these problems increases with age, and the risk of falling is directly correlated with the number of conditions present (70). Most falls, however, do not result in an injury, even among the elderly. Only about 5% of falls lead to a fracture, and only 1 in 100 ends in a hip fracture (71). Additional risk factors related to the mechanics of falling probably account for this (72). Thus, it was recently shown that the likelihood of hip fracture among community fallers was influenced by the orientation of the fall, the potential energy of the faller, and the amount of soft tissue padding over the hip, as well as by the bone density of the proximal femur (73).

A substantial number of case-control or cohort studies have been conducted in an attempt to identify the most important risk factors for hip, spine, and forearm fractures, but the results can best be described as inconsistent, as summarized in Table 6. As would be expected from the previous discussion, the risk factors for hip fractures include those undoubtedly associated with an increased risk of falling (e.g., hemiplegia), those probably operating through accelerated bone loss (e.g., early menopause), and those that might have either effect (e.g., immobilization). Because vertebral fractures are less closely associated with falls, it also seems reasonable that risk factors relating to bone loss are more prominent, especially corticosteroid use. Less is known about the risk factors for distal forearm fractures (23). Indeed, of a large number of potential risk factors that were evaluated among elderly women in the Study of Osteoporotic Fractures, only low bone density in the distal radius, increased distance walked each week, and earlier age at menopause were independent risk factors in a multivariate analysis (74).

Considering the complex pathophysiology of osteoporotic fractures, it is not surprising that attempts to use these epidemiologic risk factors to predict fracture risk in patients have met with limited success. For example, one risk factor score (age, lactation for more than 12 months, nulliparity, metacarpal bone mass less

Table 6 Epidemiologic Evidence for Associations of Various Factors With the Risk of Specific Age-Related Fractures (blanks indicate the absence of reliable epidemiologic evidence)

	Forearm fracture		Vertebral fracture		Hip fracture	
Risk factor	Men	Women	Men	Women	Men	Women
Age	±	+	±	+	+	+
Race	+	+	±	+	+	+
Estrogens (protective)		+		+	+	+
Obesity (protective)		±	+	+	+	+
Neuromuscular dysfunction						
Visual impairment						±
Dementia						±
Alcoholism			+			+
Family history						
Parity	NA		NA	−	NA	
Lactation (protective)	NA		NA	±	NA	±
Activity (protective)						±
Immobilization						+
Smoking			+	±	+	+
Moderate ethanol use			+	±	±	±
Calcium intake				±		−
Early menopause	NA		NA	+	NA	±
Hypogonadism			+			
Prior fracture					+	+
Diabetes mellitus					±	±
Corticosteroids			+		−	±
Rheumatoid arthritis						±
Thyroidectomy					±	±
Gastrectomy			+		+	
Hemiplegia					±	+
Psychotropic drugs						±

Key: +, reasonable evidence for association; ±, conflicting or weak evidence of association; −, evidence for no association; NA, not applicable.
Source: Ref. 84.

than 47 mm^2, height less than 160 cm, and menarche at age 16 or later) showed some ability to discriminate among 742 Dutch women aged 45–64 years who did and did not have subsequent fractures over 9 years of follow-up (75). However, sensitivity and specificity were low, both for defining fractures generally (37% and 83%, respectively) and for fractures of the forearm or vertebrae (48% and 84%, respectively). Risk factors of this sort were also unable to predict vertebral fractures among a group of 704 Japanese-American women (Table 7). The lack of specificity was demonstrated by the fact that all of the women had at least two of the risk factors and 91% had four or more of them (76). Likewise, a risk factor score was unable to identify vertebral fractures among 1,012 women in the United Kingdom (77). In this instance, if a cutoff score was selected to assure high sensitivity (91%), the specificity was only 23%, and 91 women out of 100 with a "positive" score were false positives (positive predictive value, 9%). Conversely, if specificity was increased to 94%, sensitivity fell to 15% so that 85 of every 100 women with a vertebral fracture would be missed. Worse, most of this modest predictive power was contributed by a history of vertebral fracture per se (77). Thus, no set of risk factors has been shown to predict fractures with accuracy sufficient for application to the care of individual patients.

Fortunately, a variety of techniques developed over the past few decades permit accurate and precise measurement of bone density at different skeletal sites. These measurements provide a convenient in vivo assessment of bone strength, as well as an ability to predict future fractures. Indeed, the most persuasive argument that bone mass is important in the determination of fracture risk comes from prospective studies where bone mass measurements were made and subjects were followed until fractures occurred. A number of such studies have been published, utilizing a variety of techniques to measure bone mass at different skeletal sites in order to predict a variety of subsequent fractures (78). Most recently, it was shown that each standard deviation decrease in femoral neck bone density was associated with a 2.6-fold increase in the age-adjusted risk of hip

Table 7 Risk Factor Prevalence and Relative Risk of Spine Fracture

	Prevalence	Relative risk	*P* value
Premature menopause (≤ age 40)	4.7%	1.6	NS
Family history (+ or −)	1.7%	2.7	NS
Short stature (ht ≤62 in)	87.2%	1.6	NS
Leanness (BMI ≤19.7)	14.7%	1.7	NS
Calcium deficiency (≤500 mg)	83.9%	1.2	NS
Physical activity (PAI ≤26.9)	7.8%	2.5	NS
Nulliparity (+ or −)	5.7%	1.6	NS
Smoking (+ or −)	16.8%	1.2	NS
Alcohol (≥2 g/day)	4.8%	1.7	NS
Asian ancestry (+ or −)	100.0%	—	—
Caffeine (≥300 mg/day)	29.6%	2.1	NS
Chronic gastrointestinal disease (+ or −)	4.1%	1.0	NS

Source: Ref. 76.

fracture among 8,134 women followed for 1.8 years in the Study of Osteoporotic Fractures (79). This short-term result was consistent with the 2.4-fold increase in age-adjusted hip fracture risk seen in a smaller group of 304 Rochester women followed for over 8 years when bone mineral was measured at the same site (80). These issues are reviewed in Chapter 9.

IV. CONCLUSIONS

A variety of pathophysiologic mechanisms contribute to the decline in bone density (a pathogenic trait), which causes a disproportionate decrease in bone strength (asymptomatic disease) and leads to an increase in fractures (symptomatic disease), which are the main clinical manifestations of osteoporosis. While osteoporosis is widely viewed as a major public health concern, the exact magnitude of the problem depends on how the condition is defined. Whether assessed on the basis of low bone mass or the occurrence of specific fractures, however, osteoporosis is a very common condition. Because there are no symptoms of osteoporosis until fractures occur, relatively few people are diagnosed in time for effective therapy to be administered. Consequently, a large number of individuals experience the pain, expense, disability, and decreased quality of life caused by these age-related fractures. As noted previously, the therapies for osteoporosis that are now available cannot restore skeletal strength to normal. Even if they could, fractures would continue to occur as a result of traumatic events, especially falls. Consequently, prevention of the clinical manifestations of osteoporosis will depend in large part on ultimately reducing the frequency and severity of falls. However, the only action that can be taken now to prevent fractures in the future is to preserve bone mass. This is crucial because demographic changes alone can be expected to increase the number of fractures dramatically in coming years. If the enormous costs associated with these fractures are to be reduced, increased attention must be given to the design and implementation of effective control programs.

ACKNOWLEDGMENTS

The author would like to thank Mrs. Mary Roberts for help in preparing the manuscript.

This study was supported by grants AR 27065 and AG 04875 from the National Institutes of Health, U.S. Public Health Service.

REFERENCES

1. Peck WA, Burckhardt P, Christiansen C, et al. Consensus Development Conference: Diagnosis, prophylaxis, and treatment of osteoporosis. Am J Med 1993; 94:646–650.

2. Kanis JA, Melton LJ, Christiansen C, Johnston CC, Khaltaev N. The diagnosis of osteoporosis. J Bone Miner Res 1994; 8:1137–1141.
3. Schapira D, Schapira C. Osteoporosis: the evolution of a scientific term. Osteoporosis Int 1992; 2:164–167.
4. Johnston CC Jr, Melton LJ III, Lindsay R, Eddy DM. Clinical indications for bone mass measurements: a report from the Scientific Advisory Board of the National Osteoporosis Foundation. J Bone Miner Res 1989; 4(suppl 2):1–28.
5. Riggs BL, Melton LJ III. The prevention and treatment of osteoporosis. N Engl J Med 1992; 327:620–627.
6. Melton LJ. How many women have osteoporosis now? J Bone Miner Res 1995; 10:175–177.
7. Johnston CC, Melton LJ. Bone densitometry. In: Riggs BL, Melton LJ, eds. Osteoporosis: Etiology, Diagnosis and Management, 2nd ed. Philadelphia: Lippincott-Raven Press: 1995: 275–297.
8. Riggs BL, Melton LJ III. Medical progress: involutional osteoporosis. N Engl J Med 1986; 314:1676–1686.
9. Peck WA, Riggs BL, Bell NH, Wallace RB, Johnston CC Jr, Gordon SL. Research directions in osteoporosis. Am J Med 1988; 84:275–282.
10. Hui SL, Slemenda CW, Johnston CC Jr. The contribution of bone loss to postmenopausal osteoporosis. Osteoporosis Int 1990; 1:30–34.
11. Melton LJ III. Differing patterns of osteoporosis across the world. In: Chesnut CH III, ed. Proceedings of the Second Asian Symposium on Osteoporosis—New Dimensions in Osteoporosis in the 1990s. Hong Kong: Excerpta Medica Asia; 1991:13–18.
12. Yano K, Wasnich RD, Vogel JM, Heilbrun LK. Bone mineral measurements among middle-aged and elderly Japanese residents in Hawaii. Am J Epidemiol 1984; 119: 751–764.
13. Sowers MR, Wallace RD, Lemke JH. Correlates of mid-radius bone density among postmenopausal women: a community study. Am J Clin Nutr 1985; 41:1045–1053.
14. Jensen MD, Kanaley JA, Roust LR, et al. Assessment of body composition with use of dual-energy x-ray absorptiometry: evaluation and comparison with other methods. Mayo Clin Proc 1993; 68:867–873.
15. Bauer DC, Browner WS, Cauley JA, et al. for the Study of Osteoporotic Fractures Research Group. Factors associated with appendicular bone mass in older women. Ann Intern Med 1993; 118:657–665.
16. Barrett-Connor E, Chang JC, Edelstein SL. Coffee-associated osteoporosis offset by daily milk consumption. JAMA 1994; 271:280–283.
17. Cooper C, Atkinson EJ, Wahner HW, et al. Is caffeine consumption a risk factor for osteoporosis? J Bone Miner Res 1992; 7:465–471.
18. Slemenda CW, Hui SL, Longcope C, Wellman H, Johnston CC Jr. Predictors of bone mass in perimenopausal women: a prospective study of clinical data using photon absorptiometry. Ann Intern Med 1990; 112:96–101.
19. Krall EA, Dawson-Hughes B, Papas A, Garcia RI. Tooth loss and skeletal bone density in healthy postmenopausal women. Osteoporosis Int 1994; 4:104–109.
20. Cooper A. A Treatise on Dislocations and Fractures of the Joints. Cooper BB, ed. London: John Churchill; 1842.

21. Albright F, Smith PH, Richardson AM. Postmenopausal osteoporosis. JAMA 1941; 116:2465–2474.
22. Seeley DG, Browner WS, Nevitt MC, Genant HK, Scott JC, Cummings SR, for the Study of Osteoporotic Fractures Research Group. Which fractures are associated with low appendicular bone mass in elderly women? Ann Intern Med 1991; 115:837–842.
23. Melton LJ III. Epidemiology of fractures. In: Riggs BL, Melton LJ III, eds. Osteoporosis: Etiology, Diagnosis, and Management. New York: Raven Press; 1988: 133–154.
24. Cooper C, Atkinson EJ, O'Fallon WM, Melton LJ III. Incidence of clinically diagnosed vertebral fractures: a population-based study in Rochester, Minnesota, 1985–1989. J Bone Miner Res 1992; 7:221–227.
25. Melton LJ III, Chrischilles EA, Cooper C, Lane AW, Riggs BL. How many women have osteoporosis? J Bone Miner Res 1992; 7:1005–1010.
26. Poór G, Atkinson EJ, O'Fallon WM, Melton LJ. Determinants of reduced survival following hip fracture in men: a controlled, population-based study. Clin Orthop 1995; 319:260–265.
27. Cooper C, Atkinson EJ, Jacobsen SJ, O'Fallon WM, Melton LJ III. Population-based study of survival after osteoporotic fractures. Am J Epidemiol 1993; 137:1001–1005
28. Chrischilles EA, Butler CD, Davis CS, Wallace RB. A model of lifetime osteoporosis impact. Arch Intern Med 1991; 151:2026–2032.
29. Jensen JS, Bagger J. Long-term social prognosis after hip fractures. Acta Orthop Scand 1982; 53:97–101.
30. Holbrook TL, Grazier K, Kelsey JL, Stauffer RN. The frequency of occurrence, impact and cost of selected musculoskeletal conditions in the United States. Chicago: American Academy of Orthopedic Surgeons; 1984.
31. Ettinger B, Black DM, Nevitt MC, et al. and the Study of Osteoporotic Fractures Research Group. Contribution of vertebral deformities to chronic back pain and disability. J Bone Miner Res 1992; 7:449–456.
32. Kaukonen J-P, Karaharju EO, Porras M, Lüthje P, Jakobsson A. Functional recovery after fractures of the distal forearm: analysis of radiographic and other factors affecting the outcome. Ann Chir Gynaecol 1988; 77:27–31.
33. Praemer A, Furner S, Rice DP. Musculoskeletal conditions in the United States. Park Ridge, IL: American Academy of Orthopaedic Surgeons; 1992.
34. Cooper C, Campion G, Melton LJ III. Hip fractures in the elderly: a world-wide projection. Osteoporosis Int 1992; 2:285–289.
35. Schneider EL, Guralnik JM. The aging of America: impact on health care costs. JAMA 1990; 263:2335–2340.
36. Melton LJ III, O'Fallon WM, Riggs BL. Secular trends in the incidence of hip fractures. Calcif Tissue Int 1987; 41:57–64.
37. Naessén T, Parker R, Persson I, Zack M, Adami H-O. Time trends in incidence rates of first hip fracture in the Uppsala Health Care Region, Sweden, 1965–1983. Am J Epidemiol 1989; 130:289–299.
38. Spector TD, Cooper C, Lewis AF. Trends in admissions for hip fracture in England and Wales, 1968–85. BMJ 1990; 300:1173–1174.
39. Johnell O, Gullberg B, Allender E, Kanis JA, and the MEDOS Study Group. The

apparent incidence of hip fracture in Europe: a study of national register sources. Osteoporosis Int 1992; 2:298–302.

40. Jacobsen SJ, Goldberg J, Miles TP, Brody JA, Stiers SW, Rimm AA. Regional variation in the incidence of hip fracture: US white women aged 65 years and older. JAMA 1990; 264:500–502.
41. Madhok R, Melton LJ III, Atkinson EJ, O'Fallon WM, Lewallen DG. Urban vs rural increase in hip fracture incidence: age and sex of 901 cases 1980–89 in Olmsted County, U.S.A. Acta Orthop Scand 1993; 64:543–548.
42. Stott S, Gray DH. The incidence of femoral neck fractures in New Zealand. N Z Med J 1980; 91:6–9.
43. Solomon L. Osteoporosis and fracture of the femoral neck in the South African Bantu. J Bone Joint Surg 1968; 50-B:2–13.
44. Wong PCN. Femoral neck fractures among the major racial groups in Singapore. Incidence patterns compared with non-Asian communities. No. II. Singapore Med J 1964; 5:150–157.
45. Jacobsen SJ, Goldberg J, Miles TP, Brody JA, Stiers W, Rimm AA. Hip fracture incidence among the old and very old: a population-based study of 745,435 cases. Am J Public Health 1990; 80:871–873.
46. Lau EMC, Cooper C, Wickham C, Donnan S, Barker DJP. Hip fracture in Hong Kong and Britain. Int J Epidemiol 1990; 19:1119–1121.
47. Solomon L. Bone density in aging Caucasian and African populations. Lancet 1979; 2:1326–1330.
48. Nevitt MC, Cummings SR, Kidd S, Black D. Risk factors for recurrent nonsyncopal falls. a prospective study. JAMA 1989; 261:2663–2668.
49. Ross PD, Norimatsu H, Davis JW, et al. A comparison of hip fracture incidence among native Japanese, Japanese Americans, and American Caucasians. Am J Epidemiol 1991; 133:801–809.
50. Nomura A, Wasnich RD, Heilbrun LK, Ross PD, Davis JW. Comparison of bone mineral content between Japan-born and U.S.-born Japanese subjects in Hawaii. Bone Miner 1989; 6:213–223.
51. Sugimoto T, Tsutsumi M, Fujii Y, et al. Comparison of bone mineral content among Japanese, Koreans, and Taiwanese assessed by dual-photon absorptiometry. J Bone Miner Res 1992; 7:153–159.
52. Bengnér U, Johnell O, Redlund-Johnell I. Changes in incidence and prevalence of vertebral fractures during 30 years. Calcif Tissue Int 1988; 42:293–296.
53. Härmä M, Heliävaara M, Aromaa A, Knekt P. Thoracic spine compression fractures in Finland. Clin Orthop 1986; 205:188–194.
54. Donaldson LJ, Cook A, Thomson RG. Incidence of fractures in a geographically defined population. J Epidemiol Commun Health 1990; 44:241–245.
55. Melton LJ III, Lane AW, Cooper C, Eastell R, O'Fallon WM, Riggs B. Prevalence and incidence of vertebral deformities. Osteoporosis Int 1993; 3:113–119.
56. Jensen GF, Christiansen C, Boesen J, Hegedüs V, Transbøl I. Epidemiology of postmenopausal spinal and long bone fractures: a unifying approach to postmenopausal osteoporosis. Clin Orthop 1982, 166:75–81.
57. Ross PD, Fujiwara S, Huang C, et al. Japanese women in Hiroshima have greater

vertebral fracture prevalence than Caucasians or Japanese-Americans in the U.S. Int J Epidemiol (In press.)

58. Bauer RL, Deyo RA. Low risk of vertebral fracture in Mexican American women. Arch Intern Med 1987; 147:1437–1439.
59. Johansson C, Mellström D, Rosengren K, Rundgren A. Prevalence of vertebral fractures in 85-year-olds: radiographic examination of 462 subjects. Acta Orthop Scand 1993; 64:25–27.
60. Lee TK. Update on osteoporosis in Taiwan. In: Chesnut CH III, ed. New dimensions in osteoporosis in the 1990s. Proceedings of the Second Asian Symposium on Osteoporosis, November 10, 1990. Hong Kong: Asia Pacific Congress Series No. 125; 1991:8–12.
61. Riggs BL, Melton LJ III. Evidence for two distinct syndromes of involutional osteoporosis. Am J Med 1983; 755:899–901.
62. Bernstein DS, Sadowsky N, Hegsted DM, Guri CD, Stare FJ. Prevalence of osteoporosis in high- and low-fluoride areas of North Dakota. JAMA 1966; 198:499–504.
63. Griffin MR, Ray WA, Fought RL, Melton LJ III. Black-white differences in fracture rates. Am J Epidemiol 1992; 136:1378–1385.
64. Hagino H, Yamamoto K, Teshima R, Kishimoto H, Kuranobu K, Nakamura T. The incidence of fractures of the proximal femur and the distal radius in Tottori prefecture, Japan. Arch Orthop Trauma Surg 1989; 109:43–44.
65. Horsman A, Burkinshaw L. Stochastic models of bone loss and fracture risk. In: Ring EFJ, Evans WD, Dixon AS, eds. Osteoporosis and Bone Mineral Measurement. York: Institute of Physical Sciences in Medicine; 1989:17–30.
66. Parfitt AM. Cortical porosity in postmenopausal and adolescent wrist fractures. In: Uhthoff H, Jaworski ZFG, eds. Current Concepts of Bone Fragility. Proceedings of the Conference on Bone Fragility in Orthopaedics and Medicine, Ottawa, May 16–18, 1985. Berlin: Springer-Verlag; 1986:167–172.
67. Nevitt MC, Cummings SR, and the Study of Osteoporotic Fractures Research Group. Type of fall and risk of hip and wrist fractures: the study of osteoporotic fractures. J Am Geriatr Soc 1993; 41:1226–1234.
68. Evans JG. Epidemiology of proximal femoral fractures. Rec Adv Geriatr Med 1982; 2:201–214.
69. Winner SJ, Morgan CA, Evans JG. Perimenopausal risk of falling and incidence of distal forearm fracture. BMJ 1989; 298:1486–1488.
70. Tinetti ME, Speechley M, Ginter SF. Risk factors for falls among elderly persons living in the community. N Engl J Med 1988; 319:1701–1707.
71. Gibson MJ. The prevention of falls in later life. Dan Med Bull 1987; 34(suppl 4):1–24.
72. Melton LJ III, Riggs BL. Risk factors for injury after a fall. Clin Geriatr Med 1985; 1:525–539.
73. Greenspan SL, Myers ER, Maitland LA, Resnick NM, Hayes WC. Fall severity and bone mineral density as risk factors for hip fracture in ambulatory elderly. JAMA 1994; 271:128–133.
74. Kelsey JL, Browner WS, Seeley DG, Nevitt MC, Cummings SR, for the Study of Osteoporotic Fractures Research Group. Risk factors for fractures of the distal forearm and proximal humerus. Am J Epidemiol 1992; 135:477–489.

75. Van Hemert AM, Vandenbroucke JP, Birkenhäger JC, Valkenburg HA. Prediction of osteoporotic fractures in the general population by a fracture risk score: a 9-year follow-up among middle-aged women. Am J Epidemiol 1990; 132:123–135.
76. Wasnich RD, Ross PD, MacLean CJ, Davis JW, Vogel JM. The relative strengths of osteoporotic risk factors in a prospective study of postmenopausal osteoporosis. In: Christiansen C, Johansen JS, Riis BJ, eds. Osteoporosis 1987, Vol. 1. Proceedings of the International Symposium on Osteoporosis. Copenhagen: Osteopress ApS; 1987: 394–395.
77. Cooper C, Shah S, Hand DJ, et al. (Multicentre Vertebral Fracture Study Group). Screening for vertebral osteoporosis using individual risk factors. Osteoporosis Int 1991; 2:48–53.
78. Ross PD, Davis JW, Vogel JM, Wasnich RD. A critical review of bone mass and the risk of fractures in osteoporosis. Calcif Tissue Int 1990; 46:149–161.
79. Cummings SR, Black DM, Nevitt MC, et al. for the Study of Osteoporotic Fractures Research Group. Bone density at various sites for prediction of hip fractures. Lancet 1993; 341:72–75.
80. Melton LJ III, Atkinson EJ, O'Fallon WM, Wahner HW, Riggs BL. Long-term fracture prediction by bone mineral assessed at different skeletal sites. J Bone Miner Res 1993; 8:1227–1233.
81. Riggs BL. Osteoporosis. In: Wyngaarden JB, Smith LH Jr, eds. Cecil's Textbook of Medicine. Philadelphia: WB Saunders Company; 1988:1510–1515.
82. Cooper C, Melton LJ. Epidemiology of osteoporosis. Trends Endocrinol Metab 1992; 3:224–229.
83. Tinetti ME, Speechley M. Prevention of falls among the elderly. N Engl J Med 1989; 320:1055–1059.
84. Melton LJ III, Cummings SR. Heterogeneity of age-related fractures: implications for epidemiology. Bone Miner 1987; 2:321–331

4

Biomechanical Aspects of Osteoporosis and Fractures

JOSEPH M. LANE

University of California at Los Angeles Medical Center
Los Angeles, California

ELIZABETH R. MYERS

Beth Israel Hospital and Harvard Medical School
Boston, Massachusetts

I. INTRODUCTION

Primary osteoporosis is characterized by decreased bone mass and increased susceptibility to fracture in an aging individual with no other endocrinopathy or disease state that would account for the bone mass changes (1). Osteoporosis affects more than 20 million individuals who sustain more than 1.2 million fractures annually at an estimated cost of $10 billion in 1992 (2). For a 50-year-old Caucasian woman today, the risk of hip fracture over her remaining lifetime is approximately 17% (3). The 1-year mortality rate from hip fractures varies from 15% to 25%, and the probability of the older patient regaining the previous level of function after hip fracture is 30–50%. Vertebral fractures also affect mortality; the 5-year survival after vertebral fracture is reduced to 81% (4). The consequences of osteoporosis can lead to significant morbidity including pain, depression, reclusiveness, and fear of further fracture (5). The purpose of this chapter is to discuss the biomechanical aspects of osteoporosis and the contribution of mechanics to the etiology of fracture.

Fracture represents a structural failure of bone. Engineering predictions of structural failure require information not only on the capacity of that structure to carry load but also on the forces that are applied to the structure during service (6,7). The mechanical consequences of decreased bone mass in osteoporosis are reductions in bone strength and decreased ability to carry load. The biomechanics of high-risk activities for fracture, however, are also important in understanding fracture etiology, as these activities affect the forces applied to the bone. These high-risk activities include, but are not limited to, falling for hip and wrist fracture, and lifting, bending, and falling for spine fracture. The influence of bone mass and osteoporosis on bone failure properties is first reviewed in this chapter, followed by considerations of how these reductions in strength interact with the forces applied to bones in hip and vertebral fractures.

II. OSTEOPOROSIS AND MECHANICAL PROPERTIES OF BONE

Bone is formed during childhood and reaches peak bone mass by the age of 25 years (8,9). Thereafter, bone loss occurs at the rate of 0.3–0.5% for women up to the point of menopause, at which time there is an expedited loss of bone at 2% per year for approximately 10 years (2). Trabecular bone, which has a high surface and low volume, has more rapid loss than cortical bone. Following the post-menopausal period, bone loss resumes at 0.3–0.5% per year in women. The rate of bone loss in the very old may actually increase again to a rate similar to that after menopause in women. Recent evidence from a longitudinal study indicates that women over the age of 65 lose approximately 0.9% of femoral bone annually. Moreover, the magnitude of this percent change increases with age such that the average femoral bone loss at age 90 is approximately 2.1% (10) (Fig. 1). Men lose bone at the rate of 0.3–0.5% per year and parallel women's rate of loss after the age of 65 (11).

The mechanics of fracture in both cortical and trabecular bone can be characterized by the failure strength—the maximum stress in a material under given loading conditions that often coincides with rupture. Bone strength is related to bone density, architecture, connectivity, and mineralization, with approximately 75–80% of the variance in the strength of bone accounted for by bone density (12–14). The material properties of cortical and trabecular bone decrease with increasing age, reflecting changes in bone density and microstructural arrangement. The tensile strength of cortical bone declines by about 2% per decade over the age range of 20 to 90 (15). Trabecular bone tissue exhibits larger age-related declines in failure strength. The compressive strength has been found to decrease by more than 10% per decade (16). This decline in strength is in part a reflection of the decrease in bone apparent density with age and osteoporosis. The compressive strength of trabecular bone is related to the bone apparent density by a power-law relationship, with an exponent of approximately 2 (12,17,18) (Fig. 2). Consequently, even small changes in density, such as the approximately 1% loss per year seen with age, can translate into major changes in bone strength.

Complicated structures such as the proximal femur, the vertebral body, or the

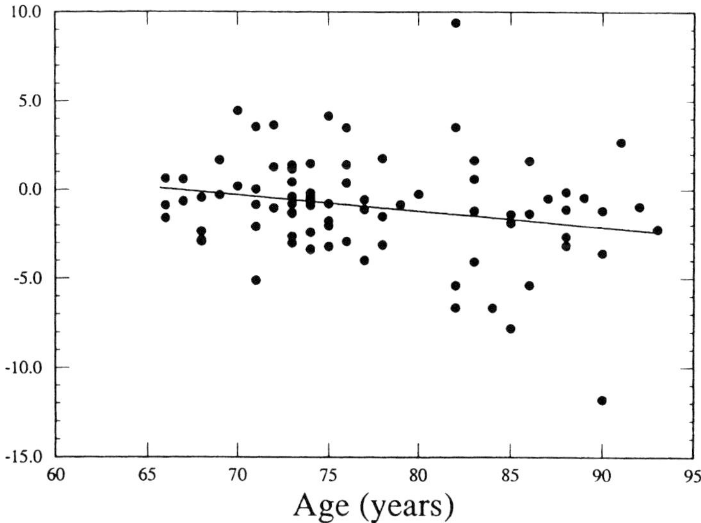

Figure 1 Dependence of percentage change in total hip bone mineral density over 1 year on age of the subjects at baseline. The subjects were women over the age of 65 (mean 77 years, range 66–93 years) from the community. Total hip bone mineral density (BMD) was assessed by DXA at two time points 1 year apart. The average change in BMD was −0.9%, but the percent change was associated significantly with age ($r = -0.23$; $P = .038$). Using an estimate from the linear regression, the change at age 90 was −2.1%. Adapted from Greenspan et al. (1994).

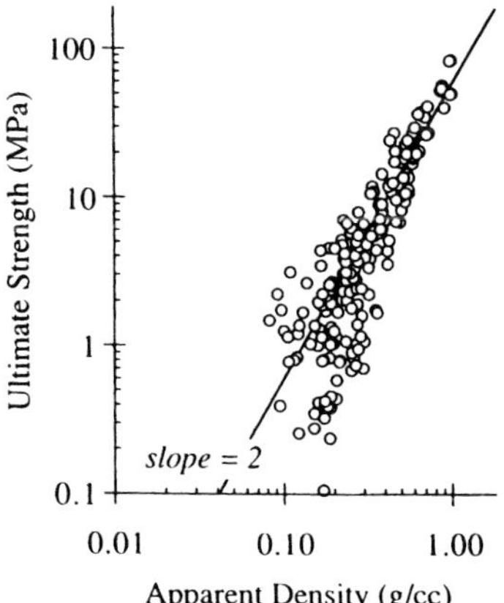

Figure 2 Compressive strength of trabecular bone as a function of apparent density. Compressive strength varies as the square of apparent density in general. From Keaveny and Hayes (1993).

bones of the wrist have failure properties that depend not only on bone strength (a material property) but also on bone geometry and the structural arrangement of bone. To capture the combined influences of the material strength and the bone geometry, the maximum force that a bone can carry is assessed under loading conditions meant to simulate clinical fracture. This force level is referred to as the structural capacity, the failure force, or the fracture load. The fracture load is specific to a certain set of loading conditions. For example, the fracture load (and the fracture pattern) of the proximal femur will be different if the hip is loaded in a configuration with side impact compared with a stance configuration. Similarly, the vertebrae fail differently if loaded in straight compression or in compression with forward flexion. Therefore, when describing results of fracture load, the results should always be placed in the context of the loading configuration.

Several studies have examined the contribution of the arrangement and structure of cortical and trabecular bone to the overall failure properties of the vertebra and femur. Biomechanical and anthropologic studies have suggested that the strength and structural capacity of bone are related to the percentage of trabecular bone and compact bone, to the architectural relationship of these various bones, to structural characteristics such as connectivity, and to bone geometry (19–22).

Noninvasive methodologies such as dual-energy x-ray densitometry (DXA) and quantitative computed tomography (QCT) give rise to an approximation of apparent density and geometry, and can be used to predict the strength and structural capacity of bone. Quantitative x-ray absorption measures the bone mineral content in a region of interest. The volumetric apparent density can then be determined by dividing the bone mineral content by volume using QCT. In a similar manner, the areal bone mineral density can be determined by dividing by projected area using DXA. Bone mineral properties derived from these methods account for 70–90% of the variance in fracture load of cadaveric hips loaded in a fall configuration (23–26) and spines in compression (21,27–30) (Fig. 3). In the elderly, a decline in bone mineral density over a decade, which could be as much as 10%, could result in a sizable decrease in spine and hip fracture loads on the order of hundreds of Newtons of force (Fig. 3). Thus, declines in bone mass and possible alterations in architecture, such as the changes that characterize osteoporosis, correspond to decreases in fracture load of the hip and spine.

III. HIP FRACTURES

About 90% of hip fractures are associated with falls (31–34), although the number of spontaneous fractures that are the source, rather than the cause, of a fall is uncertain. Only approximately 2% of falls, however, result in hip fracture (35–37). Therefore, there must be certain fall characteristics that increase the risk of hip fracture from a fall. Myers and Hayes (38) have hypothesized that the tendency to fall, the severity of a fall, including falls to the side, and bone

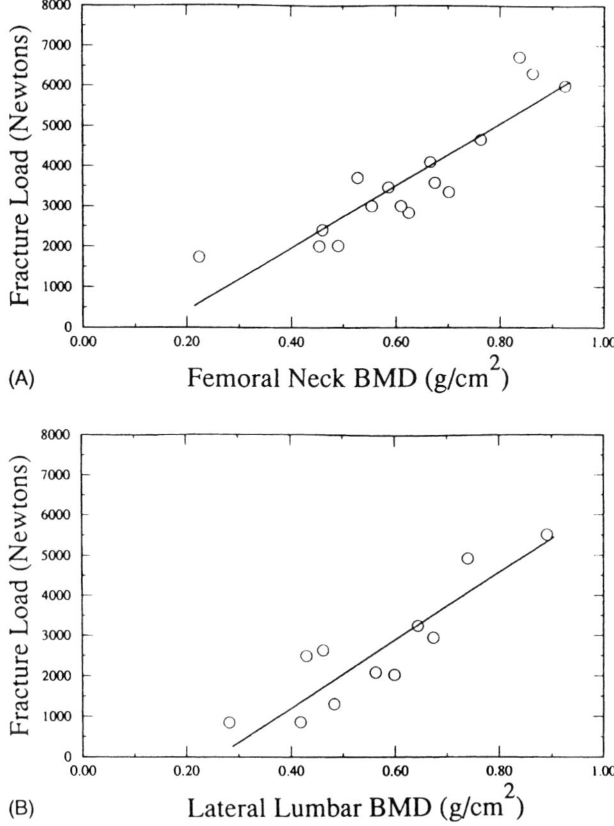

Figure 3 Fracture load as a function of BMD assessed by DXA. (A) Fracture test of the proximal femur from donors aged 59–96 years. The femur was loaded in a configuration with the side impact to the greater trochanter, and the fracture load ranged from 1,730 to 6,730 Newtons. Femoral neck BMD was measured with DXA. The fracture load was associated significantly with BMD ($r = 0.89$; $P < .001$). Adapted from Bouxsein et al. (1995). (B) Fracture test of the second lumbar vertebra from donors aged 48–87 years. Specimens were tested in compression with the first and third vertebral bodies embedded in bone cement. Fracture load ranged from 850 to 5,510 Newtons. The linear relationship between BMD and fracture load was significant ($r = 0.89$; $P < .001$). Adapted from Moro et al. (1995).

structural capacity, account for the dominant fracture risk in the area of the hip (Fig. 4).

Factors that relate to bone strength and femoral structural capacity have been noted to be associated with hip fracture, although controversy arises over the relative role of bone mass and hip fracture risk (39). Many factors other than bone density contribute to hip fractures; these include balance, frequency of falls (40), falling to the side (41), padding of the hip areas, and the structure of the femur itself. However, hip fracture incidence has long been recognized to rise steeply with age and to be higher in women than in men (42). The association of fractures with age and sex is thought to be related to the loss of bone density with age and to the lower bone density in women as compared to men (43). Decreased bone density appears to be an independent variable in terms of hip fracture risk. Cross-sectional studies have demonstrated a significantly enhanced risk associated with low bone mineral density; odds ratios are 2 to 3 for each standard deviation (SD) reduction in the femoral bone density (44–46). Cummings and associates (47) have confirmed that bone density measurements at the femoral site are superior to those at other sites for predicting future hip fracture. They noted that a decrease in bone mineral density of 1 SD, when adjusted for age, increases the fracture risk by 2.6. A 1 SD decrease in bone density in the calcaneus increases the hip fracture risk twofold, and a 1 SD decrease in the wrist bone density increases the hip fracture risk 1.6. Melton et al. (48) found that such a decrease in bone mineral density was comparable to a 13-year increase in age in terms of fracture risk. These studies and other investigations clearly identify a specific role for bone density and its relationship to increased hip fracture.

Confounding the issue of bone density is the question of connectivity and quality of bone. Estrogen and, most notably, calcium, which have a minor effect on appendicular bone mass, have a profound salutary effect on hip fracture risk. Studies performed by Chapuy and Meunier (49) demonstrate in France that a low dose of Vitamin D and calcium not only prevented loss of femoral bone mass but also decreased the rate of hip fractures in elderly persons. In that and associated studies, it was demonstrated that the secondary hyperparathyroidism was turned off with calcium supplementation and that any tendency toward a high turnover osteoporosis was thus dramatically diminished. These studies raise the issues, therefore, of minimal changes in bone mass associated with highly significant altered fracture rate presumably in the circumstances of comparable falls, balance, and weight among other aspects. Thus, the issue of density, though well documented in terms of contribution to fracture risk, must also include such elements as quality of bone that is ill-defined to date.

Factors related to fall severity affect hip fracture profoundly. Hayes and coworkers (41) have defined several distinct phases in terms of a fall: 1. instability phase that results in fall initiation; 2. descent phase; 3. impact phase; and 4. post-impact phase, during which the faller comes to rest. Cummings and Nevitt (50)

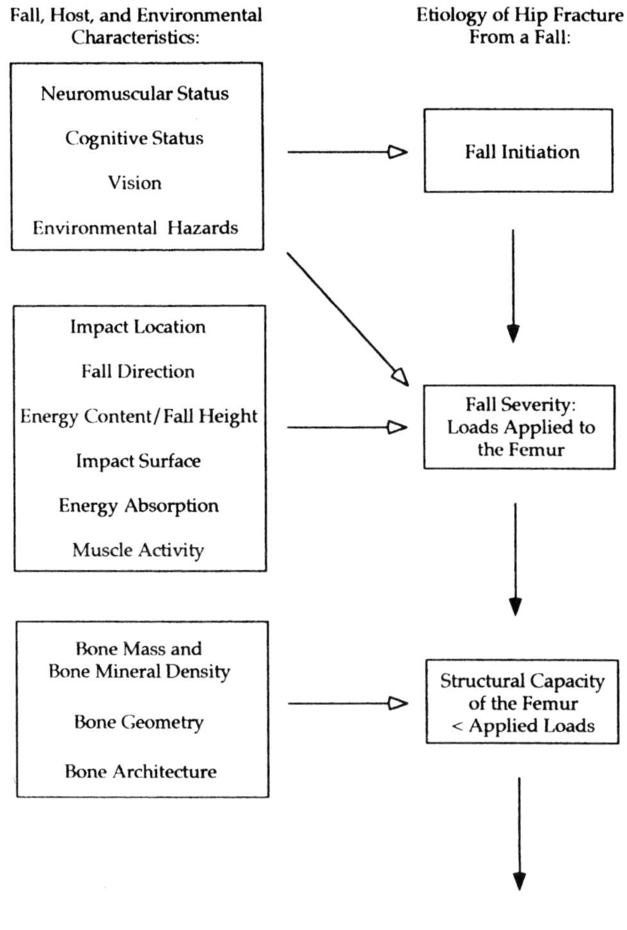

Figure 4 Possible factors in the origin of hip fracture from a fall. Falls must first be initiated and then must be of a certain severity for the impact forces to exceed the structural capacity of the femur. Fall severity seems to depend on impact location, fall direction, height of the fall, and energy absorption mechanisms. Femoral structural capacity or fracture load depends on bone geometry and bone strength, which in turn depend on density and architecture. Adapted from Myers and Hayes (1994).

have proposed that an injurious fall would include 1. impact on or near the hip, 2. lack of protective mechanism such as the use of an outstretched arm to break the fall, and 3. insufficient energy absorption by local soft tissues.

Hayes and co-workers (41) identified significant associations among fall characteristics of the descent and impact phases and hip fractures in nursing home residents (Table 1). Fallers with hip fracture fell to the side in 60% of cases and reported impact on the side of the leg in 59% of cases. In contrast, only 23% of falls that did not result in fracture were to the side, and only 6% had impact near the hip or side of the leg. Impact on the hip or the side of the leg had an adjusted odds ratio of 21.7 in multiple logistic regression. Low body mass index, as determined by weight divided by the square of the height, had an adjusted odd ratio of 4.2 for 1 SD decrease, and potential energy of fall resulted in an adjusted odds ratio of 3.3 for each standard deviation increase in energy.

Similar results were found in a nested case-control analysis of a large, prospective cohort of women in the community (51). Those who suffered a hip fracture were more likely to have fallen sideways and to have landed near the hip. Among women who fell on the hip, those with hip fracture were less likely to have landed on a hand, less likely to have grabbed an object during the fall, and more likely to have landed on a hard surface.

Greenspan et al. (46) conducted a study of risk factors associated with hip fractures in the ambulatory elderly, including both fall characteristics and bone mineral properties of the femur, and noted that the adjusted odds ratio for fracture was 5.7 for a fall to the side and 2.7 for a decrease of 1 SD in femoral neck bone mineral density (Table 2). Among hip fracture cases, 69% fell to the side, whereas only 31% of control falls were to the side. Potential energy of the fall and low body mass index were also significantly related to the frequency of hip fracture in subjects over 65 in the community (Table 2).

These studies suggest a characterization of a high-risk fall for hip fracture and help to explain why only a small portion of falls result in fracture. Falls to the side with impact near the hip strongly increase the likelihood of hip fracture. If energy is absorbed by getting the hand out or by grabbing a support, fracture is less likely.

Table 1 Comparison of Fall Characteristics Between Hip Fracture Cases and Control Subjects in the Nursing Home (Data from Hayes et al., 1993)

Fall characteristic	Fracture cases (%)[a]	Fall controls (%)[a]	Significance
Fall to side	60	23	<0.001
Impact to hip or side of leg	59	6	<0.001
Walking at time of fall	59	35	<0.001
Fall from standing height or higher	81	73	0.21

[a]Percent of subjects with positive response over total number of cases or controls who answered question.

Table 2 Independent Factors Associated With Hip Fracture in a Case-Control Study of Fallers in the Community (Data from Greenspan et al., 1994)

Factor	Adjusted odds ratio	95% Confidence interval	Significance
Fall to side	5.7	2.3–14	<0.001
Bone mineral density of femoral neck	2.7[a]	1.6–4.6	<0.001
Fall energy	2.8[b]	1.5–5.2	<0.001
Body mass index	2.2[a]	1.2–3.8	0.003

[a]Odds for 1 SD decrease.
[b]Odds for 1 SD increase.

These fall severity characteristics touch on a domain of fracture risk that is independent of bone mineral density (Table 2) and is therefore missed by assessments of femoral failure properties by DXA or QCT.

In addition to fall direction and impact location, the severity of a fall may be influenced by body habitus. Low body weight and low body mass index increase the risk of hip fracture (32,46,52,53). The influence of low body mass index may be because the local properties of the tissue adjacent to the hip play a critical role. Body mass index has been found to correlate directly with trochanteric soft-tissue thickness measured by ultrasound in women with a mean age of 72 years (54). In addition, the thickness of soft tissues overlying the greater trochanter correlates inversely with the impact force to the femur in laboratory studies (55) and may therefore blunt or divert impact energy from the femoral trochanter. Therefore, fall impact forces to the femur and the resulting fall severity may be raised in those who have thin soft tissues and low body mass index.

Mathematical models and laboratory studies of a fall with side impact allow for estimations of the impact force and energy. Robinovitch and associates (56) used a simple experiment that releases the pelvis of volunteers lying on their sides to simulate a fall onto the lateral aspect of the hip. Based on a mass-spring-damper model of the effective moving mass of the body, they were able to estimate impact forces for a fall from standing height. Predicted peak forces in men were 6,100 Newtons in a relaxed muscle state and 12,000 Newtons in an active muscle state. Corresponding values for women were 5,050 Newtons and 6,370 Newtons. These results indicate that the state of muscle activity is important in determining the impact force during a side fall. They also support the anecdotal idea that falling in a relaxed state may protect against injury. Moreover, this study provides values of peak impact force that can be compared directly with laboratory tests of the proximal femur in a fall configuration. Such fracture loads of the femur can range from approximately 1,700 Newtons to 6,700 Newtons for elderly cadaveric specimens (24) (Fig. 3A). Consequently, the impact force may often exceed the fracture load of the hip in falls to the side, indicating that fracture would be likely to occur.

The prevalence of fracture of the hip rises exponentially with age. Ninety percent of fractures of the hip occur in individuals who are more than 70 years of age, and more than 90% of these fractures are the result of simple falls from a standing height or less. To understand the importance of age in determining hip fracture, Courtney et al. (25) tested hips from comparatively young and old donors in a fall configuration. Comparison of Courtney's values for the fracture load (Fig. 5) against the estimated impact forces on the hip during falls from standing height in a relaxed state (56) indicates that, on average, impact forces exceed the fracture load of the femur in the older individuals but are less than the fracture load of the femur in the younger individuals. These findings help to explain the lower prevalence of fractures among younger adults. However, because only 2% of all falls result in a fracture of the hip, these studies also emphasize that other factors, such as the direction of fall, the site of the impact, and the use of passive and active

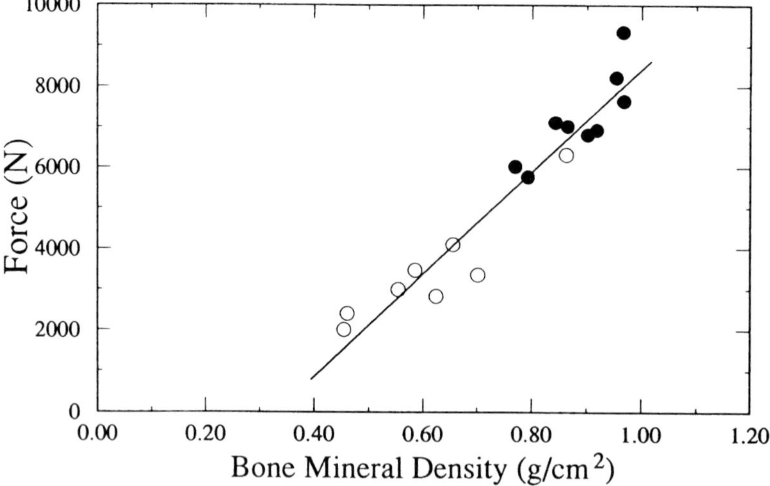

Figure 5 Fracture load of the proximal femur from comparatively older (mean 74 years, range 59–83) and younger (mean 33 years, range 17–50) donors. The mean fracture load for the young group (solid circles) was 7,200 ± 1,090 (SD) Newtons, and that for the older group (open circles) was 3,440 ± 1,330 Newtons. Bone mineral density of the femoral neck was associated significantly with fracture load, and most of the variation in fracture load with age could be explained by variation in bone mineral density. The correlation coefficient between fracture load and bone mineral density was $r = 0.95$ ($P < .001$). Adapted from Courtney et al. (1995).

energy mechanisms, must be important determinants of the risk of such a fracture. These data suggest that both fall severity and bone failure properties are important determinants of hip fracture.

In summary, fall initiation, fall severity, and the structure capacity of the proximal femoral are all important determinants of hip fracture risk. Moreover, each of these primary determinants is associated with a set of bone mass, fall, and environmental characteristics. The relative importance of these characteristics is the subject of much current research and will provide a basis for new interventional strategies. Hip fracture is the outcome of both a disease process of osteoporosis and a traumatic event related to the biomechanics of the fall (57), and prevention efforts should therefore focus on each of these factors.

IV. VERTEBRAL FRACTURES

Just as falls are associated with hip fracture, there are high-risk activities that are associated with age-related, nonburst fractures of the spine. Approximately 40% of symptomatic vertebral fractures occur after a fall, and an additional 10% are associated with lifting a heavy object (58). Thus, the biomechanics of falling and lifting in terms of loads on the spine could be important in the understanding of age-related vertebral fractures. Hayes and Myers (59) have proposed that excess mechanical force due to falling, lifting, and bending and the structural capacity of the vertebra in compression and forward flexion may account for the dominant fracture risk of the spine.

Vertebral fractures are often detected by a loss of vertebral height, resulting in a classification scheme that is open to interpretation and that contrasts sharply with fractures of the appendicular skeleton, which tend to be clear events. The distinction between vertebral fracture and vertebral deformation is ill-defined. The implications of this controversy are significant in that, as fracture definition is expanded to include other minor changes, the efficacy of drug intervention becomes clouded. Thus, the definition of the fracture is critical to the entrance and end-point criteria used in trials of osteoporosis treatments. Consensus meetings have noted radiographic definition, even with a height loss from 20–30%, is not always due to a vertebral fracture. Kleerekoper and Nelson (60) have indicated the problematic nature of deformation. Only 25% of significant radiographic deformations of the spine were associated with clinical symptoms and included nucleotide uptake. Association with a true clinical fracture occurred only when vertebral deformations crossed a 30% loss of height. Thus, it is unclear whether deformations up to 30% are indicative of osteoporosis and represent risk of vertebral fractures. Storm and associates (61) and Watts and associates (62), in their articles on the determination of the efficacy of Etidronate, define fracture as a 20–25% reduction in the anterior, middle, or posterior height accompanied by reduction of an area of approximately 10–20%. Riggs and associates (63), on the other hand, accepted a 15% change within the vertebral body as evidence of a fracture.

Bone density measurements that look at correlations between density and fracture risk in clinical studies have a much higher correlation at 20–25% vertebral body deformation and a very weak correlation between 15% and 25%. Drug trials using the latter criterion are placed in question. In addition, with the 15% definition, lack of precision between multiple readings makes it very difficult to identify these minor changes with consistency. The issues of deformation and fractures, entrance criteria for studies, and changes that would demonstrate efficacy of treatment have not yet been agreed to by either the investigators or the U.S. government.

Definitions of vertebral fracture are further clouded by the potential of the vertebra to recover some of the compressive deformation after so-called failure. In cadaveric vertebrae tested in a combined compression and flexion test, specimens compressed by an average of 18% at the anterior margin regained height after a recovery time period to a permanent deformation level of 13% (64) (Fig. 6). These results suggest that vertebral fracture could disappear in longitudinal studies

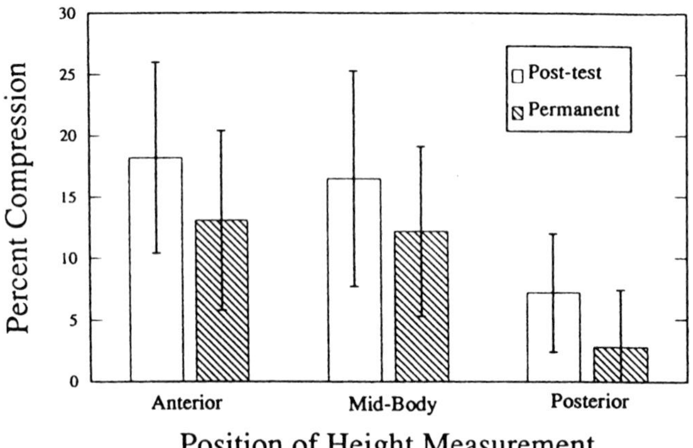

Figure 6 Recovery of vertebral bodies after compressive deformation ex vivo. Nine lumbar vertebral bodies (from donors aged 76–99 years) were tested in a mechanical test under compression and forward flexion. Radiographs were taken immediately after the test (posttest) and after a recovery time period (permanent). Six points marking the anterior, midbody, and posterior heights were measured on x-rays with a digitizing tablet. The specimens had a slight wedge deformity (anterior height was compressed more than posterior height) in the posttest radiographs. Specimens showed some recovery of height after the recovery time period. Bars are mean values for percent compression, and error bars are standard deviations.

because of transient vertebral deformities. However, a study of this type of rebound phenomenon in a clinical trial indicated that the recovery was the result of measurement error (65). Thus, the definition of vertebral fracture remains a controversial area of research.

Using standard definitions of fracture, low bone mineral density of the spine has been found to be a strong risk factor for vertebral fracture. Bone mineral density of the whole lumbar vertebrae correlates strongly with the fracture load of vertebrae in the lumbar and thoracic regions tested in compression (27,28) (Fig. 3B), and has also been found to associate significantly with the prevalence and incidence of spine fracture. In cross-sectional studies of vertebral fracture, odds ratios calculated for a change of 2 SD in lumbar bone mineral density range from 2 to 100 (66). Some of this variability could be due to the uncertainties over the definition of fracture or to varying definitions of the control group. If the severity of the loads applied to the spine are not taken into account, then the independent effect of low bone mineral density might be difficult to discriminate. Despite this large range in odds ratios, there is significant stratification of fracture and control groups based on bone mineral density, and the odds of fracture being present in patients with low bone mineral density is at least twice that in patients with bone mineral density 2 SD greater. In addition, in longitudinal studies, low lumbar bone mineral density is associated with a significant increased risk for new vertebral fractures (67–69).

Surveys similar to those performed on hip fracture subjects and control fallers, which contrast fall severity and bone mineral properties between the two groups, have not been performed for subjects with vertebral fracture. Therefore, the interaction between spinal loads during high-risk activities and the strength and fracture load of the vertebra is uncertain. In spite of this uncertainty, it seems reasonable to consider that spinal loading may be influential in these bony failures.

Compressive loads on the spine have been calculated using a variety of mathematical models (70–74) and have been validated by measurements of intradiscal pressure and myoelectric signals (75). Some of these models, originally intended for back injuries in the work place, focus on standing, twisting, bending, and lifting. Compressive forces at the third lumbar vertebral body estimated from these models (75) range from 440 Newtons for standing in a relaxed state to 2,350 Newtons for holding the body flexed forward at 30° and holding 8 kg with the arms extended. These values of compressive force can be compared with laboratory tests of the lumbar vertebrae in compression. Fracture loads of whole lumbar vertebrae can range from approximately 850 Newtons to 5,500 Newtons for elderly cadaveric specimens (27) (Fig. 3B). Comparison of these force values indicates that the compression due to a simple activity such as lifting 8 kg can exceed the structural capacity of the vertebra in a subject with low bone mineral density. It emphasizes the importance of considering the forces applied to the spine when determining fracture risk.

Models of fall impact forces and configurations for falls straight down or to the back have not been developed to estimate the compressive forces on the vertebrae. Because approximately 40% of vertebral fractures may be the result of such falls, this is an important area of research for understanding the mechanics of spine fracture.

V. SUMMARY AND CONCLUSIONS

The role of mechanics in the assessment of osteoporotic fractures is two-sided: 1. The mechanical properties of bones are affected by osteoporosis and age-related bone loss, resulting in diminished strength and structural capacity; and 2. the mechanical forces applied to bones during falls and other activities are important in determining the likelihood of fracture. The complex interactions between loading conditions and skeletal fragility lead to the conclusion that fractures are the consequence of both osteoporosis and injury. Such fractures represent a structural failure of the bone in which the forces applied during falls or other potentially high-risk activities exceed the fracture load of the bone under those loading conditions.

ACKNOWLEDGMENTS

This work was supported by grants from the National Institutes of Health (AG11985, AG12349) and the Centers for Disease Control (CCR109053). The authors thank Connie Garcia and Jeanine Goodwin for assistance in manuscript preparation.

REFERENCES

1. Consensus development conference: diagnosis, prophylaxis, and treatment. Am J Med 1993; 94:646–650.
2. Riggs B, Melton L. The prevention and treatment of osteoporosis. N Engl J Med 1992; 3:620–627.
3. Meunier P. Prevention of hip fractures. Am J Med 1993; 95:75S–78S.
4. Cooper C, Atkinson E, Jacobsen S, O'Fallon W, Melton L. Population-based study of survival after osteoporotic fractures. Am J Epidemiol 1993; 137:1001–1005.
5. Lane J, Riley E. New advances in osteoporosis: Editorial review. Curr Opin Orthop 1994; 5:1–8.
6. Hayes WC. Biomechanics of cortical and trabecular bone: implications for assessment of fracture risk. In: Mow V, Hayes WC, eds. Basic Orthopaedic Biomechanics. New York: Raven Press; 1991:93–142.
7. Hayes WC, Piazza SJ, Zysset PK. Boimechanics of fracture risk prediction of the hip and spine by quantitative computed tomography. In: Rosenthal DI, ed. Radiologic Clinics of North America. Philadelphia: WB Saunders Company; 1991:1–18.

8. Matkovic V, Fontana D, Tominac C. Factors that influence peak bone mass formation: a study of calcium balance and the inheritance of bone mass in adolescent females. Am J Clin Nutr 1990; 52:878–888.
9. Slemenda C, Hui S, Johnston C. Patterns of bone loss and physiologic growing: prospects for prevention of osteoporosis by attainment of greater peak bone mass. In: Christiansen C, Overgaard K, eds. Proceedings of the Third International Symposium on Osteoporosis. Copenhagen, Denmark: Osteopress ApS; 1990:948–953.
10. Greenspan S, Maitland L, Myers ER, Krasnow M, Kido T. Femoral bone loss progresses with age: a longitudinal study in women over age 65. J Bone Miner Res 1994; 9:1959–1965.
11. Lane J. Osteoporosis: cause of geriatric fractures. In: Brighton C, Friedlaender G, Lane J, eds. Bone Formation and Repair. American Academy of Orthopaedic Surgeons Symposium; 1995:471.
12. Carter DR, Hayes WC. Bone compressive strength: the influence of density and strain rate. Science 1976; 194:1174–1176.
13. Keaveny T, Hayes WC. A 20-year perspective on the mechanical properties of trabecular bone. J Biomechanical Eng 1993; 115:534–542.
14. Einhorn T. Bone strength: the bottom line. Calcif Tissue Int 1992; 51:333–339.
15. Burstein AH, Reilly DT, Martens M. Aging of bone tissue: mechanical properties. J Bone Joint Surg [Am] 1976; 58:82–86.
16. Mosekilde L, Danielsen CC. Biomechanical compctence of vertebral trabecular bone in relation to ask density and age in normal individuals. Bone 1987; 8:79–85.
17. Keaveny T, Hayes WC. Mechanical properties of cortical and trabecular bone. In: Hall B, ed. Bone, Vol. VII: Bone Growth-B. Boca Raton: CRC Press; 1992:285–344.
18. Gibson LJ, Ashby MF. Cellular Solids: Structure and Properties. New York: Pergamon Press; 1988.
19. Mazess R. Fracture risk. A role for compact bone. Calcif Tissue Int 1990; 47: 191–193.
20. Ruff CB, Hayes WC. Subperiosteal expansion and cortical remodeling of the human femur and tibia with aging. Science 1982; 217:945–948.
21. Brinckmann P, Biggemann M, Hilweg D. Prediction of the compressive strength of human lumbar vertebrae. Spine 1989; 14:606–610.
22. Faulkner KG, Cann CE, Hasegawa BH. Effect of bone distribution on vertebral strength: assessment with patient-specific nonlinear finite element analysis. Radiology 1991; 179:669–674.
23. Lotz JC, Hayes WC. The use of quantitative computed tomography to estimate risk of fracture of the hip from falls. J Bone Joint Surg [Am] 1990; 72:689–700.
24. Bouxsein M, Courtney A, Hayes WC. Ultrasound and densitometry of the calcaneus correlate with the failure loads of cadaveric femurs. Calcif Tissue Int 1995; 56: 99–103.
25. Courtney A, Wachtel E, Myers ER, Hayes WC. Age-related reductions in the strength of the femur tested in a fall loading configuration. J Bone Joint Surg [Am] 1995; 77:387–395.
26. Courtney A, Wachtel E, Myers ER, Hayes WC. Effects of loading rate on strength of the proximal femur. Calcif Tissue Int 1994; 55:53–58.

27. Moro M, Hecker A, Bouxsein M, Myers ER. Failure load of thoracic vertebrae correlates with lumbar bone mineral density measured by DXA. Calcif Tissue Int 1995; 56:206–209.
28. Myers B, Arbogast K, Lobaugh B, Harper K, Richardson W, Drezner M. Improved assessment of lumbar vertebral body strength using supine lateral dual-energy x-ray absorptiometry. J Bone Miner Res 1994; 9:687–693.
29. Cody DD, Goldstein SA, Flynn MJ, Brown EB. Correlations between vertebral regional bone mineral density (rBMD) and whole bone fracture load. Spine 1991; 16: 146–154.
30. McBroom RJ, Hayes WC, Edwards WT, Goldberg RP, White AA III. Prediction of vertebral body compressive fracture using quantitative computed tomography. J Bone Joint Surg [Am] 1985; 67:1206–1214.
31. Melton LJ, Chao EYS, Lane J. Biomechanical aspects of fractures. In: Riggs BL, Melton LJ, eds. Osteoporosis: Etiology, Diagnosis and Management. New York: Raven Press; 1988:111–131.
32. Grisso JA, Kelsey JL, Strom BL, et al. Risk factors for falls as a cause of hip fracture in women. N Engl J Med 1991; 324:1326–1331.
33. Michelson J, Myers A, Jinnah R, Cox Q, Van Natta M. Epidemiology of hip fractures among the elderly. Clin Orthop Rel Res 1995; 311:129–135.
34. Cummings SR, Black DM, Nevitt MC, et al. Appendicular bone density and age predict hip fracture in women. JAMA 1990; 263:665–668.
35. Campbell AJ, Borrie MJ, Spears GF, Jackson SL, Brown JS, Fitzgerald JL. Circumstances and consequences of falls experienced by a community population 70 years and over during a prospective study. Age Ageing 1990; 19:136–141.
36. Tinetti ME, Speechley M, Ginter SF. Risk factors for falls among elderly persons living in the community. N Engl J Med 1988; 319:1701–1707.
37. Nevitt MC, Cummings SR, Kidd S, Black D. Risk factors for recurrent nonsyncopal falls: a prospective study. JAMA 1989; 261:2663–2668.
38. Myers ER, Hayes WC. Age-related hip fractures. Curr Opin Orthop 1994; 5:9–15.
39. Cummings SR. Are patients with hip fractures more osteoporotic? Am J Med 1985; 78:487–493.
40. Nevitt M, Cummings S, Hudes E. Risk factors for injurious falls. A prospective study. J Gerontol Med Sci 1991; 46:M164–M170.
41. Hayes WC, Myers ER, Morris JN, Gerhart TN, Yett HS, Lipsitz LA. Impact near the hip dominates fracture risk in elderly nursing home residents who fall. Calcif Tissue Int 1993; 52:192–198.
42. Cummings S, Kelsey J, Nevitt M, O'Dowd K. Epidemiology of osteoporosis and osteoporotic fractures. Epidemiol Rev 1985; 7:178–208.
43. Kanis J. The incidence of hip fracture in Europe. Osteoporosis Int 1993; 3:10–15.
44. Mazess RB, Barden H, Ettinger B, Schultz E. Bone density of the radius, spine and proximal femur in osteoporosis. J Bone Miner Res 1988; 3:13–18.
45. Aloia JF, McGowan D, Erens E, Miele G. Hip fracture patients have generalized osteopenia with a preferential deficit in the femur. Osteoporosis Int 1992; 2:88–93.
46. Greenspan S, Myers ER, Maitland L, Resnick N, Hayes WC. Fall severity and bone

mineral density as risk factors for hip fracture in ambulatory elderly. JAMA 1994; 271:128–133.
47. Cummings S, Black D, Nevitt M, et al. Bone density at various sites for prediction of hip fractures. Lancet 1993; 341:72–89.
48. Melton L, Atkinson E, O'Fallon W, Wahner H, Riggs B. Long-term fracture prediction by bone mineral assessed at different skeletal sites. J Bone Miner Res 1993; 8:1227–1233.
49. Chapuy M, Meunier P. Calcium et vitamine D3, une prevention des fractures du col du femur chez les femmes agees. Presse Med 1993; 22:615–616.
50. Cummings SR, Nevitt MC. A hypothesis: the causes of hip fracture. J Gerontol 1989; 44:M107–M111.
51. Nevitt M, Cummings S. Type of fall and risk of hip and wrist fractures: the study of osteoporotic fractures. J Am Geriatr Soc 1993; 41:1226–1234.
52. Pruzansky ME, Turano M, Luckey M, Senie R. Low body weight as a risk factor for hip fracture in both black and white women. J Orthop Res 1989; 7:192–197.
53. Farmer ME, Harris T, Madans JH, Wallace RB, Coroni-Huntley J, White LR. Anthropometric indicators and hip fracture: the NHANES I epidemiologic follow-up study. J Am Geriatr Soc 1989; 37:9–16.
54. Maitland L, Hipp J, Myers ER, Hayes WC, Greenspan S. Read my hips: measuring trochanteric soft tissue thickness. Calcif Tissue Int 1993; 52:85–89.
55. Robinovitch S, McMahon T, Hayes WC. Force attenuation in trochanteric soft tissues during impact from a fall. J Orthop Res. (In press.)
56. Robinovitch SN, Hayes WC, McMahon TA. Prediction of femoral impact forces in falls on the hip. J Biomech Eng 1991; 1113:366–374.
57. Melton LJ, Riggs BL. Hip fracture: a disease and an accident. In: Uhthoff HK, Stahl E, eds. Current Concepts of Bone Fragility. Berlin: Springer-Verlag; 1986:385–389.
58. Cooper C, Atkinson EJ, O'Fallon WM, Melton LJ. Incidence of clinically diagnosed vertebral fractures: a population based study in Rochester, Minnesota, 1985–1989. J Bone Miner Res 1992; 7:221–277.
59. Hayes WC, Myers ER. Biomechanics of fractures. In: Riggs B, Melton L, eds. Osteoporosis: Etiology, Diagnosis, and Management, 2nd ed. New York: Raven Press; 1995:93–114.
60. Kleerekoper M, Nelson D. Vertebral fracture or vertebral deformity? Calcif Tissue Int 1992; 50:5–6.
61. Storm T, Thamsborg G, Steiniche T. Effect of intermittent cyclical etidronate therapy on bone mass and fracture rate in women with postmenopausal osteoporosis. N Engl J Med 1990; 322:1265–1271.
62. Watts N, Harris S, Genant H. Intermittent cyclical etidronate treatment of postmenopausal osteoporosis. N Engl J Med 1990; 323:73–79.
63. Riggs BL, Hodgson SF, O'Fallon WM, et al. Effect of fluoride treatment on the fracture rate in postmenopausal women with osteoporosis. N Engl J Med 1990; 322: 802–809.
64. Myers ER, Moro M. Recovery of vertebral bodies after compressive deformation ex vivo. J Bone Miner Res. (In press.)

65. Nelson D, Kleerekoper M, Peterson E. Reversal of vertebral deformities in osteoporosis: measurement error or "rebound"? J Bone Miner Res 1994; 9:977–982.
66. Ross PD, Davis JW, Vogel JM, Wasnich R. A critical review of bone mass and the risk of fractures in osteoporosis. Calcif Tissue Int 1990; 46:149–161.
67. Black DM, Cummings SR, Genant HK, et al. Axial and appendicular bone density predict fractures in older women. J Bone Miner Res 1992; 7:633–638.
68. Ross PD, Davis JW, Epstein RS, Wasnich RD. Pre-existing fractures and bone mass predict vertebral fracture incidence in women. Ann Intern Med 1991; 114:919–923.
69. Wasnich R, Ross P, Davis J, Vogel J. A comparison of single and multi-site BMC measurements for assessment of spine fracture probability. J Nucl Med 1989; 30: 1166–1171.
70. Andersson G, Ortengren R, Schultz A. Analysis and measurement of the loads on the lumbar spine during work at a table. J Biomech 1980; 13:513–520.
71. Bean J, Chaffin D. Biomechanical model calculation of muscle contraction forces: a double linear programming method. J Biomech 1988; 21:59–66.
72. McGill S, Norman R. Dynamically and statically determined low back moments during lifting. J Biomech 1985; 18:877–885.
73. Schultz A, Andersson G, Haderspeck K, Ortengren R, Nordin M, Bjork R. Analysis and measurement of lumbar trunk loads in tasks involving bends and twists. J Biomech 1982; 15:669–675.
74. Schultz A, Andersson G, Ortengren R, Bjork R, Nordin M. Analysis and quantitative myoelectric measurements of loads on the lumbar spine when holding weights in standing postures. Spine 1982; 7:390–397.
75. Schultz A, Andersson G, Ortengren R, Haderspeck K, Nachemson A. Loads on the lumbar spine. Validation of a biomechanical analysis by measurements of intradiscal pressures and myoelectric signals. J Bone Joint Surg [Am] 1982; 64:713–720.

5

Orthopedic Aspects of Osteoporosis

EARL BRIEN

University of California at Irvine
Orange, California
and University of Southern California
Los Angeles, California

JOHN H. HEALEY

Memorial Sloan-Kettering Cancer Center
and Cornell University Medical College
New York, New York

I. INTRODUCTION

Primary osteoporosis, localized or generalized, is an age-related disease characterized by normal bone composition with a decrease in the quantity of osseous tissue per unit volume and increased fracture risk. As bone density decreases, the compressive strength diminishes exponentially by a factor of 2 (1). Once the fracture threshold in this structurally weakened bone is surpassed, a pathologic fracture occurs. It is always important to remember that osteoporosis may also be secondary to tumor, metabolic, or endocrinologic causes. Bone biopsy may be needed to diagnose unusual cases and evaluate dynamic parameters such as bone turnover or mineralization rate.

Osteoporosis is expensive economically and emotionally. The staggering cost of osteoporosis and its complications is related principally to fracture management (acute and chronic). Fracture management is costly, especially in the surgically treated elderly hip fracture patient who needs hospitalization and extensive rehabilitation. Osteoporotic spine fractures are usually treated in a less expensive, outpatient setting, but the relapsing nature of the condition contributes to a large cumulative cost in managing the recurrent bouts of back pain. The loss of self-esteem is immeasurably costly. Lost wages grossly underestimate the impact of osteoporotic fracture care social costs since few elderly women work outside the home. Women are routinely unable to resume their premorbid level of activity or work inside or outside the home.

Osteoporosis is unfortunately common, affecting over 20 million people in the United States alone (2). Patients with symptoms related to pathologic fracture will confront the orthopedic surgeon, family practitioner, obstetrician, or internist. Diagnosis of osteoporosis is rarely obvious, and treatment may be delayed. Every effort should be made to diagnose the condition before the patient sustains a fracture. Clinical history, family history, and bone densitometry are indispensable in this endeavor. Osteoporosis is thus a host of diseases with a final common pathway—bone loss and fracture. Nevertheless, the syndrome treatment must be individualized to achieve the best results for patients. All practitioners should be able to diagnose and treat the common forms of the disease. Fracture care should be given in the context of overall osteoporosis management.

Knowledge regarding the etiology and natural history of osteoporosis is critical in the appropriate management of these patients. However, one must understand the structure and homeostasis of normal bone before proceeding to a discussion of osteoporosis. The information detailed elsewhere in this volume will be summarized here to highlight the interaction between the structure and physiology of bone. It provides a basis to manipulate bone and fracture biology.

II. BONE STRUCTURE AND HOMEOSTASIS

The function of bone is to provide support, protection, and critical ions for cellular activity. Inorganic matrix composes 70% of normal bone, and organic matrix constitutes 30%. The inorganic or mineral component is primarily in the form of hydroxyapatite [$Ca_{10}(PO_4)6(OH)_2$]. Hydroxyapatite, an insoluble crystalline mineral, is the primary structural component of bone and provides compression strength. Its principal components, calcium and phosphorus, have important physiologic functions. Calcium is the most widespread inorganic component of the skeleton and is predominantly extracellular. Ionized free calcium has both intracellular and extracellular functions. Phosphorus is found primarily intracellularly. Carbonate, chloride, magnesium, fluoride, sodium, and potassium also contribute to the inorganic component and provide metabolic and structural functions. Hydroxyapatite crystals are large and irregular when young and rapidly deposited. They become denser and more organized with increasing age. Mineral maturation in fracture callus parallels these normal physiologic changes.

The gastrointestinal tract, kidneys, and systemic hormones are critical factors affecting the destiny of ingested calcium. They balance dietary calcium intake, fecal calcium output, and urinary loss. Once calcium has passed from the lumen of the gut to the circulation by means of either active transport in the duodenum or passive diffusion in the jejunum, extracellular and intracellular homeostasis must be maintained. Approximately 40% of the extracellular calcium is bound to protein, primarily albumin, and the remainder of the extracellular calcium is either ionized or complexed with an acid. The distribution between these forms is partially controlled by the pH of the serum, whereby protein binding is increased with an increase in pH. An ionic pump and exchange mechanism in the mitochondria, endoplasmic reticulum, and plasma membrane regulates intracellular homeostasis to provide a low intracellular calcium concentration overall, but focally increased concentrations. The changing extracellular and intracellular calcium levels are linked by the cyclic adenosine monophosphate (cAMP) messenger system, which influences hormonal effects on calcium homeostasis.

The three major calcium-regulating hormones are parathyroid hormone (PTH), vitamin D, and calcitonin. In bone, PTH directly acts on osteoblasts to stimulate bone formation. It exploits various cytokines to communicate with osteoclasts and induce resorption. PTH in the kidney decreases reabsorption of phosphate, and increases net reabsorption of calcium and urinary excretion of bicarbonate. It indirectly increases calcium absorption by stimulating renal 25-hydroxyvitamin D-1 hydroxylase and elevates circulating $1,25(OH)_2D_3$.

1,25(OH)2-D is involved in osteoblastic synthesis of bone and normal mineralization and paradoxically promotes osteoclast recruitment and osteoclastic activation. Calcium absorption in the intestine is stimulated by increasing the synthesis of calcium-binding protein. In addition, 1,25(OH)-D has a negative feedback effect on the parathyroid gland. Calcitonin inhibits the action of the 1-alpha-hydroxylase enzyme and promotes hydroxylation at the 24 site. Calcitonin also decreases calcium and phosphorus reabsorption in the kidney and inhibits osteoclastic bone resorption by activating the cAMP messenger system.

The organic component of bone is composed primarily of hypomineralized matrix or osteoid (98%) and cells (2%). The three cell types are osteoclast, osteoblast, and osteocyte. Osteoclasts are mononuclear or multinucleated cells derived from pluripotent hematopoietic stem cell which stain positive for acid phosphatase. Responsible for bone resorption, they have a ruffled border surrounded by a clear zone thought to be related to acidification. Active osteoblasts are cuboidal, basophilic cells derived from mesenchymal cells that stain positive for alkaline phosphatase and synthesize the organic bone matrix. As the matrix surrounds the osteoblasts, the osteoblast becomes an osteocyte which is located in lacunae interconnecting other osteoblasts and osteocytes through canaliculi. To maintain normal functioning bone, cells must be continuously recruited to provide the dynamic process of activation, resorption, a reversal phase, and a formation phase (3).

The structural protein, type I collagen, is the predominant component of osteoid (85–90%) and provides tensile strength to bone (4). The collagen macromolecule is a triple helix composed of three tropocollagen molecules, one alpha-2 and two alpha-1 chains. Each of these chains is approximately 1,000 amino acids long with a common repeating tripeptide of glycine, proline, and hydroxyproline. Intramolecular and intermolecular crosslinking adds to the strength and insolubility to this structure. Bone type I collagen has different crosslinking patterns than soft tissue (skin type 1 collagen). Cartilaginous and short-chain collagens are also present in small quantities. Limited amounts of basement membrane and vascular collagens can also be found. The remainder of the matrix is composed of noncollagenous proteins including bone morphogenic protein (BMP), osteocalcin, osteonectin, protoeglycan, proteolipid, and sialoprotein (5). BMP is a glycoprotein identified first by Urist, which induces new bone formation (6). More recently through recombinant DNA sequencing, seven BMPs have been identified (7). Osteocalcin is a bone-specific protein containing a vitamin K–dependent amino acid, gamma-carboxyl glutamic acid (GLA) (8). Its function is unknown. Its alpha helical structure aligns the 3-GLA residue to facilitate adsorption to hydroxyapatite, which may regulate the mineralization of bone. Several other noncollagenous proteins have been addressed extensively in numerous articles (9,10). The apparent ability of these proteins to induce bone formation has generated an aggressive search for compounds to speed fracture healing, enhance bone strength, improve bone ingrowth into prosthesis, and substitute for auto- and allogeneic bone graft. The large number of candidate proteins and the complexity of the bone regeneration cascade have limited progress to date. Understanding the complexed interrelationship of these components and the dynamics of bone homeostasis provides the framework in diagnosing and treating osteoporosis.

III. BONE DEVELOPMENT

Skeletal development begins in utero by either endochondral or intramembranous ossification. Endochondral ossification provides longitudinal growth and essentially terminates in the second decade of life, whereas intramembranous ossification is involved in cortical thickening by subperiosteal deposition of bone throughout life. Through this process, the macroscopic organization of bone consist of approximately 80% cortical or compact bone and 20% cancellous or trabecular bone. Microscopically, the precursor of adult bone is first seen in the embryo and consists of large, randomly arranged collagen fibers, and is irregularly calcified and termed immature or woven bone. Mature or lamellar bone differs in that collagen fibers lie parallel to each other, forming a three-dimensional calcified structure of cylindrical and circumferential layers. The tertiary organization provides vascular channels for organ-systemic interaction and structural support to the body.

The skeleton is regulated by systemic and local processes that are probably genetically programmed to provide an equilibrium between bone formation and bone resorption. Collagen type and production vary, and mRNA analyses have demonstrated a probable genetic basis for familial cases of osteoporosis. An apparently distinct genetic mechanism governs the vitamin D receptor and is reported to be the strongest predictor of bone density in recent studies. Receptors may transmit signals across cell membrane, or messenger molecules may be involved in the hormone receptor interaction. Intracellular cAMP levels are controlled by stimulation of cell membrane receptors with hormones such as calcitonin, parathyroid, glucagon, epinephrine, and norepinephrine. Several other hormones, including estrogens, thyroid hormone, and androgens, cross cell membranes and alter the cell regulation through intracellular receptors located in the nucleus. Osteoclast and osteoblast must be directly or indirectly stimulated or inhibited to alter bone resorption and formation. For example, calcitonin inhibits bone resorption by binding to receptors on osteoclast, unlike parathyroid hormone and 1,25(OH)2D_3, which indirectly stimulate osteoclast through osteoblast-like cells.

Generally, normal levels of growth hormone, thyroid hormone, estrogen, testosterone stimulate a net increase in bone formation. In distinction, glucocorticoids, parathyroid, and excess thyroid hormone are systemic factors that promote net bone resorption.

Bone formation and resorption can be influenced by local humeral and biophysical factors in addition to systemic hormones (11). For example, remodeling can be influenced by electrical fields. When bone is subjected to bending strain, the concave side is under compression and the convex side is under distraction. The concave electronegative surface is associated with osteoblastic activity, while the convex electropositive surface is rich in osteoclastic activity. Electrical charges are thought to be the signals by which mechanical forces on bone are translated into physiologic cellular activity. Wolff's law refers to bone architecture changes occurring following bone loading. Bone is formed where it is needed in response to compression and lost where it is less valuable as reflected by reduced or negative compression. By this and other mechanisms, cellular changes determine how physical signals are converted to chemical signals that influence new bone deposition. This is the physiologic basis for the aphorism "form follows function."

IV. MATERIAL AND STRUCTURAL CHANGES IN BONE

Bone mass is predictive of bone strength. Compressive strength exponentially correlates to density with an exponent of 2, and bone stiffness correlates to the density with an exponent of 3. The mechanical properties of bone are inexorably linked to bone density. These relationships have been shown to apply in cadaveric systems when bone density, measured by QCT, also predicts strength and stiffness of bone (12,13). The microstructure of bone is also important. The "connectivity" or interconnectedness of trabeculae influences bone strength, amplifying changes in the overall bone mineral content (14,15).

Bone undergoes material microstructural and gross structural changes in osteoporosis (1,14,16–23). Hydroxyapatite crystals are larger and more uniform in osteoporotics than in controls, perhaps due to maturation of the crystals without effective remodeling of the bone (16,24). Gross volumetric changes also occur in osteoporotic bone, contributing to fragility of bones comprised principally of cancellous bone. Bone material properties change with aging. Bone becomes less elastic and absorbs less energy before fracturing (25). Structural properties attempt to compensate for the changes in material properties. Bone dimensions progressively enlarge with aging. Periosteal bone deposition and endosteal erosion lead to greater bone diameters, wider medullary canals, and greater moments of inertia that help to mitigate worsening fracture risks (23,26).

Altered bone mechanics influences the pattern, not only the incidence, of fractures. Patients with the poorest bone quality and quantity were shown to sustain more comminution and have more three- and four-part intertrochanteric fractures (27). In osteoporosis fracture fragments are typically smaller and more difficult to manage. Foltin found that lateral tibial plateau fragments were narrower and shorter in patients with radiographic osteopenia (28).

V. EFFECT ON INTERNAL FIXATION

Bone fragility impairs fracture fixation. Dorsal comminution of distal radial fractures often makes it impossible to hold fracture reduction. Screws lack purchase in osteoporotic bone, contributing to loss of fixation and implant failure (29,30). Although the outcome is too well known, few studies evaluate the phenomenon systematically (31). Sublaminar and pedicle hooks are stronger than pedicle screws in severely osteoporotic bone (32). Similarly, Soshi et al. found that pedicle screw pull-out strength diminishes with osteoporosis severity, but can be enhanced by increasing thread diameter and supplementing fixation with cement (33). Yet, in very severe osteoporosis, nothing was effective to augment screw fixation. Clinically, Arnold found that fixation and clinical failure of pinned femoral neck fractures were inversely correlated with bone mass and mineralization as measured by histomorphometry (34). Thus, bone quantity and quality seem to affect implant fixation and clinical outcome.

Bone density certainly relates to fracture incidence even though, just as certainly, other factors of strength, body composition, coordination, and environment play a major role (26,35,36). Clinically, the translation of densitometry data into accurate predictions of fracture remains a problem since there is significant overlap in density between fracture and nonfracture patients. Recently, investigators analyzed a 24-year study of women at high risk for fracture and found that the Z score of their bone density translated into a relative fracture risk of 1.62 even though at any give time z score did not identify who may have already sustained a fracture (37). Even in children, fractures occur in those whose bone content is on average below the mean (38,39). Orthopedic focus on fracture prevention must include efforts to maximize bone mass by encouraging bone accretion and discouraging bone loss. Training for muscle strength and coordination is also very important.

VI. FRACTURE PREVENTION AND BONE DENSITOMETRY

Education is critical to establish proper dietary and exercise habits. Theoretically this is the best way to promote bone formation and to prevent bone loss. During childhood and adolescence, skeletal mass and calcium stores increase rapidly until a peak bone mass is attained by the third or early fourth decade (40). It is uncertain whether calcium supplementation during childhood can affect the peak bone mass, but calcium supplementation in prepubertal children can increase spine bone mass. However, Fehily et al. found that 2 years of milk supplements did not alter bone mineral density of the distal forearm in children who were followed for 14 years (41), suggesting that appendicular peak bone mass may not be altered by calcium supplements. A balanced diet with green vegetables and dairy products should provide enough calcium to achieve peak bone mass; however, calcium requirements vary among individuals. Pregnant women and growing children require more calcium than young adults, and lactating women have the greatest calcium requirements. Vitamin D obtained in diet or by sunlight exposure is essential for calcium to be adequately absorbed in the gastrointestinal tract. The recommended daily dietary allowance is 400 IU in adults, 800 IU for the elderly. Alcoholism and diet deficient in protein and vitamin C may also lead to generalized osteoporosis.

Not only are calcium and vitamin D essential in obtaining and sustaining a healthy skeleton, but daily weight-bearing creates bioelectric signals which promote bone development and modeling. The amount and type of exercise that work most effectively on the skeleton remain controversial. Generally speaking, exercise that builds muscle mass (weight bearing, strengthening) builds bone mass as well. Indeed, muscle mass (measured by potassium balance studies) correlates with bone mass with an $r = 0.7$. Multiple regression analysis shows that strength correlates with bone density, not just in the adjacent bone but also at remote sites (42). Programs of high- and low-impact exercise seem equivalent in preventing bone loss (43). Most studies show that strength building exercise can even ameliorate postmenopausal bone loss (44). Walking alone seems to only contribute to bone preservation if it is over the anaerobic threshold (45). Generalized osteoporosis has been seen with prolonged inactivity, paralysis, and weightlessness while localized osteoporosis is common with prolonged immobilization and increased blood flow.

Secondary forms of osteoporosis are also well recognized and require specific intervention. Prolonged steroid, diuretics, aluminum antacids, dilantin, methotrexate, and heparin treatment may cause osteoporosis. In addition, rheumatoid arthritis, neoplasms, cirrhosis, renal failure, and other chronic diseases similar to genetic conditions such as osteogenesis imperfecta and homocystinuria make patients at risk for osteoporosis. The identification of "at-risk" patients by the physician is the first step in the prevention of osteoporosis.

Even with adequate education and early preventive intervention, involutional osteoporosis in either the axial or the appendicular skeleton may occur insidiously. The primary physician, either the family practitioner or obstetrician/gynecologist, must identify the high-risk patient and diagnose osteoporosis early. Regional osteoporosis clinics may also be valuable in early diagnosis and treatment prior to symptoms related to pathologic fractures. A careful history, baseline laboratory tests, and plain radiographs should be performed routinely in symptomatic patients in addition to studies evaluating the more common endocrine abnormalities and neoplastic conditions such as hyperthyroid, hyperparathyroid, and myeloma. Moreover, in osteomalacia where the bone matrix is hypomineralized, osteopenia and fractures may be interpreted as osteoporosis.

To characterize and quantitate bone morphology, undecalcified bone biopsy can distinguish among many diseases causing osteopenia, including the more common osteoporosis, osteomalacia, hyperthyroidism, and hyperparathyroidism. Sequential tetracycline labeling is a dynamic study evaluating mineralization rates by administering sequential doses which may differentiate the two types of involutional osteoporosis by assessing bone resorption and formation. Using a trocar to obtain a bicortical specimen from the iliac crest bone histomorphology can be evaluated after undecalcified preparation. High turnover characterized by increases osteoclast and abnormal lacunar spacing, increased osteoid production, and abnormal mineralization and marrow elements can be analyzed by light microscopy. The current role for bone biopsy is controversial. In our experience only 3% of osteoporosis cases will show histomorphometric changes that influence treatment not found by blood and urine biochemical tests. New measures of bone turnover may reflect systemic disease even better than localized bone biopsy (46). We limit biopsy to patients who have unusual chemical presentations, fail to respond to conventional therapy, or are to enter treatment with agents that potentially interfere with bone mineralization (e.g., fluoride).

Bone density analysis, which has been discussed in the text, should be performed at menopause in patients at risk for osteoporosis. Such risk factors include early menopause or oophorectomy, slender sedentary Caucasian and Asian females, women with a history of late or no childbearing, alcohol or smoking history, pathologic fractures related to osteoporosis, and family history of osteoporosis. We prefer DEXA to CT scan because of reduced cost and radiation exposure without sacrificing quality and reproducibility. A diagnosis of osteoporosis is made if a patient is below 2 standard deviations from normal premenopausal controls.

Reduction or elimination of risk factors that lead to osteoporosis should be the primary approach to prevention of osteoporosis. Early activity and adequate calcium intake may increase the peak skeletal mass and combat bone loss later in life. Proper lifestyle is important. Smoking cessation and alcohol moderation are crucial and should be prompted by encouraging physicians regardless of the complaint that brought patients to medical attention. Estrogen replacement therapy (ERT) is critical in high-risk postmenopausal patients with low bone mass or patients with established osteoporosis. Coupled with a progressive resistive exercise program, ERT will actually augment bone mass (47). ERT not only increases bone density, it appears to reduce fracture rates in the spine and appendicular skeleton. ERT is especially suitable for patients who suffer from appendicular osteoporosis and fractures since other treatments have little benefit for the peripheral skeleton. Bone loss can be further combated with the use of calcitonin and diphosphonates, discussed below.

Even when fractures have already occurred, it is not too late to assess risk factors, counsel women, and initiate antiosteoporosis therapy. One recent report noted that 50% of premenopausal women attending fracture clinic had lifestyle risk factors that could potentially be changed, and 90% of the pre- and postmenopausal women were candidates for hormone replacement therapy. The majority of patients were calcium deficient, and only 7% of patients who should be on HRT were receiving it (48). Osteoporotic fractures may predict a high chance of subsequent hip fractures. Relative hip fracture risk is increased 4.8 (lumbar), 4.1 (elbow), 3.5 (knee), and 1.5 times (ankle). These patients are at high risk and warrant aggressive treatment.

VII. CLINICAL AND RADIOLOGIC MANIFESTATIONS OF OSTEOPOROSIS

The three-dimensional network of adult normal bone composed of marrow, trabecular bone, cortical bone, and periosteum provides essential minerals, protection, and strength. In a net resorptive process like osteoporosis, calcium is mobilized from the honeycomb trabeculae where a high surface-to-volume ratio is present. Bones that are predominantly trabecular include the vertebral body, distal radius, ankle, and proximal humerus, and these sites are commonly fractured in early osteoporosis. Other bones commonly fractured in osteoporosis include proximal femur, pubic rami, foot, and ribs. Vertebral compression fractures are the most common, followed by hip fractures and wrist fractures (49–51).

The patient who presents with osteoporosis is classically a postmenopausal, slender, fair, white female with a sedentary lifestyle and either ethanol or smoking abuse. Clinical manifestations of spine fractures include loss of height, increased scoliosis or kyphosis, significant back pain with sitting or standing, and limited spinal range of motion. Scoliosis is correlated with diminished bone density (half of osteoporotics have scoliosis and half of scolitotics have osteoporosis). It is easy and cost-effective to identify these structural changes related to and predictive of osteoporosis with clinical examination alone. Progressive thoracic kyphosis may lead to increased visceral pressure and abdominal distension with circumferential skin folds where ribs contact the iliac wing. Constipation and loss of waistline are common complaints. Pain on percussion and paravertebral spasm with tenderness may be present early after fracture; however, the most consistent finding in acute fractures is pain with axial loading. This is performed by having a patient drop to her heels from a full toe raise while standing. Pain-free intervals can be expected, and neurologic findings are uncommon. Spinal alignment deteriorates in osteoporotic patients. There might be kyphosis of greater than 70°. Patients must restore the center of gravity over their feet and improve posture stability by combinations of the following mechanisms: 1. compensating cervical and lumbar lordosis; 2. thoracic extension muscle tension; 3. widening of the lower limb base; and 4. pelvic, hip, and knee flexion. When cervical arthritis is present, radiculopathy and vertebrobasilar insufficiency may become symptomatic. Lumbar lordosis may be blocked by hypertrophic or ankylosed facets. Spinal stenosis is exacerbated when the spinal canal is narrowed by spinal extension or lordosis. For this reason, loss of lordosis and pain or restriction from lumbar extension are routinely seen in stenosis and spondylosis patients. When lumbar stenosis or spondylosis is present, it is not possible to compensate for the thoracic kyphosis with lumbar lordosis. Attempts to do so produce paravertebral lumbar muscle spasm and pain. Thoracic kyphosis seems to encourage lumbar rotatory subluxation in scoliotic patients neuropathy may ensue (Sills AK. J Spinal Dis 6:269–270, 1993). All of these alignment problems contribute to poor balance and falls in the severely osteoporotic patient.

Laboratory studies should include a complete blood count and differential, blood chemistry, 24-hour urinary calcium and creatinine excretion, and studies assessing other diseases such as serum electrophoresis, erythrocyte sedimentation rate and thyroid function tests. In patients with active resorption, urine pyridinium crosslinks may be analyzed with more specificity than urinary hydroxyproline. Lateral and anteroposterior radiographs of the thoracic and lumbar spine should be obtained. Early radiological signs include generalized osteopenia, loss of transverse trabeculae, and accentuated vertical trabecular striation. Vertebral body compression fracture follows (Fig. 1). The standing full-length radiograph should also be analyzed for increased kyphosis and scoliosis (Figs. 2, 3) in addition to thoracic and lumbar fractures (Figs. 4, 5, 6).

Other common fractures include the distal radius, proximal femur, proximal humerus, pubic rami, and ankle and foot fractures. Distal radius fractures should be assessed with anteroposterior, oblique, and lateral views in addition to the forearm and elbow. Careful assessment of length, intra-articular displacement, angulation, and distal ulna involvement should be performed (Figs. 7, 8). Femoral neck and intertrochanteric fractures should be evaluated by anteroposterior views obtained with the patella directed anterior in addition to cross table lateral by elevating the contralateral limb to avoid motion at the fracture site. Proximal humerus fractures should be assessed with AP and axillary views to evaluate displacement and to rule out dislocation. Insufficiency fractures of the pubic rami are often missed because of the subtle radiographic findings seen on AP view. Foot and ankle fractures should be assessed with three views (AP, lateral, and oblique).

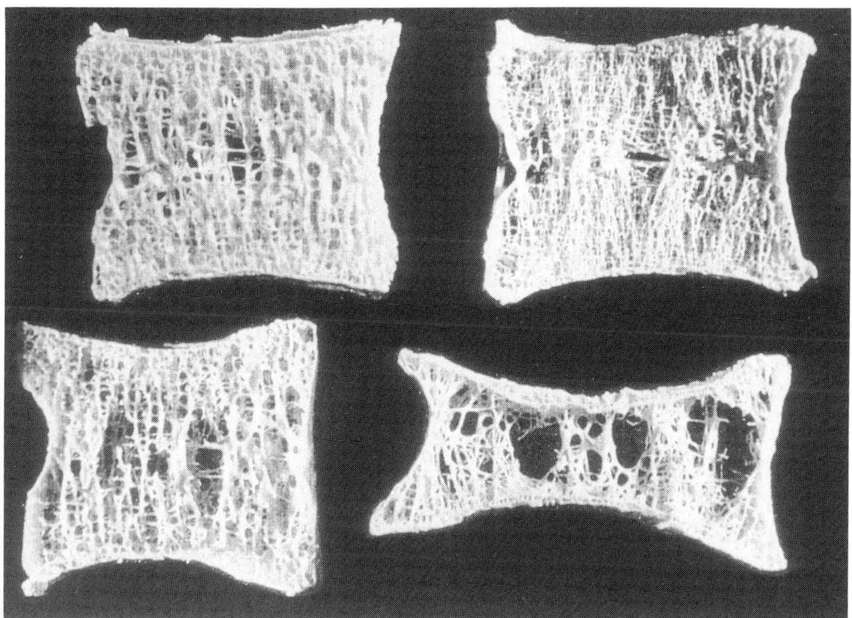

Figure 1 Progression from a normal vertebral body to a body with severe osteoporosis.

VIII. FRACTURE HEALING

Fractures may occur in pathologic bone; however, a normal repair process will ensue (11). The repair process attempts to reconstitute osseous continuity along stress lines through osteoinduction, osteoconduction, and recruitment of osteoprogenitor cells. Osteoinduction, regulated by humeral, chemical, and physical properties, stimulates cellular elements into functional osteoblasts and chondroblasts near a fracture (41). Osteoconduction requires an appropriate biologic environment for osteoprogenitor cells to function. Osteoconductive properties are present on bone surface and other substances (52,53). Osteoprogenitor cells, such as primitive mesenchymal cells, pericytes, or uncommitted bone marrow elements, can be induced to initiate fracture repair under adequate biologic conditions (54).

The four types of fracture repair include primary callus, external bridging callus, late medullary callus, and primary cortical healing. Primary callus response occurs in all fractures under most conditions. External bridging callous formation requires fracture motion and intact soft tissues, and is under humeral and mechanical control. Late medullary callus formation bridges gaps slowly; however, minimal motion at the fracture site is required and, similar to the first two repair

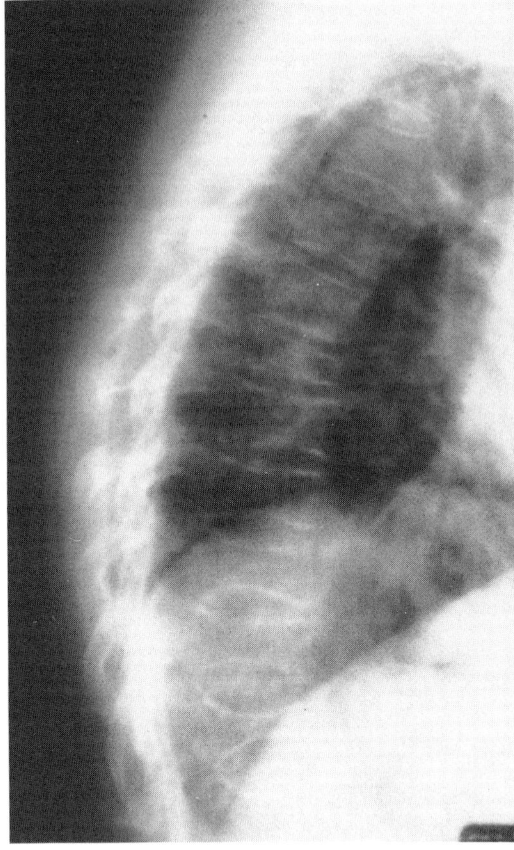

Figure 2 Multiple vertebral body fractures in the thoracic vertebrae with kyphosis.

process, it involves enchondral ossification (55). Primary cortical healing requires absolute rigidity and heals by osteoclastic resorption followed by osteoblastic formation. Local and systemic efforts to accelerate fracture healing have been unsuccessful to date. Promoters of early cell differentiation may impair remodeling necessary to convert callus into mechanically-sound cortical bone. Fluoride, electricity, growth hormone, and other agents enhance early (3 weeks) healing in animal models of fracture healing, but by 6 weeks no differences persist. Cytokines, such as TGFB and BMP, enhance healing frequency and extent in nonunion models. Major problems remain regarding drug delivery systems, appropriate dosage (most have biphasic response), and drug timing. Before any agent can be considered for clinical use, extensive testing is required. Surprising results can be found. For example, calcitonin, recognized to accelerate symptomatic resolution

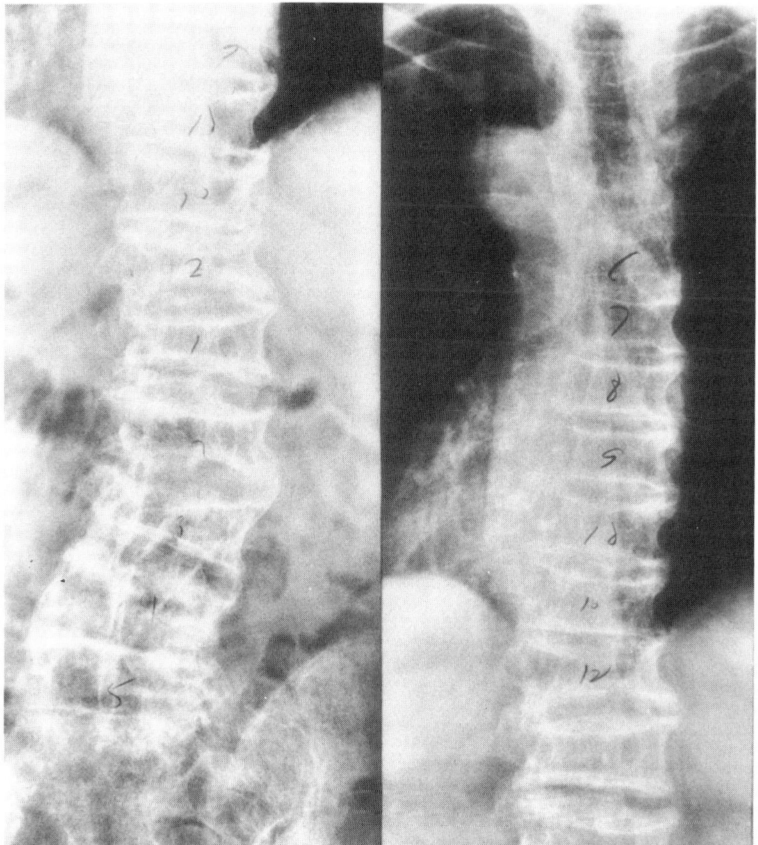

Figure 3 Lumbar scoliosis after fracture from osteoporosis.

in acute vertebral compression fractures, retards healing in animal models as measured by mechanical testing, and it has failed to improve clinical or radiographic parameters in Colle's fracture patients.

Systemic research has moved from hormonal agents to targeted drugs. New-generation bisphosphonates are undergoing intensive study, and preliminary results are encouraging in animal models (56). These agents that diminish bone resorption are relatively neutral toward bone formation and mineralization. Nevertheless, they share the theoretic disadvantage of preempting bone formation that is coupled to preliminary bone resorption. Etidronate, the only oral bisposphonate currently available, impairs fracture healing even though it seems to prevent spinal compression fractures.

Experts debate the role of calcium supplementation in patients with acute

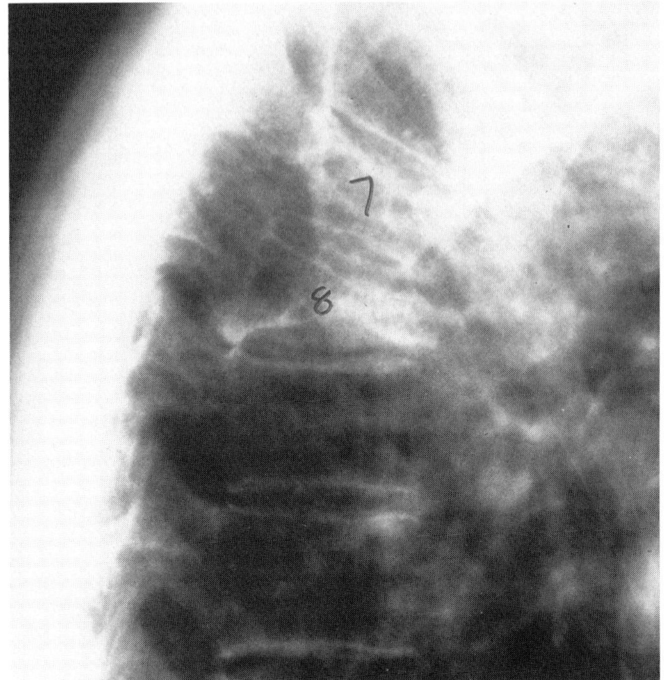

Figure 4 Significant wedge fracture of the eighth vertebrae.

fractures. Calcium certainly does not accelerate fracture healing, and sufficient calcium will be obtained from other skeleton sources. Calcium supplements reduce the need to cannibalize material and may help to prevent subsequent fractures. They certainly do not harm, and patients are very receptive to starting advisable nutritional supplements when suffering an acute fracture.

IX. TREATMENT OF COMMON OSTEOPOROTIC FRACTURES

Reduced bone mineral is the major cause of bone fragility in elderly women and men. Several authors have shown that bones with reduced mineral content fractures are being stressed with smaller loads than normal bone (18–20,57,58). The strength of cancellous bone seems to be more affected by a loss of density than cortical bone (58,59). Similarly, Ross et al. concluded that reduced bone mass was responsible for an increased risk of fracture in patients with osteoporosis (21,60). Approximately 50% of the females over age 50 and 33% of males over 70 years will develop a fracture related to osteoporosis, accounting for over 1.5 million fractures per year. The hip, radius, and spine are the most common locations where

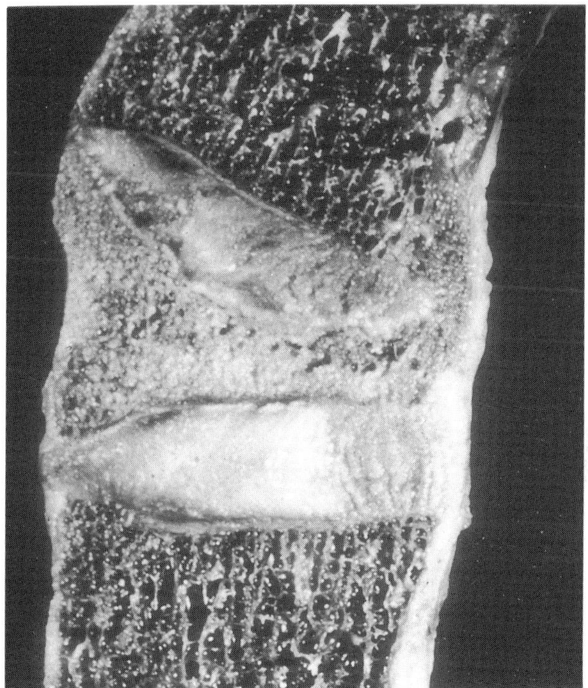

Figure 5 Gross specimen of the vertebrae with a compression fracture secondary to osteoporosis.

osteoporosis-related fractures occur. Prior to treatment for these fractures in commonly debilitated osteoporotic patients, surgical complications and difficulty obtaining secure fixation should be considered (61–63). The clinically significant fractures will be discussed individually below.

A. Hip Fractures

Frightening statistics from Malmo, Gottenberg, and other centers show that the age-adjusted rate of hip fractures has doubled in the last 30 years. Coupled with the aging of our population, the incidence of hip fractures will spiral higher and be an increasing orthopedic, geriatric, and financial problem in the U.S. Hip fractures are the most common fractures that affect the quality of life and impact survival. Two-thirds of patients sustaining hip fractures will not return to their previous functional level, and approximately 40% will not survive over 2 years (so-called "excess mortality," that greater than the age-adjusted rate, is 10–20%). Femoral neck and intertrochanteric fractures are the most common types of hip fractures in patients with osteoporosis, and both require early treatment. Because patients are

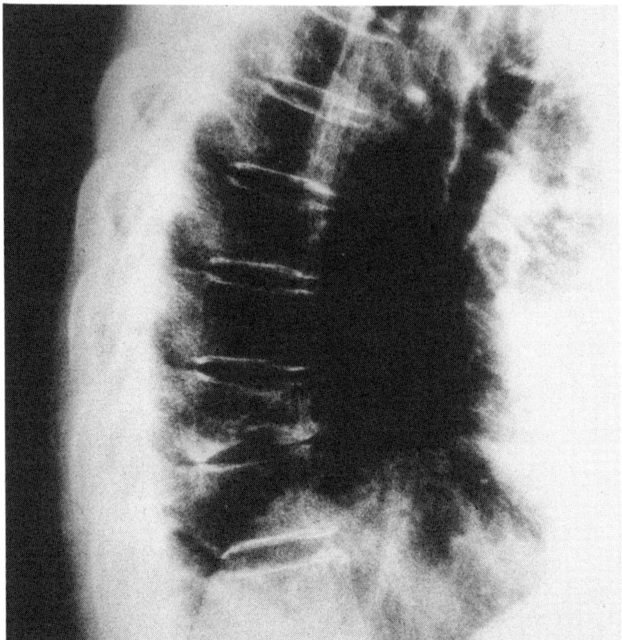

Figure 6 Collapsed anterior vertebral body with the posterior longitudinal ligament intact.

often elderly (median age 79 years) (64) and debilitated, preoperative medical evaluation and treatment of other problems should be initially performed (31). Once the patient is medically stable, fractures require either stabilization or hemiarthroplasty.

Fracture displacement and comminution of the posterior cortex of the femoral neck (65,66) have been reported to be greater in older, osteoporotic patients despite the fact that most of these fractures are a result of low-energy injuries (67). The common mechanisms of injury that have been postulated include a direct blow to the greater trochanter after a fall (68), a lateral rotation injury, and cyclical loading producing micro- and macrofractures (69). Alho et al. found that in femoral neck fractures comminution was not age-related (70). Regardless, standard fixation may lead to further comminution and be inadequate to hold the bone (71). Consequently, the use of nuts and washers with screws and supporting fixation with adjuncts such as polymethylmethacrylate (72,73) or cerclage wires has been advocated. A higher failure rate should be expected in elderly patients because of this problem (70).

It is uncommon for young patients with normal bone to sustain a femoral neck fracture (74,75) and for older patients without osteoporosis, such as Afro-Americans (76). Unlike these groups of patients, some degree of osteoporosis is seen in 84% of the patients with femoral neck fractures (77). Several theories have been proposed as to why femoral neck fractures in older patients occur. These include: By age 85, women have a bone mineral content below the fracture threshold (78); with advancing age, there is an increase in osteoporosis (79); inactivity and secondary disease lead to osteoporosis and femoral neck fracture; and patients living in urban areas have decreased cortical and trabecular bone mass.

Patients with femoral neck fractures present with pain; however, the degree of pain may vary. A nondisplaced, incomplete fracture or a complete, impacted fracture may elicit only minimal pain which does not significantly affect ambulation (Garden I). A nondisplaced, complete fracture (Garden II) is inherently unstable and more painful than the Garden I type fracture. Radiographs may not reveal a fracture line even with appropriate transgroin lateral and internal rotation films. Frog lateral films should generally be avoided to prevent displacement of a femoral neck fracture. Diagnosis must be made by physical examination followed by either bone scan or magnetic resonance imaging (MRI) in the nondisplaced fractures. The complete fracture, with either partial or complete displacement (Garden III or IV), usually does not allow the patient to ambulate and is associated with more severe pain. This clinical spectrum can be seen in the patient with osteoporosis who sustains femoral neck fractures.

The treatment options for femoral neck fractures include multiple screw fixation, sliding compression screw, hemiarthroplasty, or total hip replacement. Patients with incomplete or complete nondisplaced fractures (Garden I and II) are usually best treated with internal fixation with multiple screws. Increased osteoid production was found in 33%, 25% had increased metabolic turnover indices, and marked trabecular bone loss was present in 40% of patients (22). These metabolic changes may account for the high incidence of nonunion in older patients with femoral neck fractures.

With femoral neck displacement (Garden III or IV), hemiarthroplasty in elderly patients provides the most predictable outcome because it eliminates the risk of nonunion, fixation failure, and malunion (80). An interference fit between bone and prosthesis can be used in most cases, but in patients with severe osteoporosis, methylmethacrylate provides immediate stabilization in cases where an interference fit fails (81). Total hip arthroplasty in an active patient with significant osteoporosis and a stress fracture (82) or in mild osteoporosis with preexisting osteoarthritis in the ipsilateral or contralateral hip joint should be performed (83).

It is reported that the more common intertrochanteric fractures (Fig. 9) occur on an average in patients 10 years older than intracapsular femoral neck fractures (84,85). Similar to femoral neck fractures, it has been proposed that the mechanism of injury is either direct or indirect forces. Numerous authors have shown that intertrochanteric fractures commonly occur through osteoporotic bone (86–

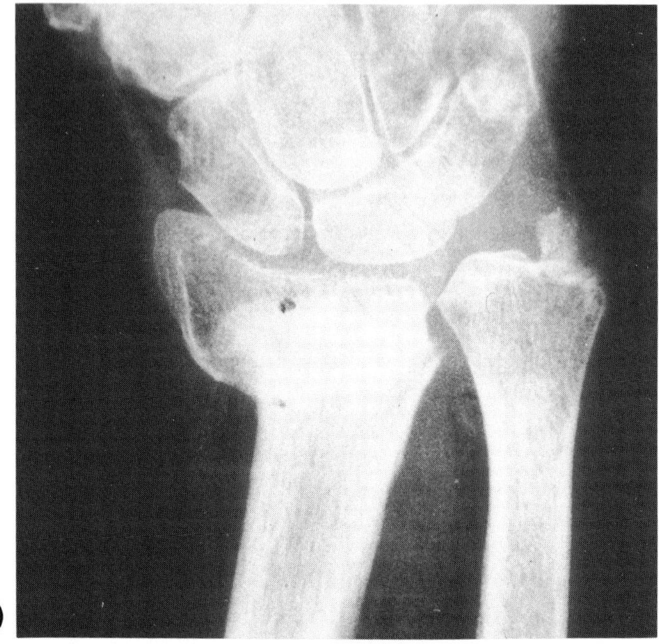

(7)

Figures 7 and 8 Anteroposterior and lateral views of a distal radius fracture secondary to osteoporosis with significant shortening and dorsal angulation.

88). However, Hayes has shown that the energy from a fall from the standing position is sufficient to produce an intertrochanteric fracture regardless of bone density. Other factors such as diminished coordination, muscle strength, and soft tissue to dissipate the energy of impact contribute to falls and fracture in the elderly. Fall prevention should be stressed when caring for older patients. Avoidance of benzodiazopenes, provision of adequate lighting, use of stable footwear, elimination of throw rugs and phone cords, and implementation of other practical measures should be standard practice.

These fractures consistently heal because of the well vascular metaphyseal bone. Shortening and external rotation deformities are common sequelae. However, failure of fixation and loss of reduction may occur in severely osteoporotic bone.

To identify patients at high risk for hardware failure and loss of reduction, Singh graded the degree of osteoporosis by evaluating the trabecular lines on the anteroposterior radiograph in the proximal femur (grade 1–6) (89). Patients with a Singh index of 3 or less (Figs. 10, 11) had a higher complication rate with hardware failure than patients with greater bone stock (grade 4–6) (Figs. 12, 13).

(8) 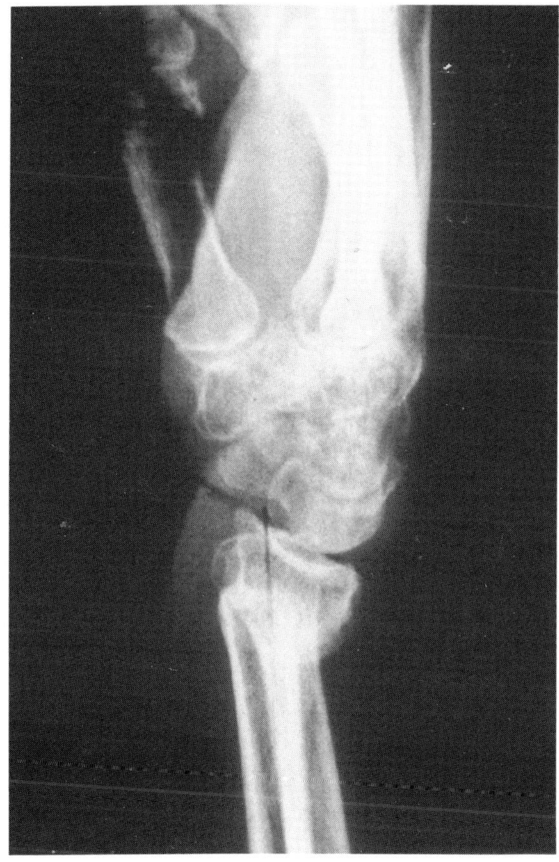

The radiologic findings correlate with the histologic findings, as seen in Figures 14 and 15.

Similar to femoral neck fractures, intertrochanteric fractures are urgent procedures that need prompt attention. Once the decision to operate has been made, not only is it important to determine the degree of osteoporosis, but it also essential to determine the stability of the fracture. In cases where the fracture pattern is unstable and severe osteoporosis is present (Singh 1, 2, or 3), strict attention in placement of internal fixation is needed (62). Medial and posterior bony contact must be reestablished for fracture stability. Placing the internal fixation screw just inferior and posterior to the center of the femoral head is best to stabilize the fracture while awaiting healing. Discriminate use of methylmethacrylate may be

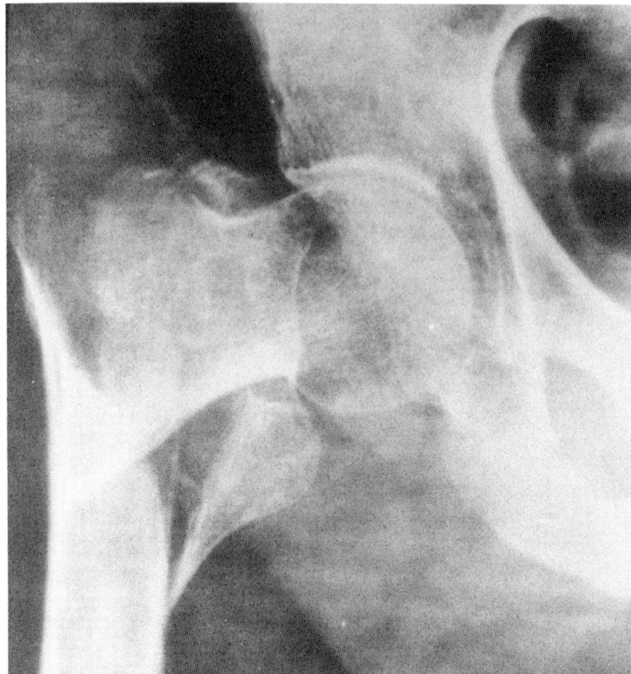

Figure 9 Comminuted intertrochanteric fracture of the right femur in an elderly patient with osteoporosis.

indicated (if the screw lacks purchase in the osteoporotic bone). Only in patients with severe osteoporosis where proximal fixation could not be achieved should a hemiarthroplasty be considered.

Fractures of the lesser trochanter are infrequently seen in patients with osteoporosis (90), and metastatic disease should be considered even in the elderly patient. These rare fractures occur when the iliopsoas muscle pulls off the osteoporotic lesser trochanter. Similarly, isolated fractures of the greater trochanter are uncommon and do not require open reduction and internal fixation in this group of patients. Strictly enforced partial weight-bearing for 6 weeks prevents extension or displacement of the fracture by neutralizing abductor muscle pull on the greater trochanter and reducing joint reactive forces. MRI is very helpful to define the extent of the fracture and confirm that it is confined to the greater trochanter.

B. Radius Fractures

The distal radius is the most common upper-extremity fracture in patients with osteoporosis (Figs. 16, 17). The mechanism of injury occurs primarily from a fall

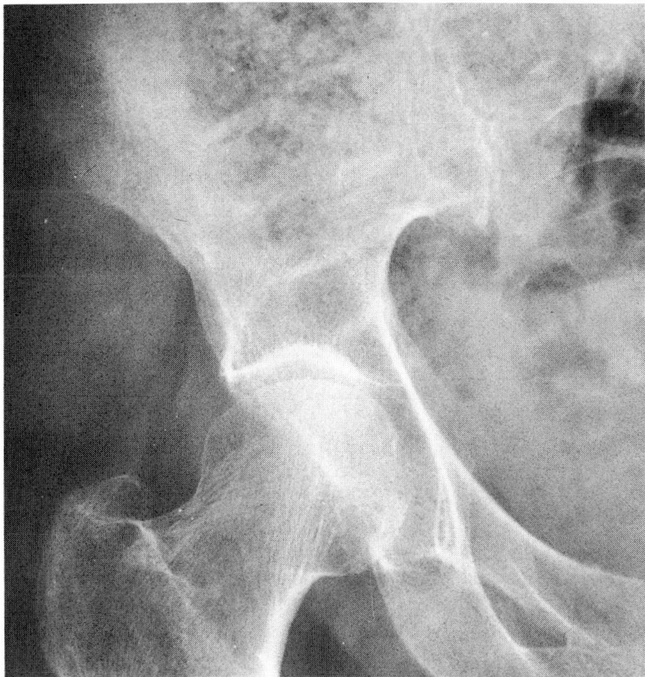

Figure 10 Radiograph demonstrating grade III (Singh's index), where there is a break opposite the greater trochanter in the continuity of the principal tensile trabeculae.

on an outstretched hand. The volar aspect is the tension side and the dorsal aspect of the radius is the compression side resulting in dorsal compression, angulation, and displacement (Colles' fracture). This may be associated with ligamentous injuries volarly.

In the elderly, extra-articular metaphyseal fractures occur because of the thin cortical bone and osteoporotic metaphysis. Early reduction with bony contact of the volar cortex, a long arm cast for 10–14 days followed by short arm cast for 4 weeks is the treatment of choice of most distal radius fractures. Postreduction radiographs evaluating shortening, angulation, and intra-articular involvement will determine if additional treatment is required. If cast immobilization cannot maintain an adequate reduction because of severely comminuted, unstable fracture patterns, external fixation has been advocated (91). Pin loosening, finger stiffness, and pin tract infection are the primary problems with this technique. Other techniques used in the treatment of distal radius fractures include percutaneous pin fixation with external immobilization (92,93) and open reduction and internal fixation, primarily for displaced intraarticular fractures (94,95).

Stiffness of the elbow and hand is a common complication with immobilization

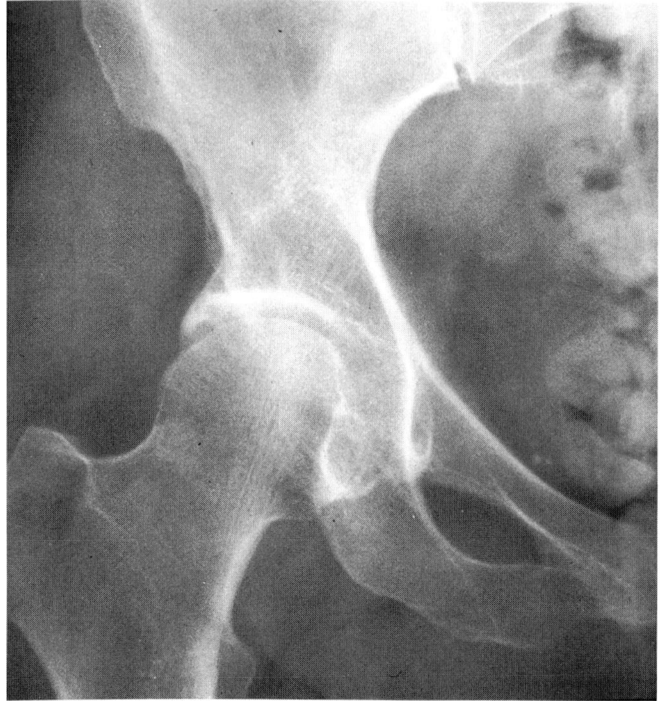

Figure 11 Only the principal compressive trabeculae can be seen, characterizing a grade II.

in the elderly. Elevation and range of motion exercises of the hand should be started early to decrease hand swelling and avoid late stiffness.

C. Compression Fractures of the Spine

Compression fractures of the spine are commonplace, occurring in about 20% of all women, yet they often pose a diagnostic dilemma. The most common location for spinal fractures secondary to osteoporosis is the thoracic and thoracolumbar junction (Fig. 18). Fractures may be due to primary osteoporosis or bone loss secondary to a neoplasm or marrow dyscrasia. It is particularly difficult to discern the etiology of fracture in patients with a history of breast cancer since both bony metastasis and osteoporosis are prevalent in this patient population with metastatic carcinoma and myeloma.

Fractures at atypical locations (e.g., above T5) are suspicious for harboring malignancy. At initial presentation, a careful history, physical examination, plain radiographs, and laboratory studies (including immunoelectrophoresis and acid

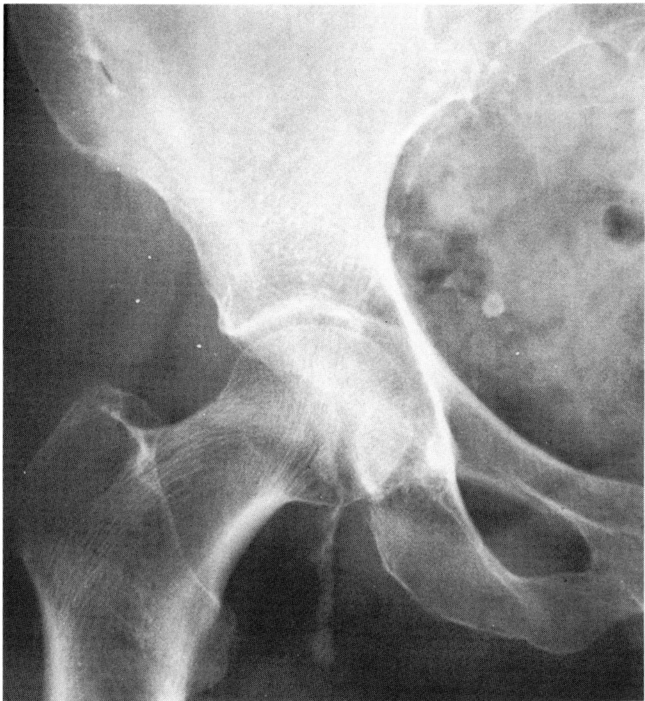

Figure 12 Grade V, where Ward's triangle appears prominent because the principal tensile and compressive trabeculae are accentuated.

phosphatase) should be performed followed by imaging studies (i.e., bone scan and MRI). Bone densitometry is superfluous. Findings suggestive of metastatic disease include complete vertebral body involvement with an intact disk, multiple levels of involvement, and pedicle or soft-tissue involvement. In addition, if axial compression pain does not resolve in 6–12 weeks, radiographs show progression of disease, or treatment is ineffective, metastatic disease should be considered and a biopsy is recommended. Fracture secondary to osteoporosis is a diagnosis of exclusion and should be made only after metastatic disease is ruled out.

Over 90% of patients with osteopenia will develop a compression fracture of the spine (96). Minor trauma of daily activities may cause fracture of this pathologic bone. The most useful clinical test we use to determine if a patient has a recent fracture is vertical loading of the vertebrae. This is tested by having the patient raise to their toes and then drop down on the back of their heels. The sudden load unmasks localized pain in fractured vertebra (or spinal infection) but not in arthritis, disk disease, stenosis, or muscle pulls. Radiographs may show

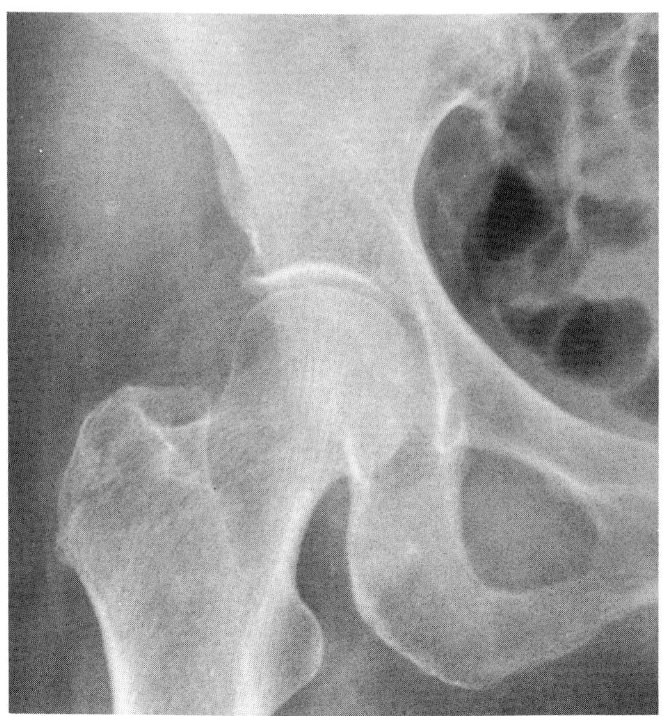

Figure 13 Grade VI, which shows all the normal trabecular groups.

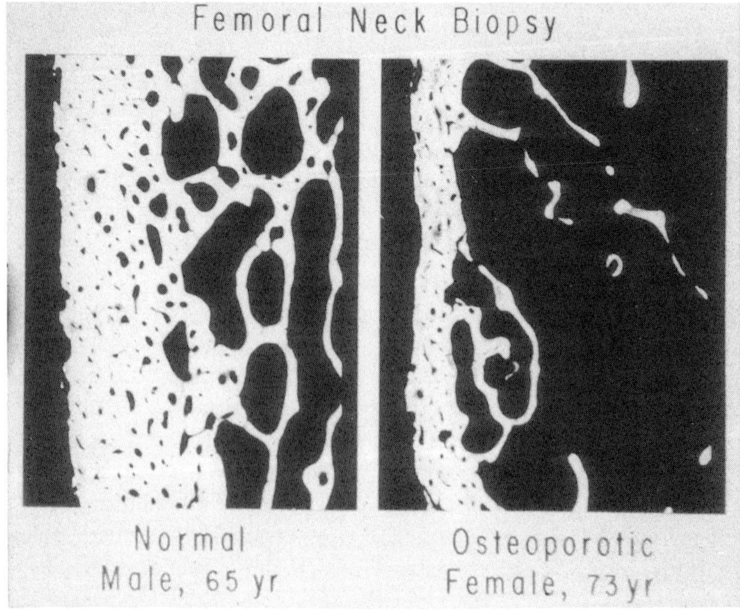

Figure 14 Femoral neck biopsy showing normal and osteoporotic trabeculae.

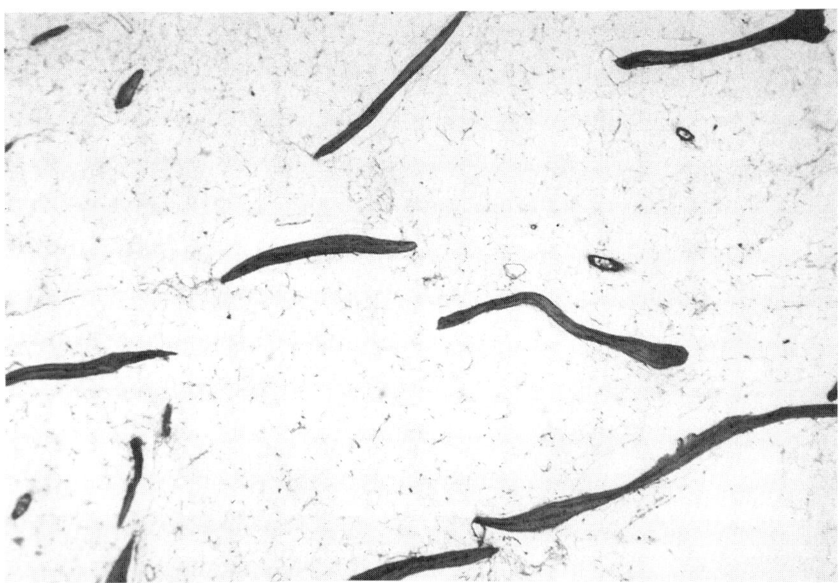

Figure 15 Severe osteoporosis characterized by sparse, thinned trabeculae and intertrabecular marrow.

subtle abnormalities such as loss of vertebral height and wedging of the vertebrae. This can be a diagnostic problem because there is no established quantitative method to diagnose spine fractures. For example, a >15% reduction in vertebral height is a sensitive measure but will have more false positives than more specific, less sensitive, strict criteria of >20% height reduction. To further complicate this dilemma, patients with >20% deformation may not recall a symptomatic event that correlates with the radiographic picture. A combination of measurements measuring the anterior, middle, and posterior heights are more accurate in determining fracture than evaluating one parameter. Multiplanar spinal deformity with increasing kyphosis and/or scoliosis may also be seen. An acute episode of fracture pain and muscle spasm followed by deformity and postural pain are the common events after fracture. Once a vertebral fracture has occurred, the risk of future spine fractures increases markedly.

Symptomatic relief is the early management of patients with spinal fractures. Ileus and, rarely, neurologic deterioration may occur after compression fracture. Bed rest, laxatives, and analgesics should be recommended immediately after fracture to relieve pain and muscle spasm aggravated by activities. Ambulation with assisted devices such as a back corset or brace and cane or walker (depending on symptoms) should be initiated after a short period of rest. Once the acute phase has passed, the fracture becomes sticky and severe pain subsides (about 3 weeks). Physical therapy focusing on thoracic extension and lumbar flexion exercises is

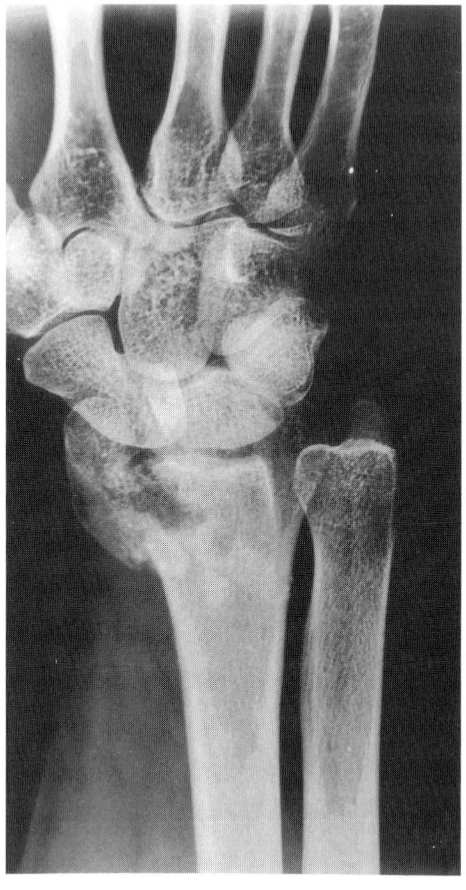

Figures 16 and 17 Anteroposterior and lateral views of a fracture of the distal radius with intra-articular involvement.

initiated to avoid chronic upper backache and stiffness and low-back pain associated with kyphotic deformity and compensatory lumbar lordosis. Exercises are very important to prevent disuse from worsening baseline osteopenia. Bracing is discontinued when axial compression pain ceases and paraspinal muscle spasm recedes. Chronic bracing is considered for patients who have 1. flexible kyphotic or scoliotic curves, or 2. chronic lumbar pain and spasm due to degenerative disk and joint disease. Flexible kyphotic deformities are corrected and supported best by braces that establish 3-point fixation with pressure over the sternum and pubis anteriorly and over the gibbus posteriorly. Polyethylene is the lightest material

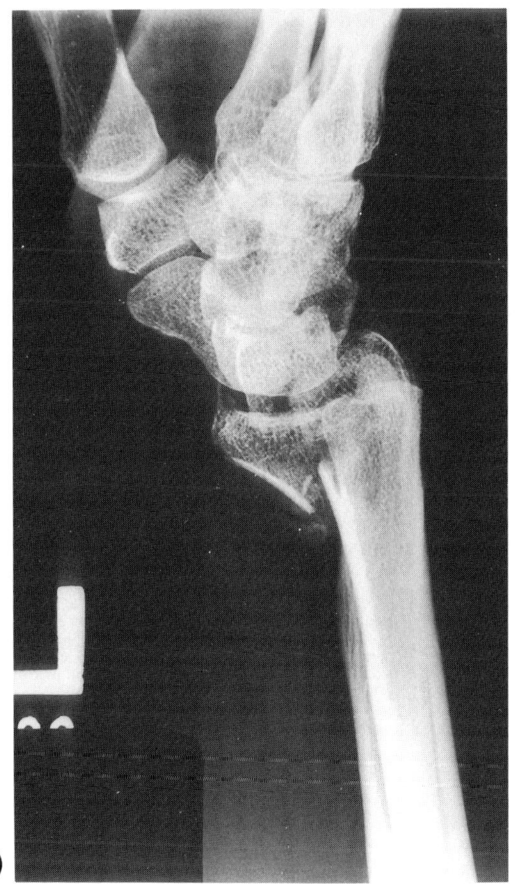

(17)

useful for supportive body jackets. While posterior opening braces retain the most support, anterior openings are the most practical to don and doff for elderly people living alone. Elastic low profile corsets work best in patients with late sequelae of low-back pain and degenerative arthritis.

Kyphosis averages 70° in osteoporotics—30° more than normal. This must be compensated by increasing cervical and lumbar lordosis proportionately in order to keep one's center of gravity stable over one's feet. When cervical and lumbar segments are flexible, this extra lordosis is easily accommodated. When spondylosis, spinal stenosis, and vertebrobasilar insufficiency coexist, it is impossible to balance the spine. Attempts at increasing lordosis lead to back pain and low-

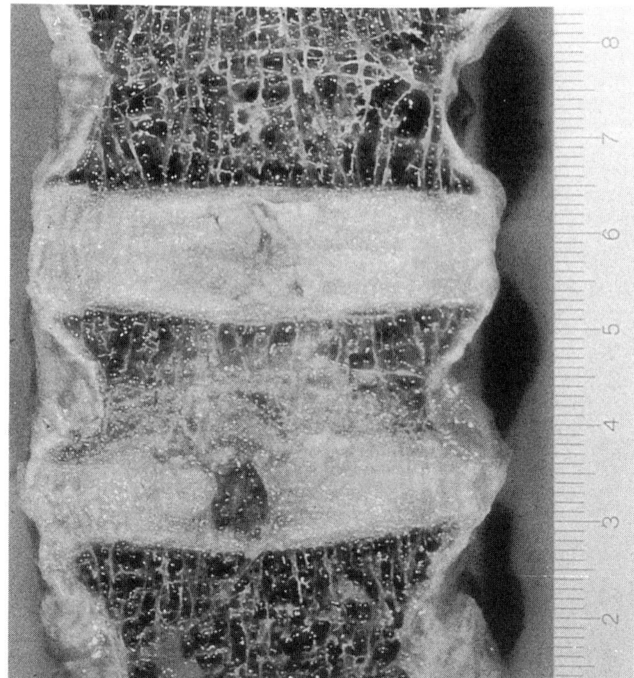

Figure 18 Wedge compression fracture of the thoracic vertebrae.

back spasm, radiculopathy, and dizziness. Around the fracture level, facet malalignment and muscle imbalance cause chronic achiness and fatigue.

In patients with neurologic deterioration from canal entrapment, preoperative MRI, CT scan, and myelogram should be performed (97). Cord compromise usually occurs in the lower thoracic level, where the canal is most narrow and can be approached easily through a transthoracic approach and stabilization with tricortical iliac crest bone graft in situ followed by rigid bracing is the treatment for this uncommon situation.

D. Treatment of Other Osteoporotic Fractures

Sacral fractures are surprisingly common. Rarely seen on plain radiographs, they are easily diagnosed by bone scan, MRI, or even CT scan. Although they heal rapidly in the sacral cancellous bone, chronic sacroiliac joint pain and foraminal encroachment with resultant sacral nerve compressionary scarring are frequent. No effective treatment exists for this problem. Rest, elastic corsets, and nonsteroidal anti-inflammatory drugs may help somewhat. Residual pelvic pain from sacral radicalopathy is unfortunately common.

E. Parasymphyseal Insufficiency Fractures

An insufficiency fracture of the os pubis may occur with mild trauma or stress (Fig. 19). Similar to spine fractures, this can be difficult to distinguish from infection and either benign and malignant tumor. The signs and symptoms of groin or anterior pelvic pain are often similar to the signs and symptoms of hip pathology, which may further obscure the diagnosis. Early radiographs reveal a lytic lesion, simulating infection or malignancy. With healing, the lytic lesion becomes blastic, and this is often bilateral. There is usually a cortical fracture, and bones within the radiograph demonstrate osteoporosis. The treatment includes rest followed by early, progressive ambulation as tolerated.

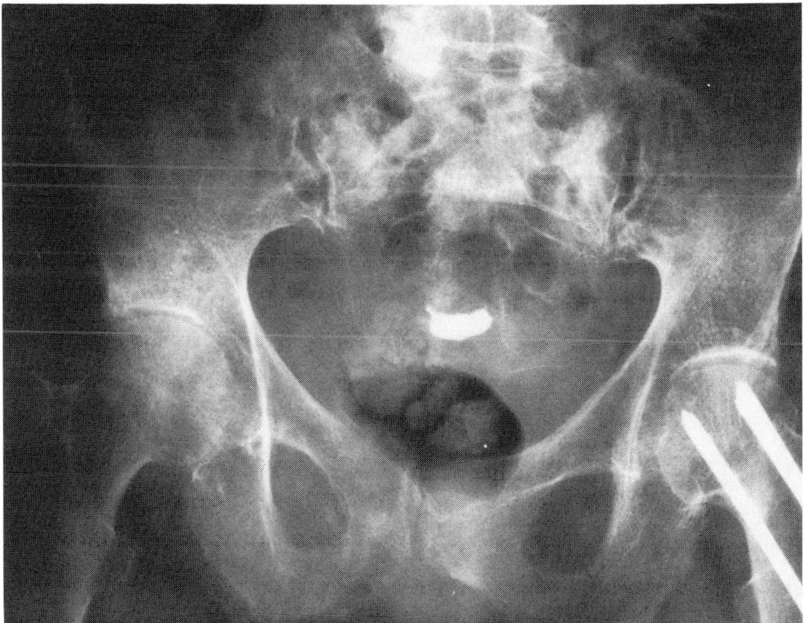

Figure 19 AP pelvis in a patient with osteoporosis, pubic pain, and tenderness, demonstrating an insufficiency fracture of the pubic rami.

F. Fractures About the Knee and Ankle

Supracondylar fractures of the distal femur are not uncommon in patients with osteoporosis (Fig. 20). There is a high ratio of trabecular to cortical bone in this area, which predisposes elderly patients to fractures in this region. Treatment must be individualized based on medical status and fracture pattern. Initial management should include evaluation of the neurovascular structures, skin, and a joint above and below the fracture site (as in all fractures).

Clinical and radiographic assessment of fracture stability and joint involvement is essential. An impacted, minimally displaced extraarticular fracture can be successfully treated with a cast brace with progressive range of motion of the knee. Displaced, unstable fractures require either closed reduction, traction and cast-bracing, or open reduction and internal fixation using condylar blade plates or dynamic compression screws. Fixation with these devices usually provides enough stability to allow range of motion in a soft brace, but if the fixation is felt to be inadequate, early range of motion in a cast brace can be started immediately. In patients with severe comminution, a buttress plate medially with iliac crest graft may be required (Figs. 21, 22). Both of these methods have been advocated with good success (98,99). We prefer early open reduction and internal fixation to traction and cast bracing in unstable or displaced, intra-articular distal femur

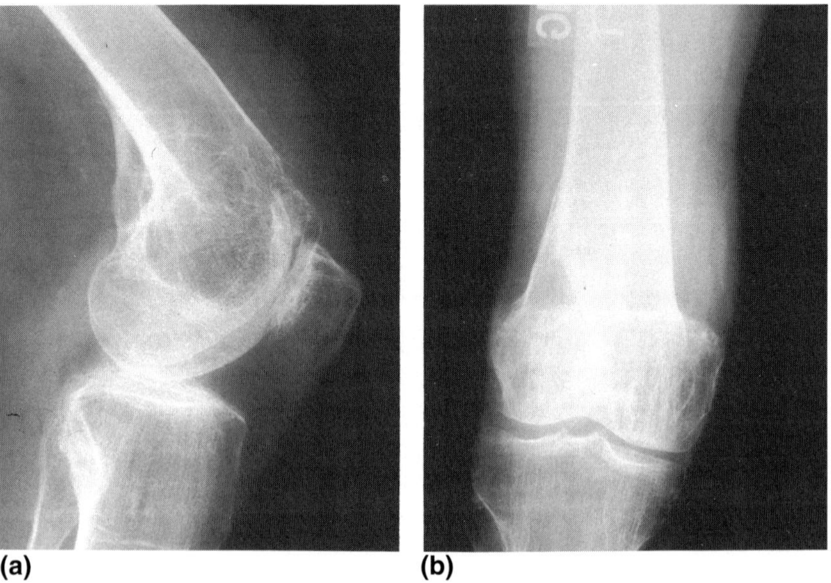

(a) (b)

Figure 20 Supracondylar fracture in an elderly male with senile osteoporosis.

fractures because of the complications related to prolonged bedrest and immobility, which include deep venous thrombosis, pulmonary embolus, bed sores, knee stiffness, and malunion.

Nondisplaced fractures of the tibial plateau are best treated with cast immobilization, early range of motion (2–3 weeks), and late weight bearing (6–8 weeks). Displacement of more than 8–10 mm or 5–10 ° of varus/valgus instability should be treated with open reduction and internal fixation and bone grafting. Displaced ankle fractures resulting in a widened mortise require open reduction and internal fixation as well. With severe ankle fracture dislocation (Figs. 23, 24), following open reduction and internal fixation, a transfixion pin may be required to maintain the talus within the mortise (Figs. 25, 26). Careful handling of the soft tissues and osteoporotic bone is critical to avoid postoperative wound breakdown, unnecessary bone sacrifice, and fracture instability.

Standard orthopedic methods should be tailored to bone quality. Fracture callus and clot debridement should be done with a dental pick or scalpel point. Bone should be cleansed with gentle irrigation rather than vigorous pulsatile lavage to avoid disrupting fragile cancellous bone. Bone grafting should be done whenever there is doubt about a fracture's healing potential. Patients who suffer from severe osteoporosis, particularly when due to steroid use or alcoholism, may not have sufficient autologous bone available from common (iliac) donor sites. Allograft and/or synthetic bone substitutes may be necessary to obtain a sufficient quantity to supplement large defects. Preoperative planning will anticipate this need.

G. Fractures of the Humerus and Olecranon

Less than 10% of all fractures related to osteoporosis occur in the humerus, and when they do occur, the proximal metaphysis is usually involved. Our initial management of impacted stable fractures utilizes a sling and swathe for a period of 2–3 weeks followed by a cast brace with a shoulder extension originally described by Balfour. This permits early, controlled range of shoulder and elbow motion, and avoids the late complication of shoulder stiffness and a frozen shoulder. In displaced proximal humeral fractures, a collar and cuff can often achieve adequate reduction and provide enough stability for union to occur. Two-part fractures involving the greater tuberosity can be treated nonoperatively; however, if there is displacement, then open reduction and internal fixation are recommended in an attempt to reattach the rotator cuff and fragment to the humeral head. This is best achieved with sutures or tension band wiring passed through the tendon of the cuff and fixed distally through drill holes in the cortical bone. Plates, screws, and pins do not provide adequate fixation in the cancellous bone fragment. Three- and four-part fractures of the humerus in elderly, osteoporotic patients are best managed with hemiarthroplasty.

Humeral shaft fractures are nearly always initially managed closed. We recom-

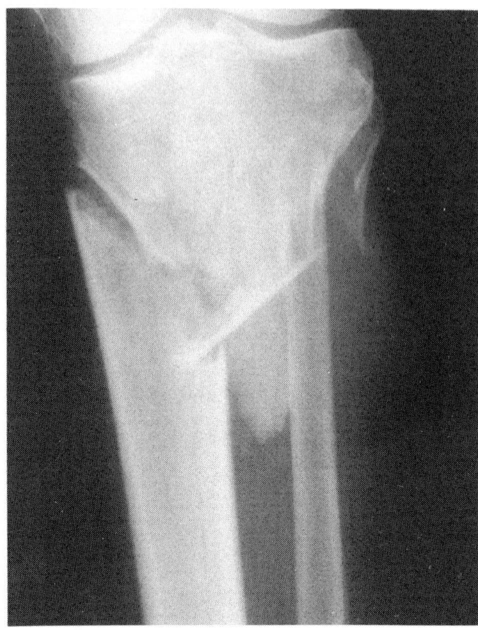
(21)

Figures 21 and 22 AP and lateral views of an elderly male who sustained a fracture of the proximal tibia associated with a crush to the fibula.

mend a sling and swathe for 7–10 days followed by early functional bracing. Patients must be aware that displacement and angulation can occur, particularly while sleeping, and a partial upright posture is required to allow gravity to align the fracture. Close radiographic follow-up is required with all nonoperative treatment of humerus fractures to avoid malunion and nonunion, particularly with humeral shaft fractures.

Displaced, intra-articular distal humerus fractures require anatomic reduction and rigid internal fixation. These fractures are technically demanding procedures and often result in significant disability. Early range of motion to avoid stiffness is required, and this can be best achieved when rigid fracture fixation is achieved surgically. Nondisplaced fractures of the olecranon in patients with active extension can be treated with immobilization of 60–90° for 3 weeks followed by active range of motion. Patients with severe osteopenia may have comminuted fractures, and this is best treated with excision of up to 70% of the olecranon and reattachment of the triceps tendon. Internal fixation in patients with severe osteopenia may result in hardware failure and should be selectively used in cases where greater

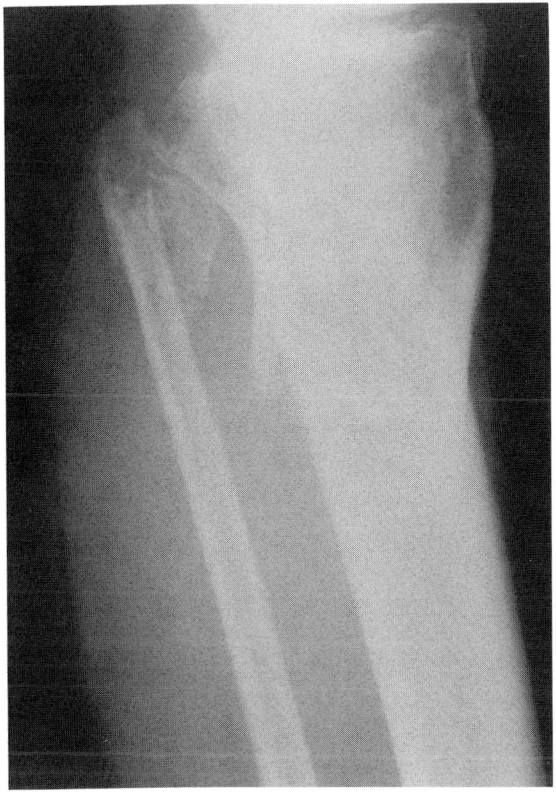

(22)

than 70–80% of the olecranon is involved, minimal comminution is present, and tension band technique would achieve adequate fixation.

H. Summary of Fracture Treatment

We have reviewed the treatment of the more common types of fractures associated with osteoporosis. The diagnosis of osteoporosis is often overlooked in patients who present with fractures. A high index of suspicion in elderly and middle-aged female patients is required to make the diagnosis of osteoporosis and pathologic fracture. This will allow prompt treatment of the underlying pathologic condition and aid the orthopedic surgeon in their treatment plan. Medical management of osteoporosis in conjunction with the orthopedic treatment of these fractures is necessary to avoid additional injuries.

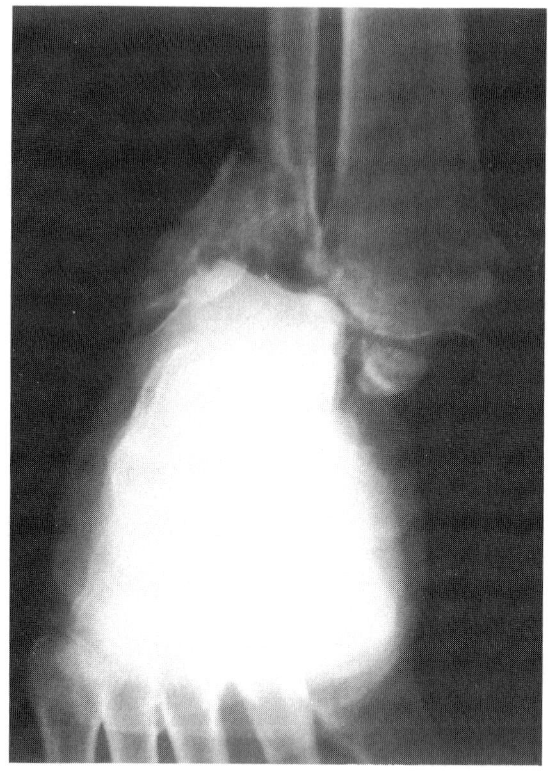

(23)

Figures 23 and 24 AP and lateral in an elderly female who sustained an open, comminuted fracture dislocation of the ankle.

X. MEDICAL TREATMENT

Most practitioners agree that calcium is essential for normal skeletal homeostasis, especially after a major fracture. Nevertheless, no agent, even calcium, accelerates healing of normal or osteoporotic bone. There is no disagreement that patients with osteoporosis should avoid drinking excessive alcohol and smoking cigarettes. Similarly, impact-loading exercises are universally accepted as being beneficial in preserving bone density compared to patients with conditions that prevent activity (100–103). This is supported by the work evaluating loss of bone mineral in astronauts, who experience weightlessness (104). The data evaluating impact-loading and exercise programs to maintain bone density are not as clear in the elderly (105,106); however, some degree of activity is required to maintain bone mass (72). Many drugs are being investigated for the treatment of osteoporosis; however, only calcium, estrogen, and calcitonin (by injection) are currently ap-

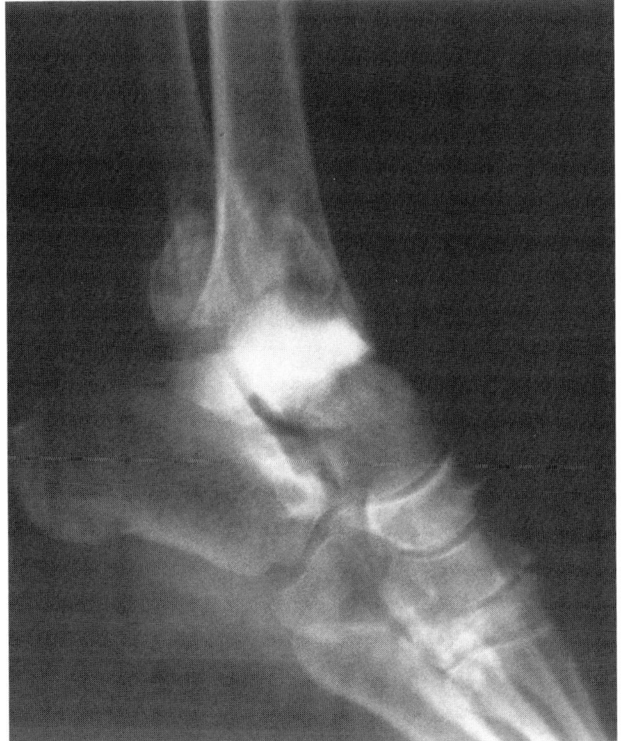
(24)

proved by the FDA for the treatment of osteoporosis. These agents are discussed more fully elsewhere in this volume.

Dietary calcium deficiency causes a negative calcium balance loss of bone density and osteoporosis. Calcium requirements in women vary. For example, a premenopausal woman requires 1,000–1,200 mg of calcium/day; a pregnant woman 1500 mg/day; and a lactating woman requires 2000 mg per day. Postmenopausal females require 1,500 mg per day for most to achieve a neutral calcium balance. The literature remains controversial on the subject of calcium supplementation in the prevention of osteoporosis. Riss et al. performed a double-blind, controlled clinical study which failed to show calcium supplementation preventing postmenopausal bone loss (107), whereas Recker et al. showed that 1,500 mg of calcium decreased the rate of bone loss (36,37). Calcium supplementation and its role in preventing loss of bone mineral may be related to menopausal status. Vitamin D is important for calcium absorption and osteoblast function.

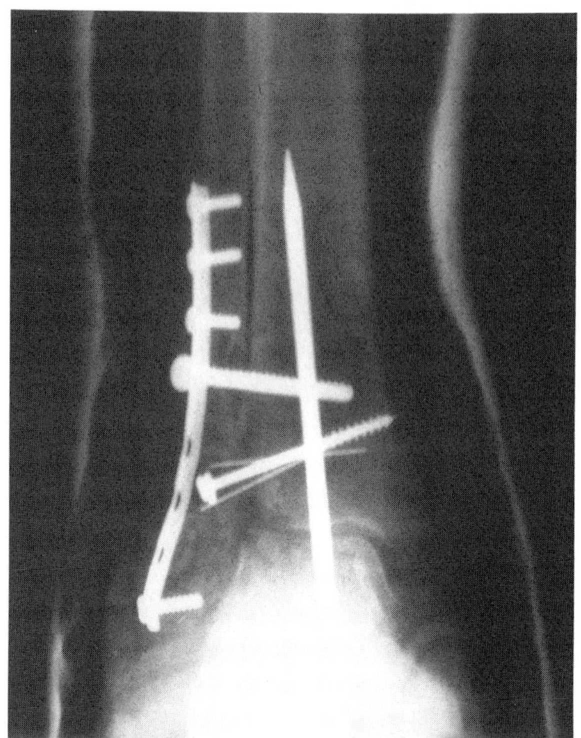

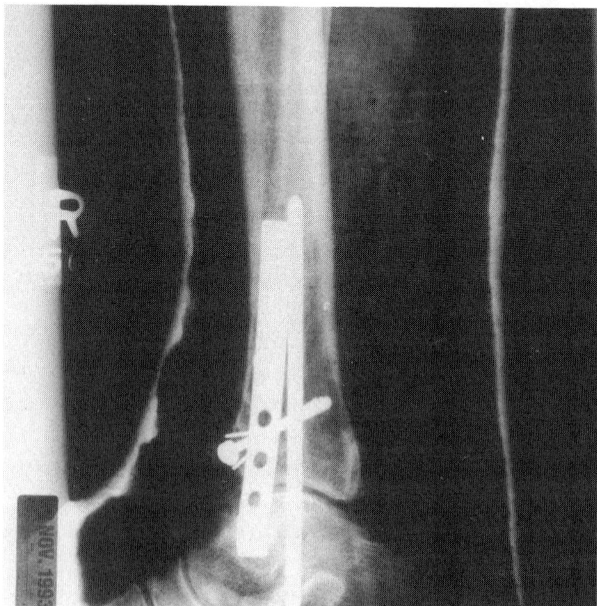

Figures 25 and 26 Treatment with open reduction and internal fixation followed by stabilization of the talus in the mortise by transarticular Steinman pin placement for a fracture dislocation of the ankle.

It is safe to conclude that calcium intake should be evaluated in all fracture patients and adequate intake ensured by dietary supplements as necessary.

Low serum vitamin D levels are often found in osteoporotic patients with fractured hips. Similarly 1,25-D3 levels in serum and bone were also low in patients with a hip fracture (108). Spine density can be increased with high-dose calcitriol (<0.6 μg/day) (109,110), and spine fractures can be reduced with even lower doses (0.5 μg/day) (111). Doses of 1 μg/day may also stabilize the spine bone mineral density (112,113).

The risks and benefits of hormonal therapy must be individualized. High-risk patients for osteoporosis include postmenopausal women (within 6 years) with accelerated bone loss, and women with premature menopause. These recommendations come from independent studies which showed that approximately 50% of postmenopausal bone loss occurs in the first 7 years (114) and the incidence of fractures and vertebral bone loss is decreased with low-dose estrogen (115,116). Both appendicular and axial bone loss are stabilized with estrogen treatment in the postmenopausal period (117) and may be effective as late as 10–20 years after menopause (118,119). All types of osteoporotic fractures can be decreased with estrogen treatment, including hip fractures (120). Perimenopausal administration of estrogen and progestin have been recommended in women under 60 who do not have contraindications to therapy by the NIH Consensus Report on Osteoporosis in 1984. Not only are there benefits in women with osteoporosis, but estrogen can decrease morbidity by lowering the risk of coronary heart disease (120,121). Absolute contraindications include patients with a diagnosis of uterine or breast carcinoma, uterine bleeding, uncontrolled hypertension, and hypertriglyceridemia. Relative contraindications include a family history of breast cancer, thromboembolic disease, and cholelithiasis. The use of progesterone in conjunction with estrogen appears to have a protective effect against uterine cancer (122); however, its effect on breast cancer is not known.

Estrogen remains the only agent to reduce the incidence of appendicular fractures. Therefore, appendicular fracture patients should be urged to consider estrogen replacement therapy (ERT). Unfortunately, many patients who suffer peripheral fractures are beyond the age when they are well to deal with resumption of their menses and other problems of ERT. Furthermore, with increasing age, the advantage of reducing cardiac disease risk diminishes. Practically, this means that ERT is rarely useful in fracture patients beyond 70 years old. Since the median age for hip fracture patients is 79 and life expectancy for women is 86 years, most fractures could be prevented by merely delaying their occurrence by 7 years. ERT may accomplish this goal.

The FDA has approved two types of calcitonin, salmon and human, for the treatment of osteoporosis. It functions by inhibiting osteoclastic function and it is thought to decrease the number of osteoclasts with long-term use. Although calcitonin has not been shown consistently to decrease the incidence of fractures, bone mass of the femoral diaphysis and lumbar spine is increased primarily in the first 6 months of treatment (123). A more recent epidemiological study showed no effect on hip fractures (124). The persuasive indication for subcutaneous calcitonin is high-turnover osteoporosis with increased number of osteoclasts seen on iliac crest bone graft and in patients with marked bone loss on successive bone densitometry who are unable to take estrogen. We use 50–100 IU T.I.W. calcitonin in conjunction with 1,500 mg of calcium and 400 U of vitamin D for 18-month periods.

Calcitonin can also be used in the acute phase of vertebral body fractures for pain management in patients with osteoporosis. Dose escalation up to 300 IU per day may reduce pain and seems to ameliorate symptoms. Flushing, nausea, and skin irritation are the most common side effects with calcitonin and can be minimized with proper technique, which is injecting into the subcutaneous tissue, not intramuscularly. Other drawbacks are the high cost of the drug and the development of antibodies and loss of effectiveness.

A more recent group of drugs effective in the treatment of osteoporosis is the bisphosphonates. Etidronate, which has been used for Paget's disease, functions by decreasing bone resorption by inhibiting osteoclastic activity and bone turnover. Use of bisphosphonates may be directed at high-turnover osteoporosis and postmenopausal and corticosteroid-induced axial osteoporosis. To avoid osteomalacia this group of drugs should be used cyclically in low dose, 400 mg for 14 days every 3 months for up to 5 years (etidronate), and an increase bone mass of 1–2% per year can be expected (125). Axial and spinal fractures decline 50–90% in randomized trials. Fractures of the appendicular skeleton are not affected by these groups of drugs, unlike the axial skeleton, possibly because the cortical osteoclasts are less responsive (126) and may even lead to paradoxical peripheral bone loss (127). Pamidronate, a second-generation bisphosphonate, may function by enhancing bone formation. A report from Europe identified increasing bone mass for up to 5 years with the use of cyclical bisphosphonates. Acute fractures are contraindications to bisphosphonate use. Calcium, vitamin D, and possibly calcitonin should be used for 3 months before starting bisphosphonates in fracture patients. Third-generation bisphosphonates, such as alendronate, are quite promising in reducing the number of spine fractures and loss of height and may not carry the risk of osteomalacia with extended use. The most common drug-related adverse effect is gastrointestinal complaints, but these are often mild.

The use of fluoride treatment in osteoporosis is considered experimental and warrants further investigation. The action of fluoride on bone to increase bone mass is probably related to stimulating activity and increasing the number of osteoblasts. Unfortunately, side effects of fluoride are common, primarily affecting the gastrointestinal tract and causing bone and joint pains. Gastric mucosal irritation and nausea are the most frequent side effects.

Several reports have shown that fluoride treatment increases bone mass 5–10% per year (128,129). With appropriate dosing, the incidence of vertebral fractures can be decreased (130–135). Animal studies have shown that fluoride-fed groups had greater shear strength and higher compressive stress in compact and trabecular bone than control groups. A more recent randomized study using high-dose fluoride alone revealed increased bone mass and increased appendicular fractures without a significant decrease in spinal fractures (136). The data on the use of fluoride in the prevention of hip fractures are even more controversial. Several reports have shown an increase in the number of nonvertebral fractures with high-dose fluoride (75 mg/day) (136,137) while others have seen no change or a decreased incidence (138). Additional trials investigating this drug are required before its use should be advocated.

A drug used for osteoporosis in Japan and Italy is ipriflavone. Early reports suggested that this drug may have a positive effect on bone; however, with the dose currently recommended (600 mg/day), this drug may not be effective (139), and additional testing for changes in bone density and mechanism of action may be required.

XI. REGIONAL OSTEOPOROSIS

Regional osteoporosis is commonly seen by the orthopedic surgeon. There are four categories: 1. Postimmobilization; 2. Sudek's posttraumatic; 3. pregnancy-associated; 4. (migratory) localized. Type 1 is most common, occurring after cast immobilization of a limb for more than 4 weeks. Ulivieri et al. have shown that statistically significant regional bone loss occurs within 1 month, and by 4 months, a full 50% of regional bone density is lost after fracture (140). This should largely resolve once immobilization is discontinued and the limb begins to function normally.

Type 2 regional osteoporosis is associated with reflex sympathetic dystrophy. Reflex sympathetic dystrophy is characterized by a swollen, painful extremity with impaired mobility and autonomic dysfunction. It is usually associated with trauma; however, a precipitating event may not be found. The stages described by Steinbocker include an acute pain aggravated by emotional disturbance and motion (stage I); osteopenia, muscle wasting, and stiffness (stage II); and severe demineralization and joint contracture (stage III). This spectrum encompasses Sudek's atrophy (Fig. 27). Immobilization of limbs and restricted weight-bearing contribute to regional osteoporosis. Certain methods of fracture management such as external fixation reportedly are more apt to produce acute localized osteoporosis (110). Treatment consists of mechanical and biologic interventions to reverse the osteoporosis vasomotor instability and prevent fracture. Types 3 and 4 are rare and beyond the scope of the discussion. All types seem to respond to similar treatment measures.

Assisted range-of-motion and intensive physical therapy is the cornerstone of treatment. Physical therapy modalities such as whirlpool massage-controlled edema, joint mobilization, and pain reduction are needed. Aggressive physical therapy must prevent fracture, especially in the lower extremity, by judicious use of crutches and graduated weight-bearing as pain diminishes. This stimulates

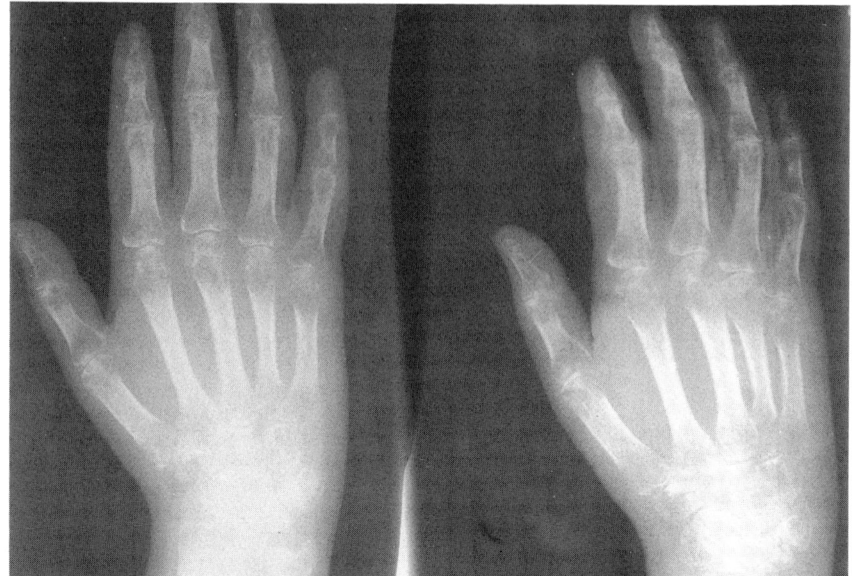

Figure 27 Following minor trauma to the hand, patient developed Sudek's atrophy and severe regional osteoporosis.

osteoblastic bone formation as well as healing the runaway osteoclastic resorption. Except during pregnancy, nonsteroidal anti-inflammatory drugs may help with pain control. Other treatments include oral prednisone for the first 4 weeks to reduce the edema and pain. Yet it should be used with caution because steroids increase bone loss and diminish bone formation, worsening the osteopenia systemically. Sympathetic blockade may also control pain. Aggressive antiresorptive therapy is advocated including calcium supplementation (1,500 mg/d). Calcitonin 100 IU SC QD and, when appropriate, estrogen are also recommended. Full correction of the cortical and cancellous loss seems to occur over the ensuing year.

XII. PERIPROSTHETIC BONE LOSS AFTER TOTAL HIP REPLACEMENT

Over 200,000 hip replacements were performed last year, primarily for degenerative joint disease. Cemented or uncemented prosthesis may be used, and both can develop loosening and periprosthetic bone loss. Bone loss commonly occurs adjacent to implants because of stress shielding. This usually occurs rapidly in 6–12 months, and 10–50% bone loss can be expected. DEXA provides the best measurement of bone loss (141,142) and is superior to CT scan and ultrasound.

The ability to quantitate periprosthetic bone loss may provide guidelines for revision surgery and long-term prognosis in these patients.

XIII. ATHLETIC AMENORRHEA AND OSTEOPENIA

Exercise in postmenopausal, sedentary women with documented osteoporosis has been found to increase bone density in vertebral bodies (143). Intense exercise, which can cause irregularity of the menstrual cycle and exercise-induced oligomenorrhea or amenorrhea, can affect nearly 50% of women in competitive sports and 20% of exercising women (144). Eumenorrheic women ran fewer miles and had higher progesterone peaks, estradiol concentrations, and prolactin levels than the amenorrheic group who often weighed less than 115 pounds or had lost more than 10 pounds.

The diagnosis of estrogen-deficient amenorrhea should only be made after a negative pregnancy test and hormonal evaluation. Amenorrheic, premenopausal women may develop cancellous bone loss similar to postmenopausal women. When amenorrheic athletes were compared with eumenorrheic women, eumenorrheic women had significantly greater vertebral body bone density, but this was not clinically significant because there was no difference in axial fracture rate between the two groups. Stress fractures are common among these patients. Treatment consists of dietary calcium supplements, maintaining adequate body fat stores, and considering estrogen supplementation.

A group of females that will be soon entering the population at risk for osteoporosis, who have not been previously studied, are women who have been nutritionally depleted at some period of their life through dietary and eating disorders. The unknown effects of diseases such as bulimia, anorexia nervosa, and severe dietary restrictions may eventually lead to a new population afflicted with osteoporosis.

REFERENCES

1. Carter DR, Hayes WC. The compressive behavior of bone as a two phase porous structure. J Bone Joint Surg 1977; 59(A):954–962.
2. National Institutes of Health Consensus Development Conference Statement on Osteoporosis. JAMA 1984; 252:799–802.
3. Frost HM. Treatment of osteoporosis by manipulating of coherent bone cell population. Clin Orthop Rel Res 1979; 143:227–244.
4. Miller EJ, Marvin GR. The collagen of bone. Clin Orthop Rel Res 1968; 195.
5. Yamauchi M, Young DR, Chandler GS, Mechanic GL. Cross-linking and new bone synthesis in immobilized and recovering primate osteoporosis. Bone 1988; 9: 415–418.
6. Urist MR, Mikulski AJ. A soluble bone morphogenic protein extracted from bone

matrix with an aqueous and non-aqueous solvent. Proc Soc Exp Biol Med 1979; 148–162.

7. Wozney JM, Rosen V, Celeste AJ, et al. Novel regulators of bone formation in molecular clones and activity. Science 1988; 1528–1533.
8. Price PA, Otsuka AS, Poser JW, et al. Characterization of a gamma-carboxy glutamic acid containing protein of bone. Proc Natl Acad Sci USA 1973; 73:1447.
9. Romberg RW, Werness PG, Lollan P, Riggs BL, Mann KG. Isolation and characterization of native adult osteonectin. J Biol Chem 1985; 260:2728–2736.
10. Gevers G, Dequecker J. Collagen and non-collaginous protein content (osteocalcin, sialoprotein, proteoglycan) in the iliac crest bone and serum osteocalcin in women with and without hand osteoarthritis. Collagen Rel Res 1987; 7(6):435–442.
11. Johnston CC, Milner JZ, Slemenda CW, Reister TK, Christian JC, Peacock M. Calcium supplementation and increases in bone mineral density in children. N Engl J Med 1992; 327:82–87.
12. McBroom RJ, Hayes WC, Edwards WT, Goldberg RP, White AA. Prediction of vertebral body compressive fracture using quantitative computed tomography. J Bone Joint Surg [AM] 1985; 67:1206–1214.
13. Woo SL, Kuei SC, Amiel D, et al. The effect of prolonged physical training on the properties of long bone: a study of Wolff's Law. J Bone Joint Surg [Am] 1981; 63: 780–787.
14. Recker RR. Architecture and vertebral fracture. Calcif Tissue Int 1993; 53(suppl 1): S139–S142.
15. Snyder BD, Piazza SJ, Edwards WT, Hayes WC. Role of trabecular morphology on the etiology of age related vertebral fracture. Calcif Tissue Int 1993; 53(suppl): s14–s22.
16. Boskey AL. Bone mineral and matrix. Are they altered in osteoporosis? Orthop Clin North Am 1990; 21:19–29.
17. Carter DR, Hayes WC, Vaes G, et al. The compressive behavior of bone as a two phase porous structure. National Institutes of Health Consensus Development Conference Statement on Osteoporosis. Biochem J Collagen Rel Res 1992; 327:82–87.
18. Hayes WC. Biomechanics of cortical and trabecular bone. Implications for assessment of fracture risk. In: Moe VC, Hayes WC eds. Basic Orthopaedic Biomechanics. New York: Raven Press; 1991:93–142.
19. Alho A, Stromsoe K, Hoiseth A. Bone mineral related to mechanical strength of cancellous bone. Trans Eur Orthop Res Soc 1992; 2:16(abstract).
20. Alho A, Husby T, Hoiseth A, Fonstelien E. Bone mineral content and mechanical strength of human femur. Finn J Orthop Traum 1985; 8:56–57.
21. Dalen N, Hellstrom LG, Jacobson B. Bone mineral content and mechanical strength of the femoral neck. Acta Orthop Scand 1976; 47(5):503–508.
22. Riggs BL, Wakner HW, Dunn WL, Mazells RB, Offord KIP, Melton JJ III. Differential changes in bone mineral density of the appendiculum and axial skeleton with aging; relationship to spinal osteoporosis. J Clin Invest 1981; 67:328.
23. Beck TJ, Ruff CB, Scott WW Jr, Plato CC, Tobin JD, Quan CA. Sex differences in geometry of the femoral neck with aging. Calcif Tissue Int 1992; 50:24–29.

24. Boskey AL. Current concepts of the physiology and biochemistry of calcification. Clin Orthop Rel Res 1981; 157:225.
25. Burstein AH, Reilly DT, Martens M. Aging of bone tissue: mechanical properties. J Bone Joint Surg [Am] 1976; 58:82–86.
26. Ruff CB, Hayes WC. Bone-mineral content in the lower limb. Relationship to cross-sectional geometry. J Bone Joint Surg [Am] 1984; 66:1024–1031.
27. Zain-Elabdien BS, Olerud S, Karlstrom G. Ender nailing of pertrochanteric fractures. Complications related to technical failures and bone quality. Acta Orthop Scand 1985; 56:138–144.
28. Foltin E. Osteoporosis and fracture patterns. A study of split compression fractures of the lateral tibial condyle. Int Orthop 1988; 12:299–303.
29. Stromsoe K, Alho A, Hoiseth A. Retention of distal femoral osteotomy fixed with AO condylar plate and Grosse Kempf locked nail related to bone mineral in cadavers. Trans Eur Res Soc 1993; 3:9.
30. Stromsoe K, Kok WL, Hoiseth A, Alho A. Holding power of the 4.5 mm AO/ASIF cortex screw in cortical bone in relation to bone mineral. Injury 1993; 24:656–659.
31. Wittenberg RH, Shea M, Swartz DE, Lee KS, White AA, Hayes WC. Importance of bone mineral density in instrumented spine fusions. Spine 1991; 16(6):647–652.
32. Coe JD, Warden KE, Herzig MA, McAfee PC. Influence of bone mineral density on the fixation of thoracolumbar implants. A comparative study of transpedicular screws, laminar hooks, and spinous process wires. Spine 1990; 15:902–907.
33. Soshi S, Shiba R, Kondo H, Murota K. An experimental study on transpedicular screw fixation in relation to osteoporosis of the lumbar spine. Spine 1991; 16:1335–1341.
34. Arnold WD. The effect of early weight-bearing on the stability of femoral neck fractures treated with Knowles pins. J Bone Joint Surg 1984; 66A:847–852.
35. Lotz JC, Hayes WC. The use of quantitative computed tomography to estimate risk of fracture of the hip from falls. J Bone Joint Surg [Am] 1990; 72:689–700.
36. Heaney RP. Bone mass, nutrition, and other lifestyle factors. Am J Med 1993; 95: 29S–33S.
37. Stegman MR, Recker RR, Davies KM, Ryan RA, Heaney RP. Fracture risk as determined by prospective and retrospective study designs. Osteoporos Int 1992; 2:290–297.
38. Hagino H, Yamamoto K, Teshima R, Kishimoto H, Nakamura T. Fracture incidence and bone mineral density of the distal radius in Japanese children. Arch Orthop Trauma Surg 1990; 109:262–264.
39. Pouilles JM, Bernard J, Tremollieres F, Louvet JP, Ribot C. Femoral bone density in young male adults with stress fractures. Bone 1989; 10:105–108.
40. Matkovic V, Ilich JZ. Calcium requirements for growth: are current recommendations adequate? Nutr Rev 1993; 51:171–180.
41. Fehily AM, Coles RJ, Evans WD, Elwood PC. Factors affecting bone density in young adults. Am J Clin Nutr 1992; 56:579–586.
42. Kritz-Silverstein D, Barrett-Connor E. Grip strength and bone mineral density in older women. J Bone Miner Res 1994; 9:45–51.

43. Grove KA, Londeree BR. Bone density in postmenopausal women: high impact vs low impact exercise. Med Sci Sports Exerc 1992; 24:1190–1194.
44. Cook DJ, Guyatt GH, Adachi JD, et al. Quality of life issues in women with vertebral fractures due to osteoporosis. Arth Rheum 1993; 36:750–756.
45. Hatori M, Hasegawa A, Adachi H, et al. The effects of walking at the anaerobic threshold level on vertebral bone loss in postmenopausal women. Calcif Tissue Int 1993; 52:411–414.
46. Delmas PD. Biochemical markers of bone turnover. I. Theoretical considerations and clinical use in osteoporosis. Am J Med 1993; 95:11S–16S.
47. Notelovitz M, Martin D, Tesar R, et al. Estrogen therapy and variable-resistance weight training increase bone mineral in surgically menopausal women [see Comments]. J Bone Miner Res 1991; 6:583–590.
48. Gundle R, Simpson AH. Should women attending fracture clinics be counselled about osteoporosis? Injury 1993; 24:441–442.
49. Melton LJ, Chrischilles EA, Cooper C, Lane AW, Riggs BL. Perspective. How many women have osteoporosis? J Bone Miner Res 1992; 7:1005–1010.
50. Melton LJ. Epidemiology of osteoporosis. Baillieres Clin Obstet Gynaecol 1991; 5: 785–805.
51. Cummings SR. Epidemiologic studies of osteoporotic fractures: methodologic issues. Calcif Tissue Int 1991; 49(suppl):S15–S20.
52. MacAusland WR, Wyman ET Jr. Management of metastatic pathologic fractures. Clin Orthop Rel Res 1970; 73:39.
53. Tuli SM, Singh AD. The osteoinductive property of decalcified bone matrix. An experimental study. J Bone Joint Surg 1978; 60(B):116–123.
54. Einhorn TA, Lane JM, Burstein AH, Kopman CR, Vigorita VJ. The healing of segmental bone defects induced by demineralized bone matrix. J Bone Joint Surg 1984; 66(A):274–279.
55. Urist MR, Lietze A, Mitzutani H, et al. A bovine low molecular weight bone morphogenetic protein (BMF fraction). Clin Orthop Rel Res 1982: 162:219–232.
56. Guy JA, Shea M, Peter CP, Morrissey R, Hayes WC. Continuous alendronate treatment throughout growth, maturation, and aging in the rat results in increases in bone mass and mechanical properties. Calcif Tissue Int 1993; 53:283–288.
57. Ashton BA, Allen TD, Howlett CR, Eaglesone CC, Hattori A, Owen M. Formation of bone and cartilage by marrow stromal cells in diffusion chambers in vivo. Clin Orthop Rel Res 1980; 151:294.
58. Lane JM, Boskey AL, Li WKP. A temporal study of collagen, proteoglycan, lipid and mineral constituents in a model of endochondral osseous repair. Metab Bone Dis 1979; 1:319–324.
59. Vose GP, Mack PB. Roentgenologic assessment of femoral neck density as related to fracturing. Am J Roentgenol 1963; 89:1296–1301.
60. Snyder SM, Schneider E. Estimation of mechanical properties of cortical bone by computed tomography. J Orthop Res 1991; 9(3):422–431.
61. Ross PD, Davis JW, Vogel JM, Wasnick RD. A critical review of bone mass and the risk of fractures in osteoporosis [see Comments]. Calcif Tissue Int 1990; 46(3):149–160.

62. Barrios C, Brostrom LA, Stark A, Walheim G. Healing complications after internal fixation of trochanteric hip fractures: the prognostic value of osteoporosis. J Orthop Trauma 1993; 7:438–442.
63. Stark A, Brostrom LA, Barrios C, Walheim G, Olsson E. A prospective randomized study of the use of sliding hip screws and Ender nails for trochanteric fractures of the femur. Int Orthop 1992; 16:359–362.
64. Hayes WC, Piazza SJ, Zysset PK. Biomechanics of fracture risk prediction of the hip and spine by quantitative computed tomography. Radiol Clin North Am 1991; 29(1):1–18.
65. Alffram PA. An epidemiologic study of cervical and trochanteric fractures of the femur in an urban population. Acta Orthop Scand 1964; 65(suppl):1–109.
66. Kenzora JE, McCarthy RE, Lowell JD, Sledge CB. Hip fracture mortality: relation to age, treatment, preoperative illness, time of surgery, and complications. Clin Orthop Rel Res 1984; 186:45–56.
67. Scheck M. Management of fractures of the femoral neck. J Bone Joint Surg 1965; 47(A):819–829.
68. Bently G. Treatment of nondisplaced fractures of the femoral neck. Clin Orthop Rel Res 1980; 152:93–101.
69. Banks HH. Factors influencing the result in fractures of the femoral neck. J Bone Joint Surg 1962; 44(A):931–964.
70. Linton P. On different types of intracapsular fractures of the femoral neck. Acta Chir Scand 1944; 90(suppl):1–122.
71. Urovitz EPM, Fornasier VL, Risen MI, MacNab I. Etiological factors in the pathogenesis of femoral trabecular fatigue fractures. Clin Orthop Rel Res 1977; 127: 275–280.
72. Alho A, Benterud JG, Ronningen H, Hoiseth A. Prediction of disturbed healing in femoral neck fracture. Radiographic analysis of 149 cases. Acta Orthop Scand 1992; 63(3):639–644.
73. Van Audekerche R, Martens M, Mulier JC, Stuyck J. Experimental study on internal fixation of femoral neck fractures. Clin Orthop Rel Res 1979; 141:203–212.
74. Sarmiento A. Unstable intertrochanteric fractures of the femur. Clin Orthop Rel Res 1973; 92:77–85.
75. Harrington KD. The use of methylmethacrylate as an adjunct in the internal fixation of unstable comminuted intertrochanteric fractures in osteoporotic patients. J Bone Joint Surg 1975; 57(A):744–750.
76. Arnoldi LL, Linderholm H. Fracture of the femoral neck. Clin Orthop Rel Res 1972; 84:116–127.
77. Fielding JW. Displaced femoral neck fractures. Orthop Rev 1973; 2:11–17.
78. Gyepes M, Mellins HZ, Katz I. The low incidence of fracture of hip in Negro. JAMA 1962; 181:1073–1074.
79. Atkin JM. Prevalence of osteoporosis in women with fracture of the femoral neck. Br Med J (Clin Res) 1984; 288:597–601.
80. Barnes R, Brown JT, Garden RS, Nicoll EA. Subcapital fractures of the femur. J Bone Joint Surg 1976; 58(B):2–24.

81. Scileppi KP, Stolberg B, Vigorita VJ. Bone histomorphometry in femoral neck fractures. Surg Forum 1981; 3:543–545.
82. Thompson RF. Vittalium intramedullary hip prosthesis: preliminary report. NY State J Med 1952; 52:3011–3020.
83. Gingras MB, Clarke J, Evarts CM. Prosthetic replacement in femoral neck fractures. Clin Orthop Rel Res 1980; 152:147–157.
84. DelaMarter R, Moreland JR. Treatment of acute femoral neck fractures with total hip arthroplasty. Clin Orthop Rel Res 1987; 218:68–74.
85. Sim FH, Stauffer RN. Management of hip fractures by total hip arthroplasty. Clin Orthop Rel Res 1980; 152:191–197.
86. Cleveland M, Bosworht DM, Thompson FR. Intertrochanteric fractures of the femur. J Bone Joint Surg 1947; 29:1049–1067.
87. Morris HD. Trochanteric fractures. South Med J 1941; 34:571–578.
88. Ganz R, Thomas RJ, Hammerle CP. Trochanteric fractures of the femur: treatment and results. Clin Orthop Rel Res 1979; 138:30–40.
89. Kaufer H. Mechanics of the treatment of hip injuries. Clin Orthop Rel Res 1980; 146:53–61.
90. Weiss NS, Ure CL, Ballard JH, Williams AR, Daling JR. Decreased risk of fractures of the hip and lower forearm with postmenopausal use of estrogen. N Engl J Med 1980; 303:1195–1198.
91. Singh M, Nagrath AR, Maini PS. Changes in trabecular pattern of the upper end of the femur as an index of osteoporosis. J Bone Joint Surg 1970; 52(A):457–467.
92. Kewenter Y. A case of isolated fracture of the lesser trochanter. Acta Orthop Scand 1931; 2:160–165.
93. Cooney WP. External fixation of distal radius fractures. Clin Orthop Rel Res 1983; 180:44–49.
94. Clancy GJ. Percutaneous Kirschner wire fixation of Colles fractures. J Bone Joint Surg 1984; 66(A):1008–1014.
95. DePalma AF. Comminuted fractures of the distal end of the radius treated by ulnar pinning. J Bone Joint Surg 1952; 34(A):51–62.
96. Bassett RL, Ray MJ. Carpal instability associated with radial styloid fracture. Orthopedics 1984; 7:1356–1361.
97. Heggenness MH. Spine fracture with neurologic defect in osteoporosis. Osteoporos Int 1993; 3:215–221.
98. Melone CP Jr. Open treatment for displaced articular fractures of the distal radius. Clin Orthop Rel Res 1986; 202:103–111.
99. Urist MR, Gurvey MS, Fareed DO. Long term observations on aged women with pathological osteoporosis. In: Barzel US, ed. Osteoporosis. New York: Grune and Stratton; 1970:3.
100. Mooney V, Nickel V, Harvey J, Snelson R. Cast brace treatment for fractures of the distal part of the femur. J Bone Joint Surg 1967; 49(A):591–613.
101. Mize RD, Bucholz RW, Grogan DP. Surgical treatment of displaced comminuted fractures of the distal end of the femur, an extensile approach. J Bone Joint Surg 1982; 64(A):871–879.

102. Krolner B, Toft B, Pors Nielson S, Tondevold E. Physical exercise as prophylaxis against involutional vertebral bone loss: a controlled trial. Clin Sci 1982; 64: 541–546.
103. Cheng S, Suominen H, Rantanen T, Parkatti T, Heikkinen E. Bone mineral density and physical activity in 50-60-year-old women. Bone Miner 1991; 12:123–132.
104. Aloia JF, Cohn SH, Ostuni JA et al. Prevention of involutional bone loss by exercise. Ann Intern Med 1978; 89:356–358.
105. Rambaut PC, Johnston JS. Prolonged weightlessness and calcium loss in man. Acta Astronautica 1979; 6:1113–1122.
106. LeBlanc AD, Schneider VS, Evans HJ, Engelbretson DA, Krebs JM. Bone mineral loss and recovery after 17 weeks of bed rest. J Bone Miner Res 1992; 5:843.
107. Meredith CN. In: Munro HSG, ed. Nutrition of the Elderly. New York: Vevy/Raven Press; 1992:169–175.
108. Gutin BKM. Can vigorous exercise play a role in osteoporosis prevention? A review. Osteoporosis Int 1992; 2:55–69.
109. Brostrom LA, Barrios C, Kronberg M, Stark A, Walheim G. Clinical features and walking ability in the early postoperative period after treatment of trochanteric hip fractures. Results with special reference to fracture type and surgical treatment. Ann Chir Gynaecol 1992; 81:66–71.
110. Smith EJ, Ward AJ, Watt I. Post-traumatic osteoporosis and algodystrophy after external fixation of tibial fractures. Injury 1993; 24:411–415.
111. Caniggia A, Nuti R, Lore F, Martini G, Turchetti V, Righi G. Long-term treatment with calcitriol in postmenopausal osteoporosis. Metabolism 1990; 39(4):43–49.
112. Gallagher JC, Goldgar D. Treatment of postmenopausal osteoporosis with high doses of synthetic calcitriol: a randomized controlled study. Ann Intern Med 1990; 113:649–655.
113. Tilyard MW, Spears GFS, Thomson J, Dovey S. Treatment of postmenopausal osteoporosis with calcitriol of calcium. N Engl J Med 1992; 326:357–362.
114. Orimo H, Shiraki M, Hayashi T, Nakamura T. Reduced occurrence of vertebral crush fractures in senile osteoporosis treated with 1(OH)-vitamin D3. Bone Miner 1987; 3:47–52.
115. Pouilles JM, Tremollieres F, Ribot C. Prevention of post-menopausal bone loss with 1-hydroxy vitamin D3. A three-year prospective study. Clin Rheumatol 1992; 11: 492–497.
116. Defazio J, Speroff L. Estrogen replacement therapy: current thinking and practice. Geriatrics 1985; 40:32–48.
117. Lindsay R, Hart DM, Aitken JM, et al. Long-term prevention of post-menopausal osteoporosis by oestrogen. Lancet 1976; 1:1038–1041.
118. Horsman A, Gallagher JC, Simpson M, Nordin BEC. Prospective trial of oestrogen and calcium in post-menopausal women. Br Med J 1977; 2:789–792.
119. Ribot C, Tremollieres F, Pouilles JM. Effect of 17β-oestradiol and norethisterone acetate on vertebral bone mass and lipid metabolism in early post-menopausal women. Maturitas 1992; 15:217–223.
120. Spector TD, Brennan P, Harris PA, Studd JWW, Silman AJ. Do current regimes of

hormone replacement therapy protect against subsequent fractures? Osteoporosis Int 1992; 2:219–224.

121. Reginster JY, Sarlet N, Deroisy R, Albert A, Gaspard U, Franchimont P. Minimal levels of serum estradiol prevent post-menopausal bone loss. Calcif Tissue Int 1992; 51:340–343.
122. Finucane FF, Madans JH, Bush TL, Wolf PH, Kleinman JC. Decreased risk of stroke among postmenopausal hormone users. Arch Intern Med 1993; 153:73–79.
123. Grady D, Rubin SM, Petitti DB, et al. Hormone therapy to prevent disease and prolong life in post-menopausal women. Ann Intern Med 1992; 117:1016–1037.
124. Gambrell RD Jr. Clinical use of progestins in the postmenopausal patient: dosage and duration. J Reprod Med 1994; 27:531.
125. Gruber HE, Ivey JL, Baylink DJ. Long-term calcitonin therapy in postmenopausal osteoporosis. Metabolism 1984; 33:295–303.
126. Kanis JA, Johnell O, Gullberg B, et al. Evidence for efficacy of drugs affecting bone metabolism in preventing hip fracture. Br Med J 1992; 305:1124–1128.
127. Storm T, Thamsborg G, Steiniche T, Genant HK, Sorensen OH. Effect of intermittent cyclical etidronate therapy on bone mass and fracture rate in women with post-menopausal osteoporosis. N Engl J Med 1990; 1265–1271.
128. Chappard D, Petitjean M, Alexandre C, Vico L, Minaire P, Riffat G. Cortical osteoclasts are less sensitive to etidronate than trabecular osteoclasts. J Bone Miner Res 1991; 6:673–680.
129. Price RI, Gutteridge DH, Stuckey BGA, et al. J Bone Miner Res 1993; 8:209–217.
130. Hansson T, Roos B. The effect of fluoride and calcium on spinal bone mineral content: a controlled perspective (3 year) study. Calcif Tissue Int 1987; 40:315.
131. Schulz EE, Engstrom H, Sauser DD. Osteoporosis: radiographic detection of fluoride induced extra-axial bone formation. Radiology 1986; 159:457–462.
132. Lane JM, Vigorita VJ, Schwartz E, Healey JH, Suda M. Is fluoride bone osteomalacic: a histomorphometric analysis. Orthop Trans 1984; 8:272–273 (abstract).
133. Lane JM, Healey JH, Schwartz E, et al. Treatment of osteoporosis with sodium fluoride and calcium: effects on vertebral fracture incidence and bone histomorphometry. Ortho Clin North Am 1984; 15:729–745.
134. Lane JM, Vigorita VJ, Eihorn TA, et al. Treatment of osteoporosis with sodium fluoride: increased bone mass and prevention of spinal fractures. Orthop Trans 1983; 7:499–500.
135. Farley SM, Wergedal JE, Farley JR, et al. Spinal fractures during fluoride therapy for osteoporosis: relationship to spinal bone density. Osteoporosis Int 1992; 2:213–218.
136. Jowsey J, Riggs BL, Kelly PJ, et al. Effect of combined therapy with sodium fluoride, vitamin D and calcium in osteoporosis. Am J Med 1972; 53:43–49.
137. Riggs BL, Seeman E, Hodgson SF. Effect of the fluoride/calcium regimen on vertebral fracture occurrence in post-menopausal osteoporosis: comparison with conventional therapy. N Engl J Med 1982; 306:446–450.
138. Riggs B, Hodgson S, O'Fallon W, Chao E. Effect of fluoride treatment on the fracture rate in postmenopausal women with osteoporosis. N Engl J Med 1990; 322: 802–809.

139. Bayley TA. Fluoride-induced fractures: relation to osteogenic effect. J Bone Miner Res 1990; S217–S222.
140. Ulivieri FM, Bossi E, Azzoni R, et al. Quantification by dual photonabsorptiometry of local bone loss after fracture. Clin Orthop Rel Res 1990; 291–296.
141. Vose GP, Keele DK, Milner AM. Effect of sodium fluoride, inorganic phosphate, and oxymetholone therapies in osteoporosis: a six year progress report. J Gerontol 1978; 33:204–212.
142. Azria M, Behhar C, Cooper S. Lack of effect of ipriflavone on osteoclast motility and bone resorption in in vitro and ex vivo studies. Calcif Tissue Int 1993; 52:16–20.
143. Krolner B, Toft B, Nielsen SP, Tondevold E. Physical exercise as prophylaxis against involutional vertebral bone loss: a controlled trial. Clin Sci 1983; 64:541–546.
144. Shangold MM. Causes, evaluation, and management of athletic oligo-amenorrhea. Med Clin North Am 1985; 69:83–95.

6

Radiographic–Pathologic Correlation

JOHN A. M. TAYLOR*

University of California, San Diego, Medical Center
San Diego, California

DONALD L. RESNICK

University of California, San Diego, School of Medicine,
and Veterans Affairs Medical Center
San Diego, California

DAVID J. SARTORIS

University of California, San Diego, School of Medicine,
and University of California, San Diego, Medical Center
San Diego, California

I. INTRODUCTION

The role of radiography in evaluating patients with osteoporosis is well established. Routine radiography, supplemented with conventional and computed tomography (CT), radionuclide bone imaging (scintigraphy), and, more recently, magnetic resonance (MR) imaging, is well suited to the assessment of the morphologic patterns, skeletal distribution, and imaging appearance of osteoporosis. Radiography also is used extensively to detect and evaluate fractures in osteoporotic patients. Although radiographs can suggest the diagnosis of osteoporosis, because 30–50% of skeletal calcium must be lost before radiographic changes

**Present affiliation*: Western States Chiropractic College, Portland, Oregon.

appear, routine radiography is not sufficiently sensitive to detect early changes (1,2). As a result of this limitation, more advanced techniques such as photon absorptiometry (3–6), quantitative computed tomography (QCT) (7–15), ultrasonography (16,17), and dual-energy x-ray absorptiometry (DXA) usually are employed for early detection and quantitative evaluation of osteoporosis (18–20). These quantitative techniques are discussed elsewhere in this book.

II. TERMINOLOGY

The term osteoporosis was defined by Pommer in 1885 as increased porosity of bone (21,22). The increased radiolucency seen on radiographs of patients with osteoporosis is termed osteopenia, meaning "poverty of bone" (Fig. 1). The terms demineralization, undermineralization, and deossification should never be used to describe radiolucency on radiographs; they are best reserved to describe specific phenomena such as osteomalacia and conditions causing accelerated bone resorption.

Diffuse osteopenia occurs in a variety of conditions, including osteoporosis, osteomalacia, neoplasm, and hyperparathyroidism. When osteopenia is detected, a careful search for specific abnormalities suggesting these other conditions is essential (Table 1). The radiographic findings in osteoporosis are often nonspecific. The diagnosis of osteoporosis, then, is frequently one of exclusion and rests on the radiographic appearance of osteopenia coupled with typical clinical and histologic features.

"Osteoporosis is established when the decrease in bone mass is greater than that expected for a person of a given age, sex and race, and when it results in structural bone failure manifested by fractures" (23). Although some authors have concluded that routine radiographs of the lumbar spine can provide a rough estimate of bone density in some subjects (24), radiologists have generally agreed that identifying osteopenia from radiographs is highly subjective and variable from film to film and from observer to observer (25,26).

Fractures associated with osteoporosis are a most serious public health concern, the magnitude of which is discussed elsewhere in this book. Such fractures occur most frequently in the spine, proximal portion of the femur, and distal part of the radius, and result from cortical or trabecular bone loss, or loss of both types of bone.

Osteoporosis is classified as generalized, regional, or localized. Generalized osteoporosis involves a large area of the skeleton and is primarily axial in distribution. Regional osteoporosis involves only one portion of the skeleton and typically affects the appendicular skeleton. Localized osteoporosis affects single or multiple focal areas (27). Additionally, the radiographic appearance of rapid bone loss differs from that of slow bone loss (28). The radiographic features combined with the skeletal distribution of osteopenia provide clues to the precise nature of the osteoporosis.

III. RADIOGRAPHIC AND PATHOLOGIC FINDINGS

A. Generalized Osteoporosis

The axial distribution of generalized osteoporosis includes the spine, pelvis, proximal portion of the femur, ribs, and sternum (Fig. 2). In more advanced cases, the tubular bones of the appendicular skeleton become involved. The skull is typically affected to a lesser extent, but extensive involvement can occur in conditions such as Cushing's disease and hyperthyroidism (27). Table 1 outlines some of the more common causes of generalized osteoporosis.

The radiologic and pathologic findings vary according to the specific site of involvement (29,30). The most characteristic radiographic findings occur in the pelvis, thorax, proximal portion of the femur, spine, and small tubular bones of the appendicular skeleton.

1. Pelvis and Thorax

The most prominent radiographic finding in generalized osteoporosis affecting the pelvis and thorax is increased radiolucency. The radiolucency often is accompanied by an apparent prominence of the trabecular pattern of the spongiosa and, in advanced cases, by thinning of cortical margins. Pathologically, the trabeculae are thin and sparse, the cortex is thin, and the spongiosa is excessively porous. Owing to overlying soft-tissue and skeletal structures, abnormalities of the ribs and sternum are not as well visualized as those of the pelvis. Consequently, evidence of osteoporosis of the thoracic cage is not evident until insufficiency fractures occur.

2. Proximal Portion of the Femur

The proximal portion of the femur is important in the study of osteoporosis because it represents one of the most frequent sites of fracture in this disorder and because analysis of the trabecular pattern in this region is useful as an index of osteoporosis (31). The trabeculae of the upper end of the femur are typically divided into five anatomic groups (Fig. 3):

a. Principal Compressive Group. The principal compressive trabeculae, the thickest and most densely packed, represent the uppermost compressive trabeculae. They arise from the cortex of the medial femoral neck and extend in a curvilinear arc to the upper portion of the femoral head.

b. Secondary Compressive Group. The secondary compressive trabeculae are thin and widely spaced and arise from the medial cortex of the femoral shaft below the principal compressive group. These trabeculae curve upward and slightly laterally toward the greater trochanter and the upper femoral neck.

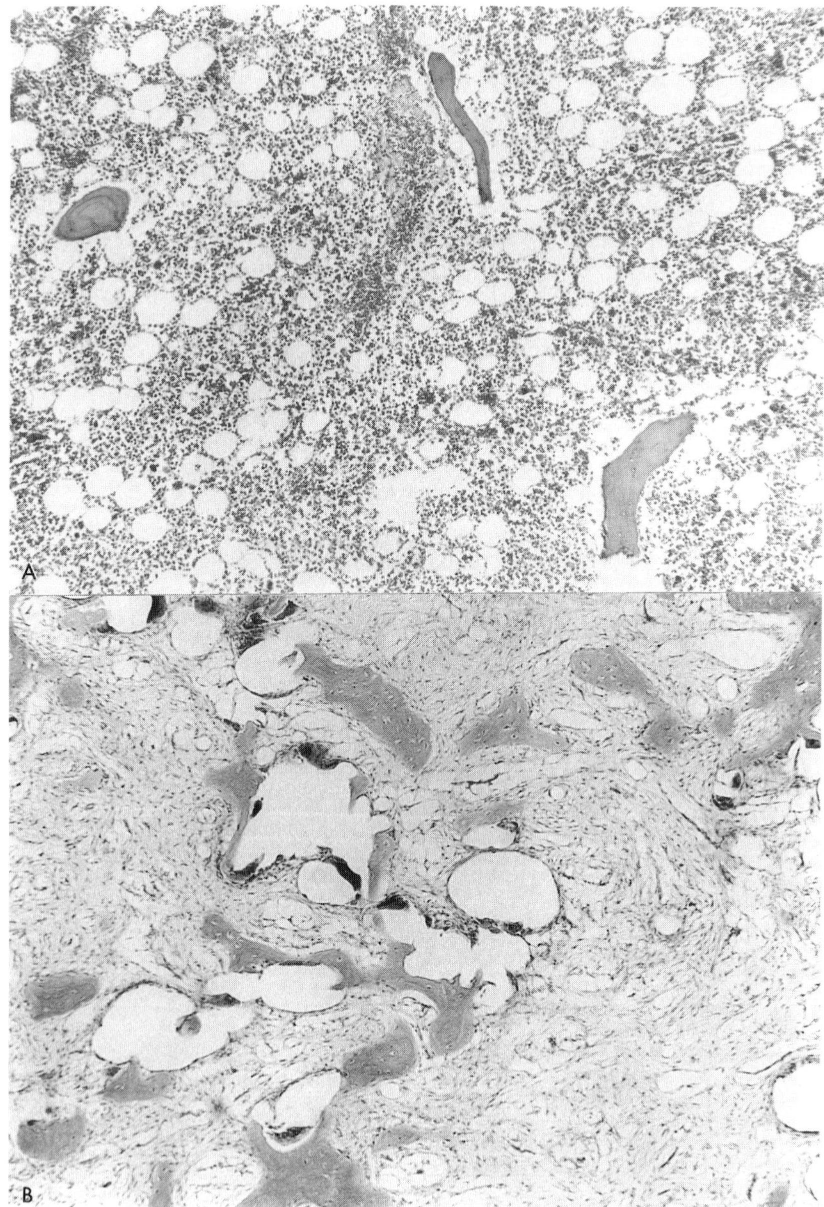

Figure 1 Osteoporosis: Pathologic abnormalities and differentiation from osteitis fibrosa cystica and osteomalacia. (A) Osteoporosis. The bone is qualitatively normal but quantitatively deficient (100×). Osteoclastosis is not a significant feature. (B) Osteitis

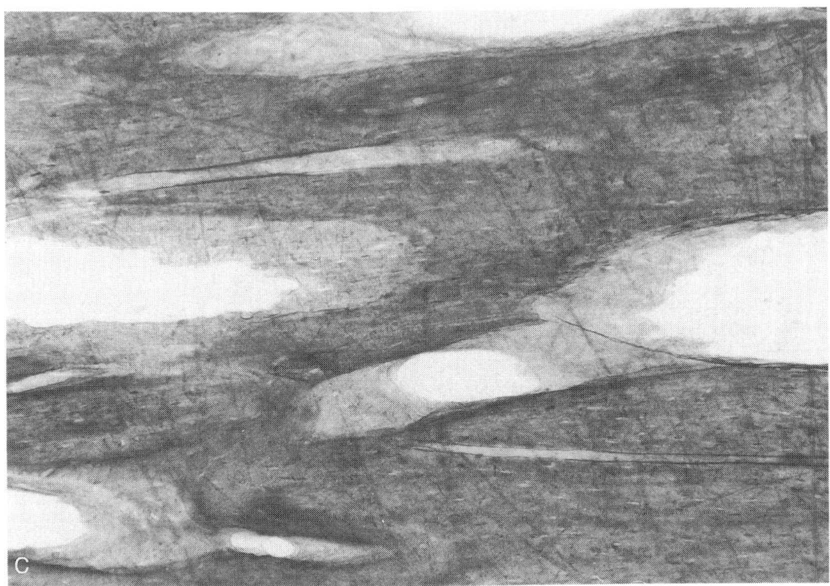

fibrosa cystica (hyperparathyroidism). Diffuse fibrosis of the stroma of the bone marrow is associated with osteoclastic resorption and new bone formation (100×). (C) Osteomalacia. Undecalcified section of bone stained for calcium reveals superficial osteoid tissue that is not so heavily stained as is the calcified bone (86×). (From Ref. 27.)

Table 1 Major Causes of Generalized Osteoporosis

Endocrine causes	Hematologic causes
Senile and postmenopausal states	Sickle cell anemia
Hyperparathyroidism	Thalassemia
Glucocorticoid-induced	Other causes
Cushing's syndrome (endogenous)	Alcoholism
Iatrogenic (exogenous)	Osteogenesis imperfecta
Hyperthyroidism	Idiopathic juvenile osteoporosis
Acromegaly	Homocystinuria
Pregnancy and related conditions	Scurvy
Diabetes mellitus	Malnutrition
Hypogonadism	

Source: Ref. 214.

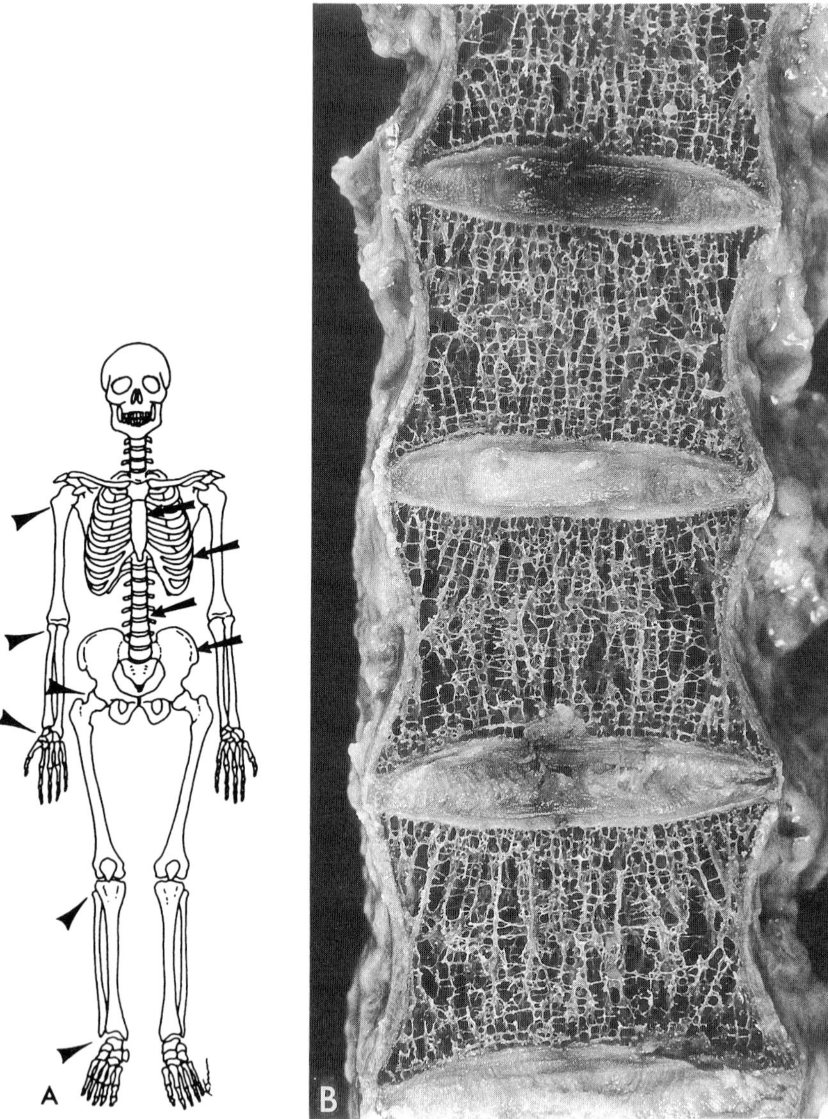

Figure 2 Osteoporosis: distribution of abnormalities. (A) Generalized versus regional osteoporosis. In generalized osteoporosis (arrows, on right half of diagram), the spine, pelvis, ribs, and sternum are most commonly affected. In regional osteoporosis (arrowheads, on left half), the appendicular skeleton is the predominant site of alterations, particularly the periarticular regions. (B–D) Generalized osteoporosis. Findings predominated in the spine (B), sternum (C), and pelvis, including the symphysis pubic (D). Note sparse trabeculae about the sternum and sternoclavicular articulations, the vertebral bodies, and pubic bones. (From Ref. 27.)

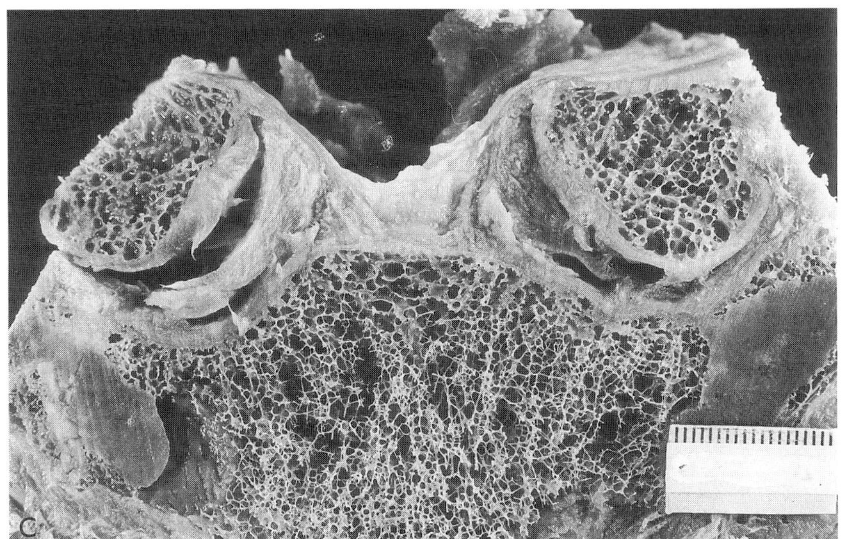

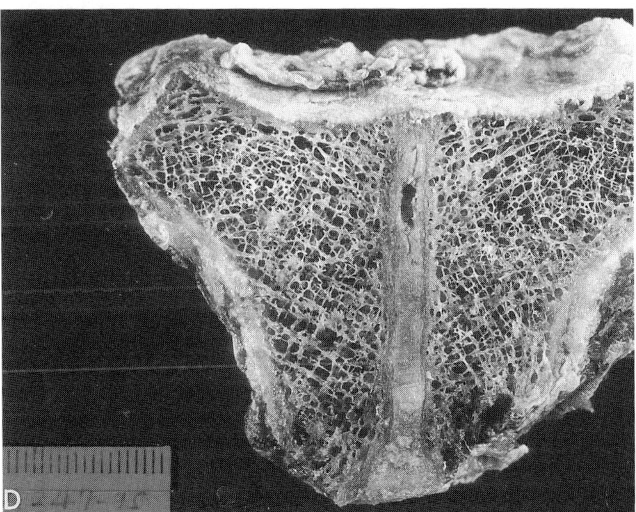

c. Greater Trochanteric Group. The greater trochanteric trabeculae are slender and poorly defined. They are tensile trabeculae that arise on the lateral portion of the femur below the greater trochanter and extend superiorly to the superior surface of the greater trochanter.

d. Principal Tensile Group. The principal tensile trabeculae are the thickest of the tensile varieties. They form a long, curvilinear arc extending through the

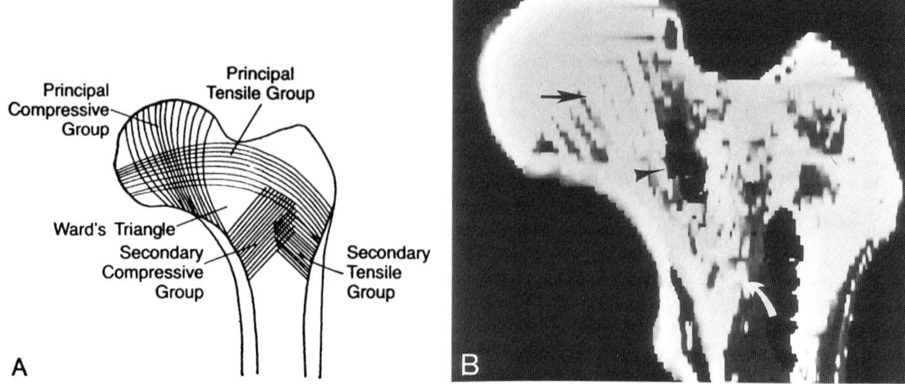

Figure 3 Proximal femur: normal trabecular pattern. (A) Four of the five anatomic groups of trabeculae are indicated in this schematic diagram. Ward's triangle lies within the neutral axis wherein compressive and tensile forces balance one another and contains thin, widely spaced trabeculae. (B) A midcoronal three-dimensional computed tomographic section of a normal macerated specimen demonstrates primary compressive trabeculae (arrow), secondary compressive trabeculae (curved arrow), and Ward's triangle (arrowhead). (C,D) A specimen photograph and radiograph of an axial section through the femoral head reveal thick, closely packed primary compressive trabeculae radiating from the center in the patten of an asterisk or stylized star. (E,F) A specimen photograph and radiograph of an axial section through the femoral neck reveal Ward's triangle (black arrows) as an area of relative paucity of trabeculae, bordered medially by primary compressive trabeculae (white arrows) and laterally by primary tensile and secondary compressive trabeculae (arrowheads). (G,H) A specimen photograph and radiograph of an axial section through the intertrochanteric region demonstrate the superior portion of the calcar femorale (arrows) arising from the posteromedial cortex. (From Ref. 27.)

femoral neck from the lateral cortex just below the greater trochanter to the inferior portion of the femoral head.

e. Secondary Tensile Group. The secondary tensile trabeculae extend superiorly and medially, arising from the lateral cortex just below the principal tensile group. They terminate just before reaching the center of the femoral neck.

Another important anatomical region in the proximal portion of the femur is Ward's triangle. This radiolucent triangular region in the inferomedial region of the femoral neck contains thin, loosely packed trabeculae. It is enclosed within the medullary cavity by trabeculae from the principal compressive, secondary compressive, and tensile groups (32).

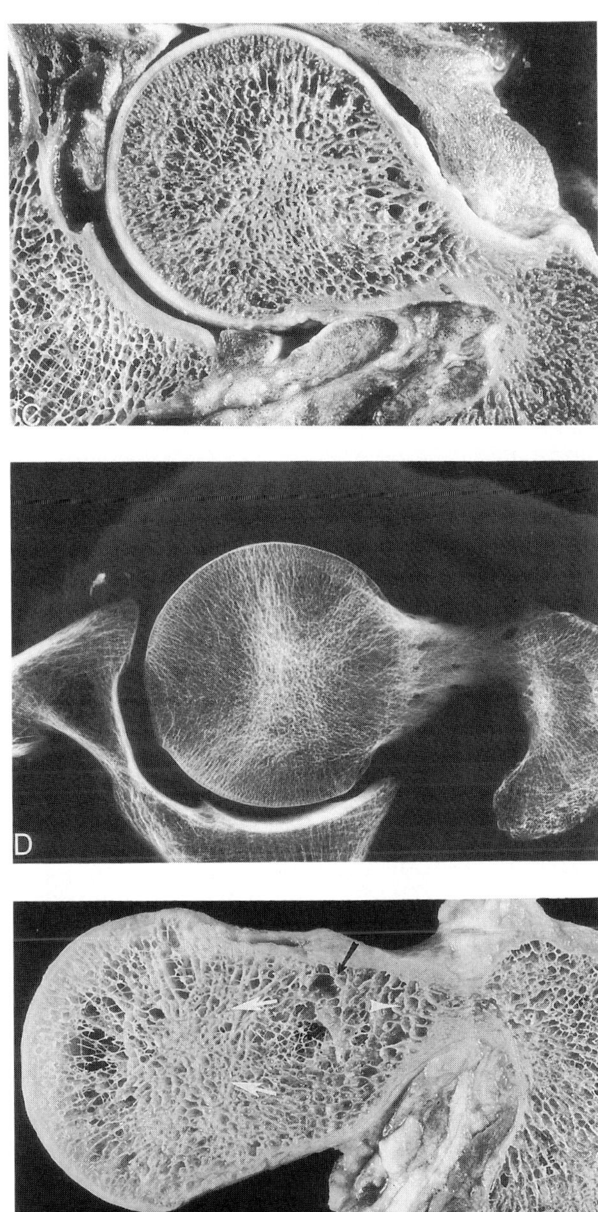
C
D
E

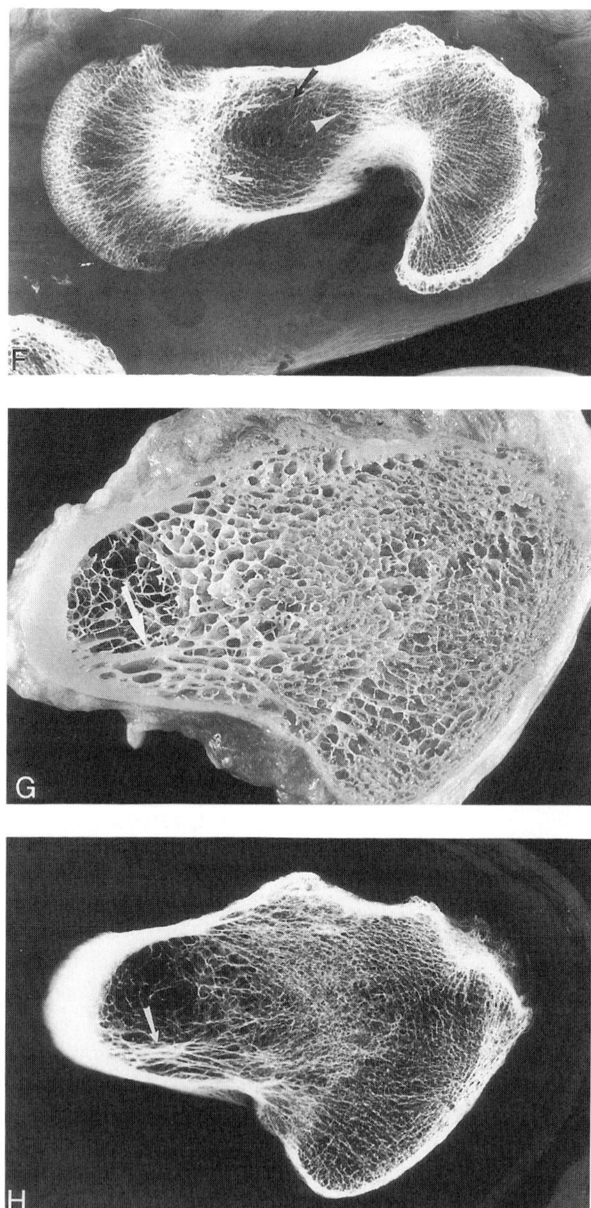

Figure 3 Continued

Kerr et al. studied the CT appearance of the proximal femoral trabecular pattern in patients with osteoporosis and osteoarthritis and described a distinctive pattern of increased radiodensity (32,33). This pattern, created by unmasking or hypertrophy of preexistent reinforcing trabeculae, can simulate a pathologic osseous condition such as enchondroma or bone infarct.

In 1970, Singh et al. correlated the severity of osteoporosis with patterns of trabecular loss seen on routine radiographs of the proximal portion of the femur. Their observations have been well documented (31) and have been formulated into the "Singh index" summarized in Table 2 and illustrated in Figure 4.

Singh et al. observed that, with early trabecular resorption, accentuation of the structure of the principal compressive and tensile groups predominates. The secondary compressive trabeculae are less distinct, and Ward's triangle appears more prominent. Accentuation and prominence of the principal trabeculae appear to be due to resorption of thin trabeculae that obscure detail of the principal groups (33,34).

As trabecular resorption advances, tensile trabeculae become reduced in number, leading to obliteration of the medial extent of the principal tensile trabeculae. The secondary tensile group of trabeculae become completely resorbed, resulting in lateral enlargement of Ward's triangle.

With further trabecular resorption, the principal tensile trabeculae on the lateral

Table 2 The Singh Index

Grade	Radiographic Appearance of Trabeculae in the Proximal Portion of the Femur
6	*No evidence of osteoporosis* All normal trabecular groups visible Proximal portion of femur appears to be completely occupied by cancellous bone
5	Principal tensile and compressive trabeculae accentuated Ward's triangle is prominent
4	*Equivocal evidence of osteoporosis* Principal tensile trabeculae reduced in number but continue to extend from lateral cortex to the femoral neck
3	*Suggests definite osteoporosis* Break in continuity of principal tensile trabeculae opposite greater trochanter
2	*Marked osteoporosis* Only the principal compressive trabeculae are seen No tensile trabeculae visible
1	*Severe osteoporosis* Marked reduction even in number of principal compressive trabeculae

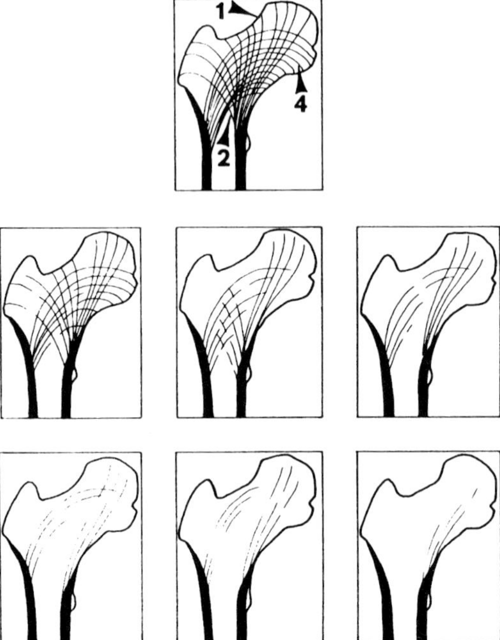

Figure 4 Osteoporosis: proximal femur—Singh index. Five groups of osseous trabeculae are seen in the proximal femur. In the normal situation, it frequently is difficult to identify all of these groups, but with increasing osteoporosis, they initially may be identifiable and subsequently may be resorbed. In the top diagram, three groups can be well seen: the principal compressive group (1); the secondary compressive group (2); and the principal tensile group (4). In the subsequent drawings, increasing degrees of osteoporosis lead to trabecular resorption. The principal compressive group is usually the last to be obliterated. (From Ref. 27.)

aspect opposite the greater trochanter disappear, a reliable radiographic sign that the patient is indeed osteoporotic.

With marked osteoporosis, all trabecular groups but the principal compressive group are resorbed. In the most severe cases of osteoporosis, even the principal compressive trabeculae are obliterated partially or completely.

On the basis of these observations and those of other investigators (35–43), classification of femoral neck trabeculae was adopted as a useful technique in evaluating osteoporotic patients. The Singh index correlates well with the amount of trabecular bone in the proximal portion of the femur and vertebrae as well as with the frequency of compression fractures of the spine (35,40) and with the risk of femoral neck fracture (39), despite the fact that fractures can develop without changes in the index (44).

The Singh index correlates poorly, however, with the cortical mineral content of the radius as determined by photon absorptiometry (45,46). Nevertheless, radiologists have generally agreed that bone mineral content of cortical bone in the extremities is not necessarily an accurate reflection of trabecular bone in the axial skeleton (47). Griffiths and Virtama (48) concluded that the Singh index of femoral neck trabecular patterns correlates well with age but not with cortical thickness. Several other authors (18,45,46,49–52) have also concluded that the Singh index is an unreliable measure of osteoporosis and that this method should not be used exclusively for screening patients with osteoporosis or for estimating fracture risk. Singh et al.'s original observations remain important, however, as a means of estimating the extent of trabecular resorption in the proximal portion of the femur.

3. Vertebral Column

The radiographic findings of osteoporosis in the spine include increased radiolucency, trabecular abnormalities, and changes in the shape of the vertebral bodies (Fig. 5).

a. Radiolucency. Before osteoporosis can be detected on spinal radiographs, approximately 30% of bone tissue must be lost. Additionally, small lesions, less than 2 cm in diameter, are often not visible radiographically. Technical factors such as over- or underexposure of film, increased bone opacity from vertebral compression and callus formation (53), and differences in patient body composition further increase the difficulty of assessing overall bone density accurately. In advanced osteoporosis, however, it is possible to identify an area in the central portion of the vertebral bodies that is more radiolucent than the vertebral end plates. In many cases, the subchondral bone of the vertebral end plate often appears more dense owing to the relative lucency of the spongiosa of the vertebral body. In fact, the subchondral end plate usually is thinned and attenuated. End-plate sclerosis, which is seen in the rugger-jersey spine of renal osteodystrophy, does not occur in osteoporosis in the absence of a healing compression fracture.

b. Trabecular Alterations (Fig. 6). The pathologic changes in osteoporosis include thinning and loss of trabeculae. The changes are more prominent in the horizontal trabeculae, presumably as a result of biomechanical or bioelectric effects of loading in compression (44). This phenomenon results in a relative prominence or accentuation of the remaining vertical trabeculae, creating a striated appearance simulating vertebral hemangioma. The trabeculae in osteoporosis, although diminished in number, remain well defined. This feature is important in distinguishing osteoporosis from osteomalacia, in which the individ-

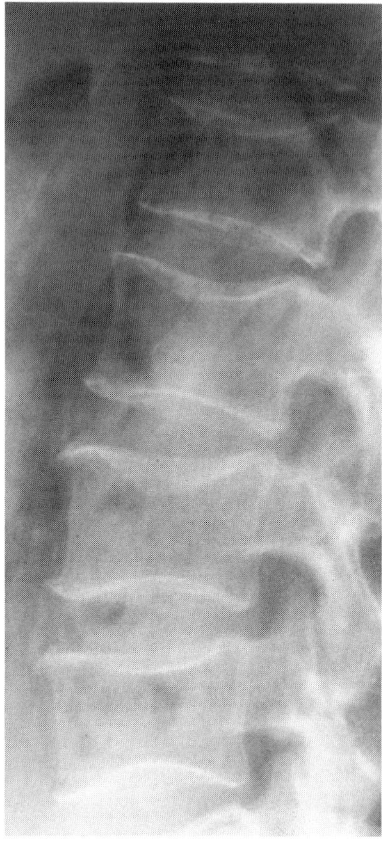

Figure 5 Senile and postmenopausal osteoporosis: spine alterations. In this elderly woman, a lateral radiograph of the lumbar spine demonstrates increased radiolucency and biconcave deformities of multiple vertebral bodies ("fish vertebrae"). (From Ref. 27.)

ual trabeculae appear indistinct and fuzzy, producing a coarsened or spongy pattern and in which bone density actually can be increased (27,44).

c. Vertebral Body Shape Alterations (Fig. 7). Alterations in the shape of vertebral bodies are characteristic in osteoporosis. Normal variations of vertebral contour and artifacts of radiographic positioning can simulate the changes typically seen in osteoporosis, however.

The posterior heights of the thoracic vertebrae normally measure 1–3 mm more than the anterior heights owing to a slight prominence just anterior to the superior rib facet (54). The prominence levels off abruptly, resulting in parallel superior and inferior end-plate surfaces anteriorly. When the posterior vertebral body, including the prominence, is measured, a difference of 4 mm or more between the anterior and the posterior vertebral body surfaces represents a true

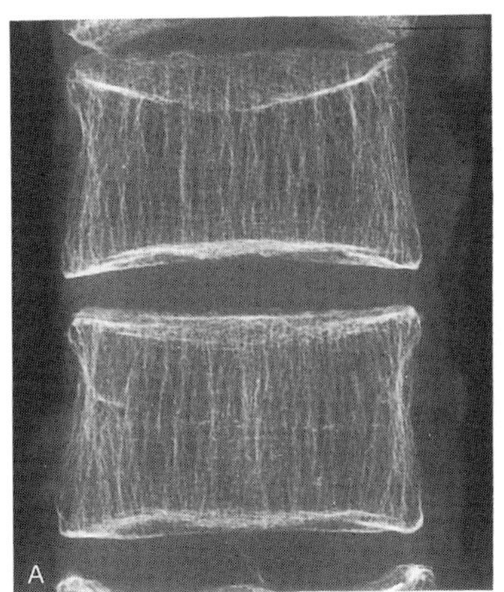

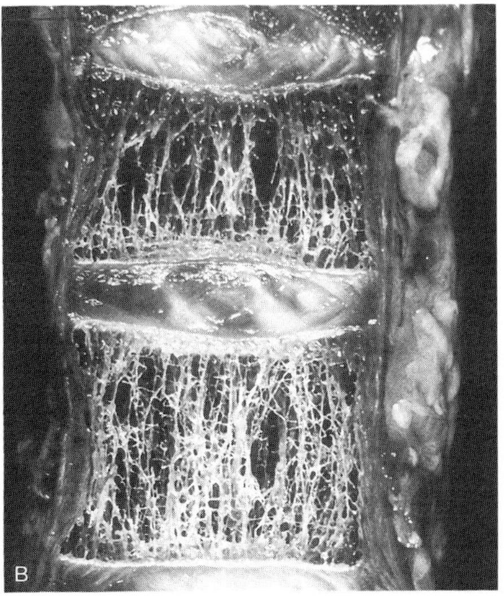

Figure 6 Osteoporosis: Spine—alterations in radiolucency and trabecular pattern. In two different cadaveric spines, observe accentuation of the vertical trabeculae with preferential resorption of horizontal trabeculae (A). Additional findings characteristic of osteoporosis are the depression of the superior margin of the vertebral body and a distinct but thinned bone plate at the superior and inferior surfaces of the vertebral bodies (B). (From Ref. 27.)

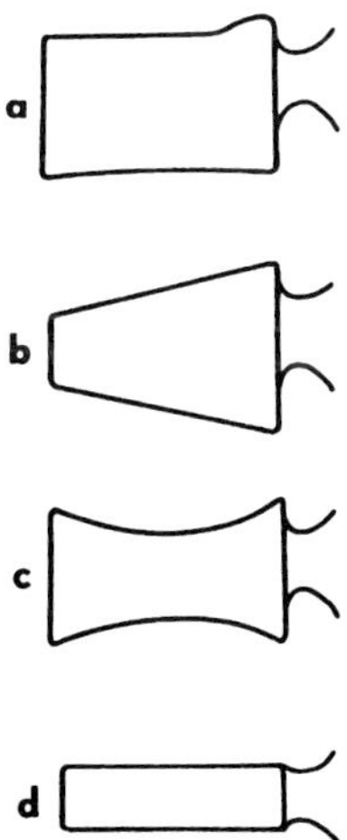

Figure 7 Osteoporosis: Spine—alterations in vertebral body shape. (a) In the normal situation, the superior and inferior vertebral outlines are relatively parallel, although a slight elevation or protuberance can be seen at the posterosuperior aspect of the vertebral bodies. (b) Wedge-shaped vertebrae relate to collapse of the anterior aspect of the vertebral body. (c) Biconcave or "fish vertebrae" are characterized by biconcave deformity of the superior and inferior surfaces of the vertebral body. (d) Flattened or "pancake" vertebrae are associated with compression of the entire vertebral body surface. (From Ref. 27.)

vertebral compression deformity. If this normal prominence is not included in the measurement, a difference of 2 mm or more is considered abnormal (54). Similar criteria can be used to measure the vertical height of the lumbar vertebrae.

In osteoporosis, several abnormal patterns of vertebral body shape can be identified alone or in combination: *wedge-shaped* vertebrae, vertebral *compression, biconcave* or "*fish*" vertebrae, and *Schmorl's cartilaginous nodes.* Both wedging and compression in osteoporosis indicate a vertebral body fracture (55), whereas biconcave or fish vertebrae are typically considered vertebral "deformities."

In wedge-shaped vertebrae, the anterior border is reduced in vertical height and the posterior border is normal. The wedge-shaped vertebra is common, especially in the thoracic spine, where the kyphotic curve predisposes to this type of abnormality and where the strong neural arches and paravertebral muscles protect the middle and posterior columns (56). Vertebral compression, in which both anterior and posterior body heights are compressed, usually represents more advanced disease, but this pattern is often combined with wedging.

"Fish vertebrae" is the term applied to vertebrae with increased concavity of the subchondral endplate (57). The term is derived from the typical biconcave appearance seen on radiographs of the vertebrae of normal fish (Fig. 8). The degree of exaggeration of the end-plate concavity can be assessed by measuring the shortest vertical height between the end plates and expressing it as a fraction of the height of the posterior vertebral body margin (58). The concavity occurring in fish vertebrae is often associated with intraosseous intradiscal displacements termed Schmorl's cartilaginous nodes. Schmorl's nodes, however, also are present in patients without osteoporosis and with no evidence of biconcave deformities. A shallow concavity at the inferior end plates of normal lower lumbar vertebrae is common and should not be considered an osteoporotic or pathologic deformity.

Biconcave vertebral body deformities (fish vertebrae) are seen in disorders characterized by diffuse weakening of bone, such as osteoporosis. However, these deformities are also apparent in osteomalacia, Paget's disease, hyperparathyroidism, and neoplasms (27). The osseous deformity in all of these diseases results from the expansile pressure of the adjacent intervertebral disks. The archlike indentations affect both the superior and inferior endplates (Fig. 9).

Pathologically, the fish vertebra reveals stretching and thinning of the cartilaginous end plates without evidence of disruption or overt fracture. Fish vertebrae are most common in the lower thoracic and lower lumbar spine. In these locations, intradiscal pressure from the nucleus pulposus is maximum in the midportion of the vertebral body, whereas the peripheral bony rim is stronger and more resistant to such pressure. In the normally kyphotic middle and upper thoracic spine, maximum pressure is exerted anteriorly, resulting in anterior osseous weakening and vertebral wedging.

In osteoporotic patients with abnormal disks that have diminished expansile

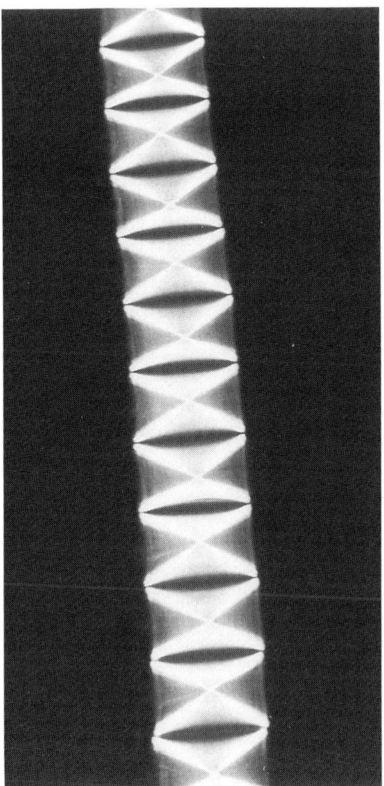

Figure 8 "Fish vertebrae." Origin of term. A radiograph of the spine of a normal fish reveals depression in the superior and inferior surfaces of each vertebral body. (From Ref. 27.)

pressure, diffuse flattening is more common than biconcave (fish vertebra) deformities (27).

In advanced osteoporosis, cartilaginous Schmorl's nodes can accompany the biconcave deformities. Cartilaginous nodes are common in osteoporosis (59–61). These nodes are visible radiographically and represent focal, angular end-plate disruptions with vertical protrusion of intervertebral disk material into the spongiosa of the vertebral body. Weak areas in the cartilaginous end plate and the adjacent subchondral bone arise from regression of the chorda dorsalis, gaps in ossification, or vascular channels (62,63), as well as numerous local and systemic bone abnormalities. Pressure from the adjacent nucleus pulposus overwhelms the weakened area, and a defect occurs (64). Because younger persons have higher intradiscal pressure, cartilaginous nodes are more prominent and progress more rapidly in young patients. Up to 38% of all spines demonstrate cartilaginous nodes

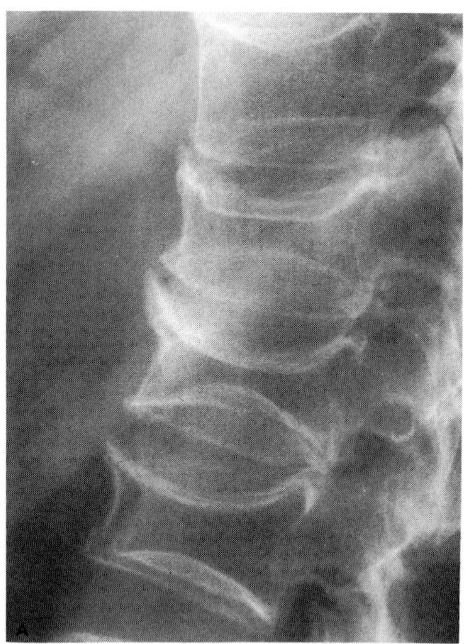

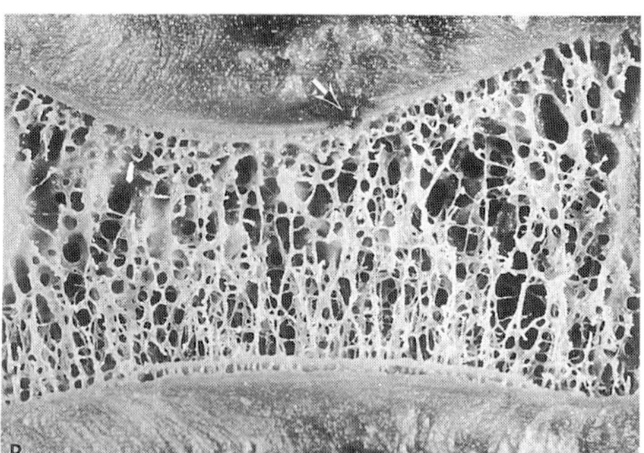

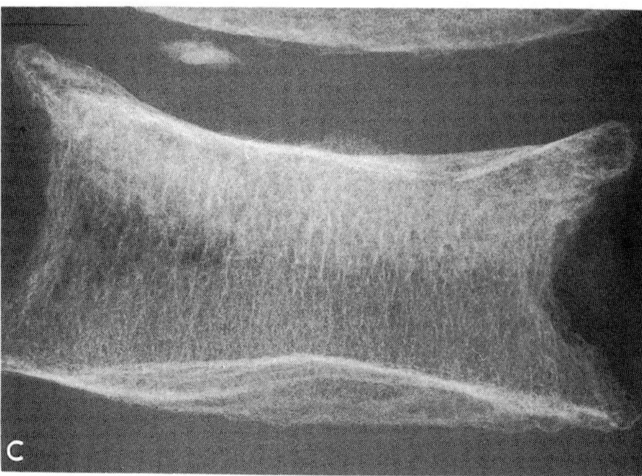

Figure 9 Osteoporosis: "fish vertebrae." (A) A lateral radiograph of the lumbar spine reveals severe osteoporosis with multiple "fish vertebrae." Note that the inferior and superior surfaces of the vertebral bodies are not involved to the same extent. Note also that the subchondral bone plates appear dense compared with the lucent central portion of the vertebral bodies. (B,C) A photograph and radiograph of coronal sections of the vertebral body outline fish vertebrae in osteoporosis. Although the indentations appear relatively smooth, the superior and inferior surfaces of the vertebral body are not involved to the same extent. A small cartilaginous (Schmorl's) node also is present (arrow). (D,E) Sagittal spin-echo magnetic resonance images (TR 0.2 s, TE 26 ms) in a 22-year-old woman reveal biconcave vertebral body deformities in the cervical (D) and lumbar (E) segments. Of interest, the precise cause of the vertebral abnormalities was not clear in this patient, as extensive clinical evaluation failed to reveal evidence of an underlying disorder. As a child, however, this patient had received corticosteroid medication for several months in a dosage sufficient to lead to Cushing-like features. (From Ref. 27. D,E, Courtesy of G. Greenway, MD, Dallas, Tex.)

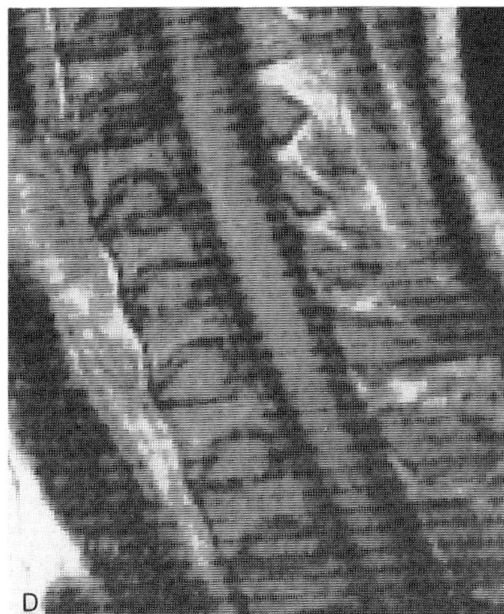

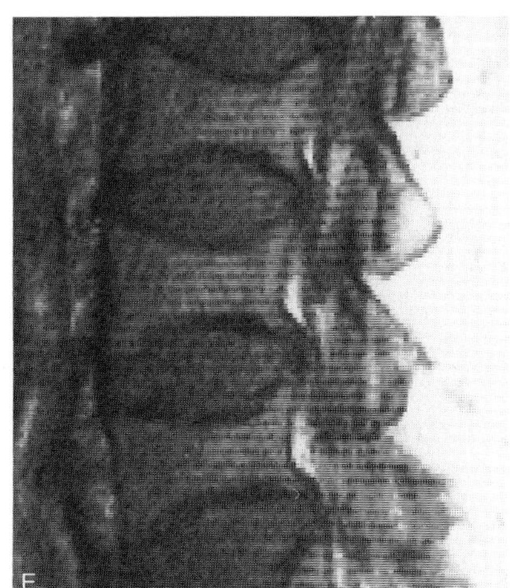

(65), and they are seen in several diverse processes affecting the vertebral end plate in addition to osteoporosis (Table 3).

The radiographic appearance of cartilaginous nodes includes a break in the subchondral bone plate, a lucent area of varying size bordering on the intervertebral disk, and minimal bone sclerosis surrounding the defect (Fig. 10). Pathologically, the break corresponds to the site of discal displacement, the lucent area corresponds to the amount of protruded disk material, and the sclerosis corresponds to condensation and thickening of the involved trabeculae. Cartilaginous nodes in osteoporosis tend to be small, are usually associated with biconcave deformities, and more frequently affect the lower vertebral end plate (27).

Pogrund et al. observed an association on routine radiographs between decrease in the width of the psoas muscle and increasing osteoporosis (66). This

Table 3 Processes Associated With Schmorl's Cartilaginous Nodes

Osteoporosis
Osteomalacia
Paget's disease
Hyperparathyroidism
Infection
Neoplasm
Intervertebral osteochondrosis
Scheuermann's disease

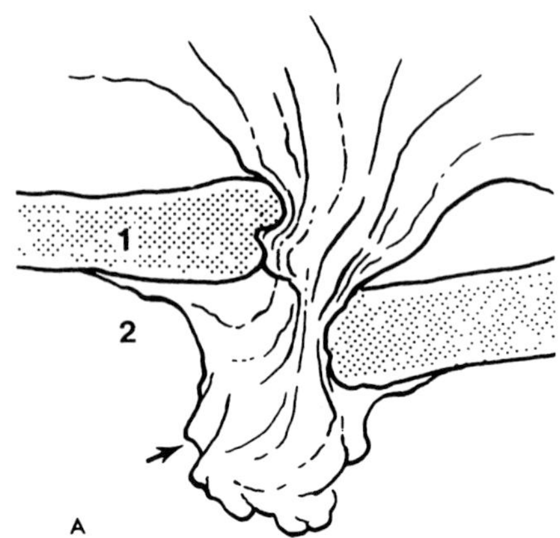

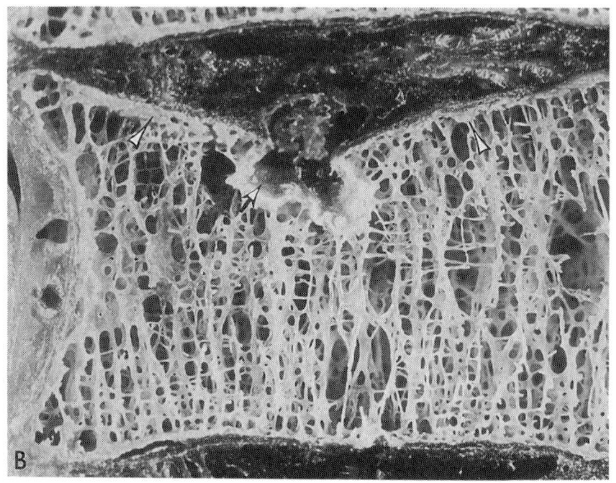

Figure 10 Osteoporosis: cartilaginous (Schmorl's) nodes. (A) Cartilaginous (Schmorl's) nodes occur when a portion of the intervertebral disk protrudes into the vertebral body (arrow) through a gap in the cartilaginous end plate (1) and subchondral bony plate (2). (B,C) a photograph and radiograph of a coronal section reveal depression of the subchondral bone (arrowheads). A cartilaginous node (arrows) has resulted from disruption of the cartilaginous and bony plates. It has created a radiolucent defect within the bone with a small rim of sclerosis. A small cartilaginous node is also noted on the on the inferior vertebral end plate. (From Ref. 59.)

observation was evident some years before radiographic evidence of osteoporosis appeared. The role of CT in comparing paraspinal muscle and bone as a correlate of osteoporosis has also been investigated (67).

The value of scintigraphy in identifying fractures in vertebral osteoporosis is well established. Although increased radioisotope uptake is present at areas of

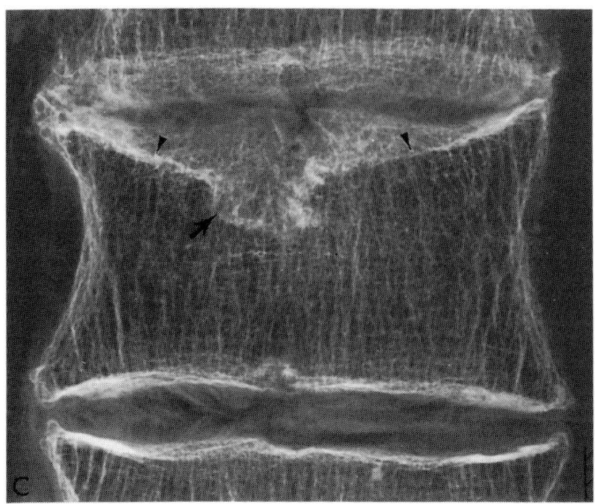

vertebral fracture, scintigraphy is not useful in differentiating between vertebral fractures that occurred in the recent past versus the remote past (68).

4. *Cortex of Tubular Bones*

The cortical bone of the appendicular skeleton has been evaluated in the investigation of osteoporosis and other metabolic bone diseases (69–79). As a general rule, combined cortical thickness should be at least 50% of the shaft diameter in the midportion of most long tubular bones (28). High-resolution radiography, sometimes employing magnification, is used to evaluate the fine bone architecture of the small tubular bones of the hand. Interpretation of these radiographs is based on the envelope theory of bone resorption (78,80).

In the envelope theory, three distinct envelopes are identified: endosteal, cortical, and periosteal. Various endocrine and metabolic diseases affect these different envelopes in unique ways. Using high-resolution radiography, it is possible to detect subtle changes in each of these regions of the tubular bones, which may provide valuable differential diagnostic clues (79) (Table 4) (Fig. 11).

Endosteal resorption results in scalloped concavities on the inner margin of the cortex with resultant enlargement of the marrow cavity. Normal remodeling changes, both bone resorption and bone formation, occur in the endosteal region. These normal changes make interpretation of subtle endosteal changes difficult. Progressive scalloping of the endosteal surface, however, should be considered pathologic (79).

Intracortical resorption is seen radiographically as prominent longitudinal striations within the cortex, usually in the subendosteal region. When examined histologically, intracortical resorption appears as a small osteoclastic focus within the compact bone. As osteoclastic proliferation advances, a resorptive tunnel is

Table 4 Patterns of Osseous Changes in Tubular Bone and Some Related Conditions

Site	Pattern	Related conditions
Cortex		
Endosteal	Diffuse cortical thinning or scalloped erosions	Osteoporosis, any metabolic disorder, neoplasms
Intracortical	Cortical radiolucent areas or striations	Rapid bone turnover states; reflex sympathetic dystrophy, disuse osteoporosis
Periosteal	Subperiosteal erosions	Hyperparathyroidism: severe; rapid bone turnover states when less advanced
Spongiosa		
Subchondral	Linear, bandlike, or spotty radiolucent areas	Immobilization states; reflex sympathetic dystrophy
Metaphyseal	Bandlike radiolucent areas	Immobilization states; reflex sympathetic dystrophy; in children can simulate infection
Diffuse	Homogeneous or spotty radiolucent areas	Postmenopausal and senile osteoporosis

created, which is associated with mesenchymal cell proliferation, leading to an increase in connective tissue and blood vessels. This can end in a reparative phase in which osteoid calcification results. Normally, bone resorption and formation proceed at the same pace. In certain metabolic diseases, high bone turnover occurs because osteoclastic activity predominates over osteoblastic activity. This leads to an increase in the number of resorptive tunnels in cortical bone (79,81,82). As these tunnels measure only 200–300 μm in diameter, they usually cannot be detected on routine radiographs but are visible with magnification radiography. The second metacarpal shaft is typically used as a reference point to grade the number and appearance of these tunnels (74,83).

The observation of several radiolucent striae deep within a localized portion of the cortex can be a normal finding. An increased number of striae with a wider distribution is indicative of a pathologic process. In some cases, abnormal linear resorption may localize to the outer cortex, simulating subperiosteal bone resorption or even periosteal bone formation—pseudoperiostitis (84).

Abnormal linear cortical radiolucent shadows can be detected in hyperparathyroidism, hyperthyroidism, acromegaly, osteomalacia, renal osteodystrophy, disuse osteoporosis, and reflex sympathetic dystrophy. Cortical lucent areas are generally not evident in low bone turnover states, such as senile or postmenopausal osteoporosis and Cushing's disease.

Subperiosteal resorption results in irregularity and poor definition of the outer surface of the cortex. Such resorption also becomes prominent in rapid bone turnover states, particularly hyperparathyroidism. Moderate to severe subperiosteal resorption is virtually specific for hyperparathyroidism. Mild subperiosteal changes, however, can be present in other diseases such as the reflex sympathetic dystrophy syndrome. Intracortical resorption in the superficial aspect of the cortex can resemble subperiosteal resorption, causing diagnostic confusion (79).

Radiographic morphometry is a procedure used with magnification radiography to quantify cortical resorption. This procedure consists of measuring cortical dimensions on a radiographic film with a suitable caliper. The metacarpal shafts, especially the second, are most commonly used for measurement (71,74,83,85, 86), but radiographs of the humerus (87), clavicle (88), radius, femur, and mandible (89,90) have also been used.

The measurements obtained are the outer bone diameter, the width of the medullary canal, and the width of the cortex. The most widely used measurement is the combined cortical thickness (CCT). The first step in obtaining this measurement is to identify the midpoint of the second metacarpal shaft. This is determined by dividing in half the length between the most distal part of the base of the bone and the most distal part of its head. Next, the outer diameter (W) and marrow cavity (m) widths are determined. The CCT represents the difference between these two measurements (CCT = W − m). The measured CCT value must then be compared with normal values, which can be found in certain published sources (74,91,92). If the measured CCT value is below the normal range for the 20- to 50-year-old age group, endosteal bone loss has been confirmed; in this age group, the causes of bone loss may include metabolic abnormalities and immobilization (74). After the age of 50 years, a low CCT value usually indicates postmenopausal or senile osteoporosis. In equivocal cases, an additional measurement, the percentage of cortical area (%CA) can be calculated. This measurement can be obtained using the following formula: $\%CA = (W^2 - m^2/w^2) \times 100$.

Measurements of the CCT usually are applied in the appraisal of endosteal resorption. However, CCT combined with other measurements, such as total width, medullary canal width, and CA, can be used to allow distinction among a variety of metabolic diseases (69).

In summary, the envelope theory of bone resorption emphasizes three potential sites of cortical lysis: endosteal, intracortical, and subperiosteal. Endosteal erosion is the least specific, occurring in any metabolic disease, including osteoporosis, and may accompany certain neoplasms, such as plasma cell myeloma. Intracortical erosion is more specific, resulting in excessive tunneling in disease states characterized by rapid bone turnover. These states include disuse osteoporosis and reflex sympathetic dystrophy. Subperiosteal resorption is the most specific pattern. When extensive, subperiosteal resorption is pathognomonic of hyperparathyroid-

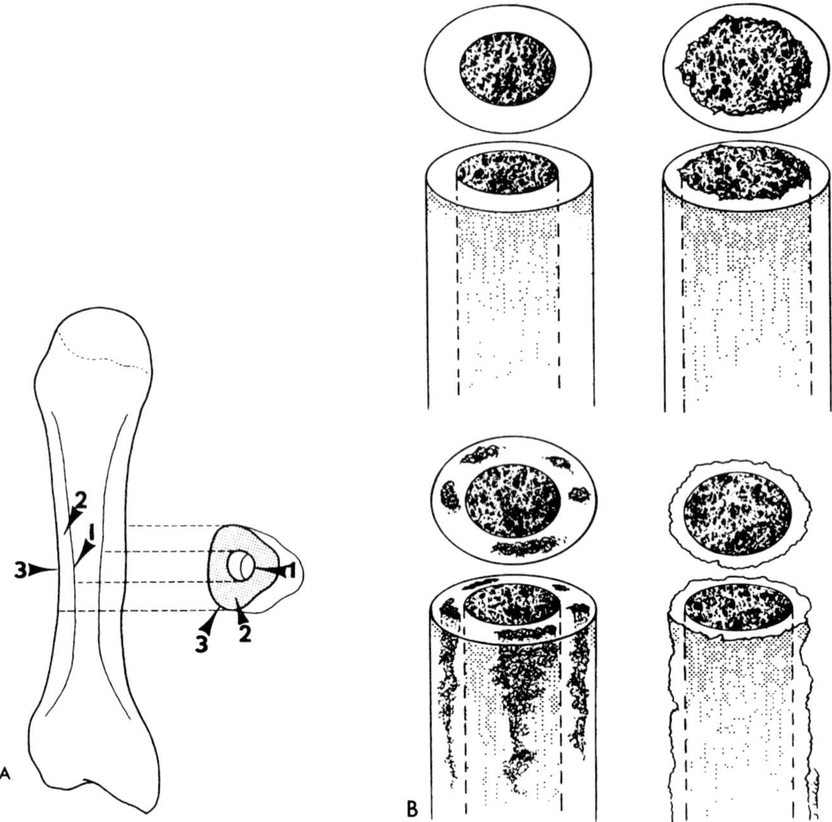

Figure 11 Cortex of tubular bones: sites of osseous resorption. (A) Three envelopes exist at which cortical resorption may occur. These are the endosteal envelope (1), the intracortical (haversian) envelope (2), and the periosteal envelope (3). (B) Diagram indicates the normal situation (top left), endosteal resorption (top right), intracortical resorption (bottom left), and subperiosteal resorption (bottom right). (C) Magnification radiograph of a phalanx in a patient with reflex sympathetic dystrophy syndrome reveals endosteal (arrowhead) and intracortical (arrow) resorption. (From Ref. 27.)

ism; however, lesser degrees may be seen in rapid bone turnover states, such as reflex sympathetic dystrophy.

5. *Spongiosa of the Appendicular Skeleton*

The spongy bone in the medullary cavity undergoes early and significant changes in osteoporosis and related metabolic conditions (Table 4). Several radiographic

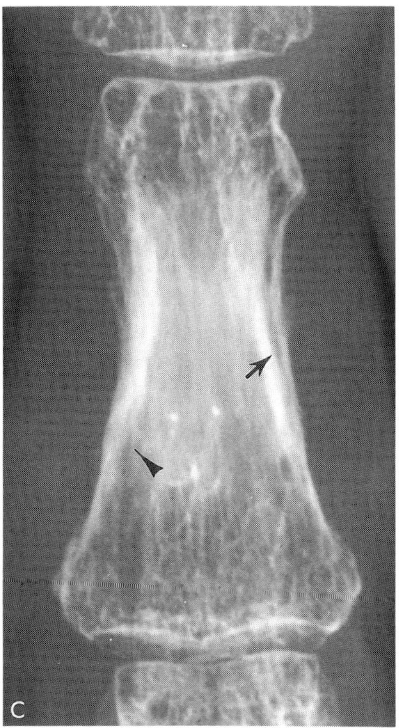

patterns can be identified in the tubular bones and the carpal and tarsal regions of the extremities. These patterns include 1. diffuse or homogenous osteoporosis; 2. speckled or spotty osteoporosis, particularly prominent in periarticular regions; and 3. bandlike subchondral and metaphyseal osteoporosis.

Although these different patterns may all be present in a single patient with osteoporosis, one or two may predominate, providing a clue to the specific diagnosis of various conditions (Figs. 12, 13) (Table 4).

The periarticular distribution of speckled or bandlike bone resorption is due to the highly vascular nature of the periarticular cancellous bone (93,94). Linear radiolucent bands in subchondral locations produce thinning of the overlying bone plate, resulting in small areas of osseous disruption. These subchondral bony defects can occur centrally or at the margins of the joint. Marginal defects can simulate the erosions typically seen in rheumatoid arthritis and other synovial inflammatory processes. Defects occurring centrally may resemble the subchondral fractures of osteonecrosis. The absence of large gaps in the subchondral bone and of joint space narrowing allows differentiation from inflammatory

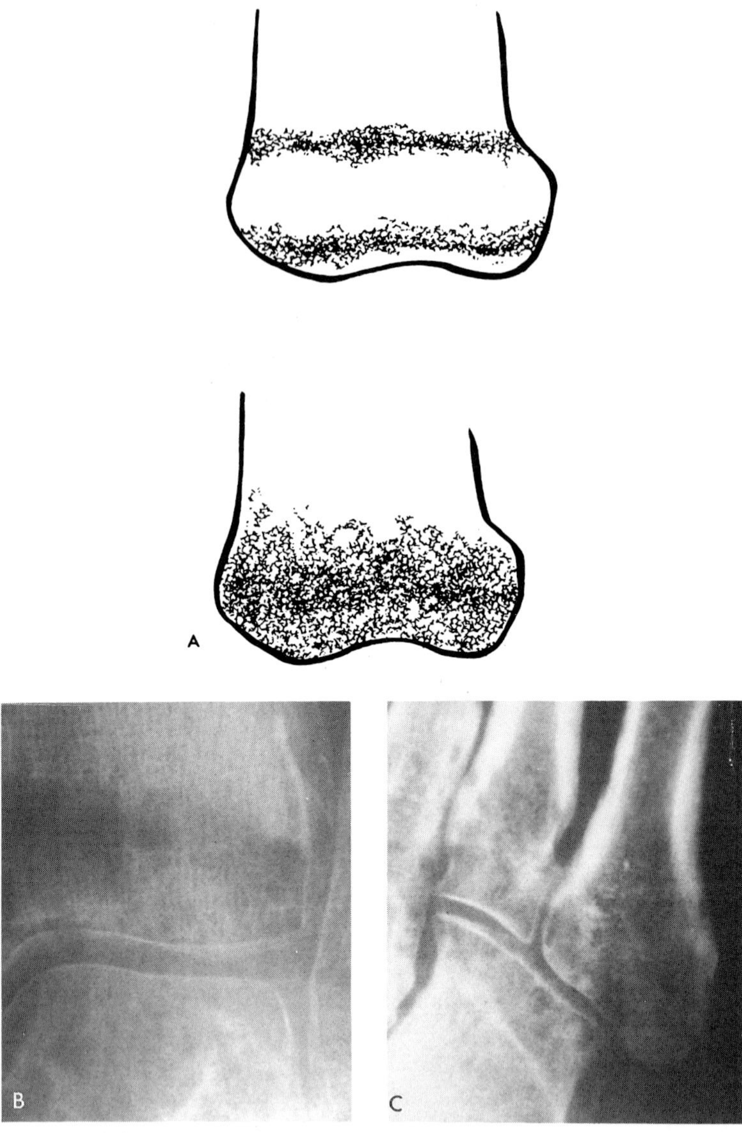

Figure 12 Spongiosa of tubular bones: sites of osseous resorption. (A) Patterns of bone loss include bandlike radiolucent areas in the metaphysis or subchondral bone (top drawing) and homogenous periarticular radiolucent areas (bottom drawing). (B) Bandlike resorption: metaphyseal and subchondral linear radiolucent areas are evident. (C) Spotty resorption: a cystic pattern is apparent. (D) Homogenous resorption: relatively uniform periarticular osteoporosis is evident. (E) Subchondral erosions: severe resorption in periarticular regions can lead to small gaps in cartilage and bone stimulating erosions of inflammatory arthritis. Defects in the subchondral bone plate of multiple metacarpal heads (arrows) are apparent in this patient with the reflex sympathetic dystrophy syndrome. (From Ref. 27.)

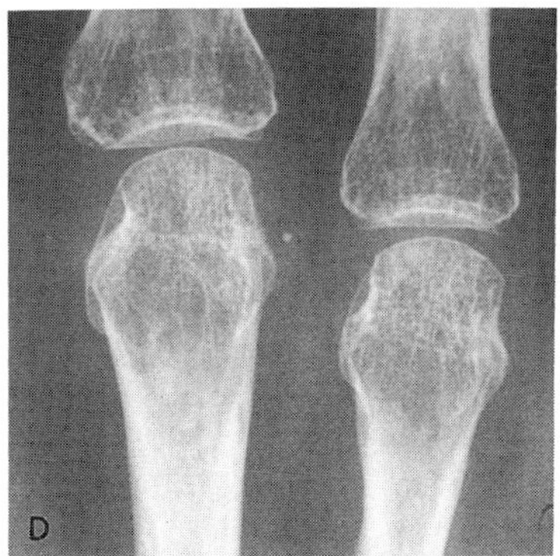

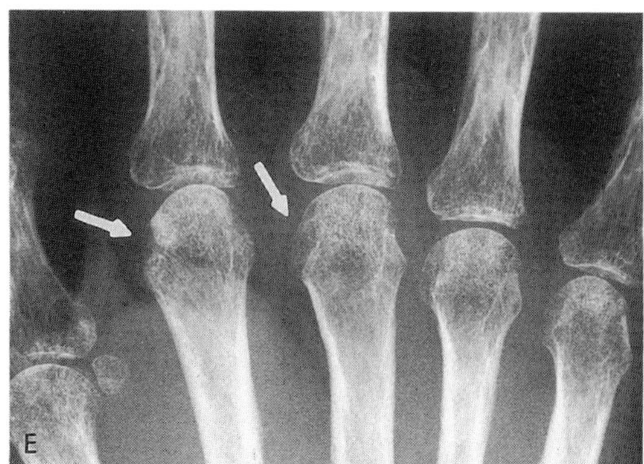

arthritis; the absence of significant bony collapse facilitates differentiation from osteonecrosis.

The degree of periarticular bone resorption in osteoporosis can be striking, and casual inspection of the radiographs may lead to an erroneous diagnosis of arthritis, infection, or neoplasm (95,96). Aggressive bone resorption in osteoporosis may be altered with time. Over a period of years, a pattern of homogeneous or diffuse osteoporosis and cortical thinning can appear identical to that in postmenopausal or senile osteoporosis (97). Pathologically an initial highly aggressive type of osteoclastic bone resorption may be transformed into a less aggressive, low remodeling state (27).

The mandible is subject to dramatic osteopenia in edentulous persons. This appears to result from mechanical factors, as no correlation is evident between mandibular bone measurements and bone measurements in other parts of the skeleton in normal controls and osteoporotic patients (98).

6. *Additional Complications and Manifestations of Osteoporosis*

a. Acute Fractures. Acute fractures are the most important complication of osteoporosis (99–101). The vertebral bodies, the neck and intertrochanteric regions of the femur, the humeral neck, and the distal portion of the radius are the most frequent sites of acute fracture in the osteoporotic patient. Although attempts have been made to define the importance of trabecular bone loss or cortical bone loss, or both, as factors contributing to such fractures, no uniform agreement has been reached on the subject. In general, it seems that trabecular bone resorption is more significant than cortical bone loss in the pathogenesis of fractures of the spine and distal portion of the radius (102). Loss of axial trabecular bone in women after menopause is also known to occur, predominantly by a reduction in the number of trabecular plates rather than by a decrease in their thickness (103). Loss of cortical bone is also important, however, especially in the proximal portion of the femur (104,105). Probably other factors are important as well. As an

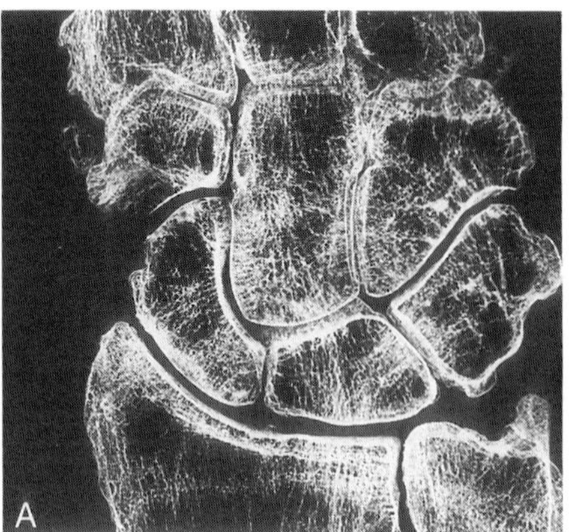

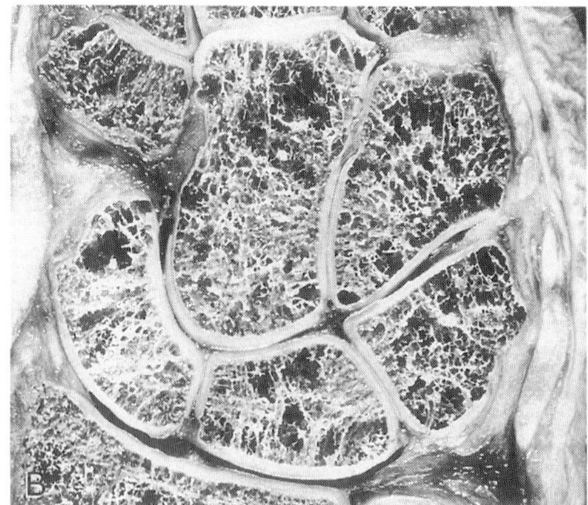

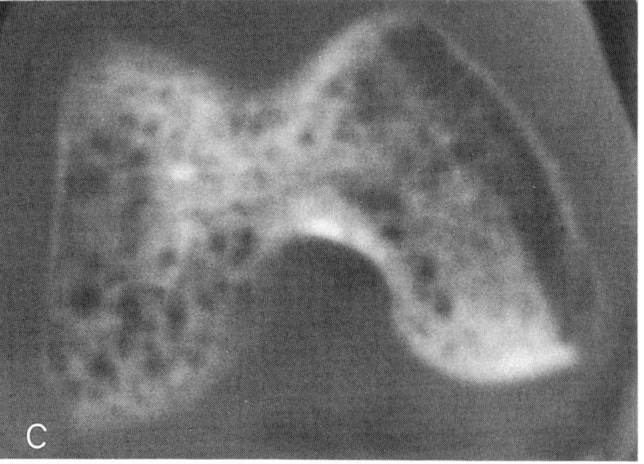

Figure 13 Spongiosa of tubular bone: spotty osteoporosis. (A,B) In a cadaveric wrist, cystic lesions in the carpal bones represent one characteristic pattern of regional osteoporosis. (C) A transaxial computed tomographic scan at the level of the femoral condyles reveals cystic osteoporosis simulating plasma cell myeloma. (From Ref. 27.)

example, some authors have postulated that, in the femur, the relatively greater number of fractures in the femoral neck than in the shaft is related to an increase in mechanical rigidity in the shaft as a consequence of progressive circumferential enlargement of bone. This increased shaft rigidity transfers stress to the proximal portion of the femur, leading to fracture. Also, despite the repeated emphasis in the literature that osteoporosis increases the likelihood of femoral neck fractures, some studies indicate that this increased risk is not very dramatic. This suggests that factors other than bone mass, such as a tendency to fall, are important determinants of which elderly patients will have fractures (106,107). Femoral neck fractures in osteoporotic patients tend to become more displaced than those in nonosteoporotic patients (108). Other disease processes leading to fracture of the femur include skeletal metastasis, which causes pathologic fracture of femoral neck and shaft, and Paget's disease, which typically causes pathologic fracture only of the femoral shaft.

Acute vertebral compression fractures in osteoporotic patients are seen most frequently at the T8, T12, L1, and L4 vertebral levels, and develop spontaneously (46%), after trivial strain (36%), or even while the patient is in bed (30%) (109). Although anterior vertebral compression fractures in osteoporotic patients result in hyperkyphosis, loss of muscle tone in these elderly persons may also contribute to hyperkyphosis, which in turn predisposes to compression fracture (110). Furthermore, many osteoporotic compression fractures are misdiagnosed initially and often require serial radiographs or scintigraphy for accurate diagnosis (109). Osteoporotic compression fractures usually result in spinal deformity, but nerve root and spinal cord compression is extremely rare (111).

Osteoporotic fractures usually heal quickly owing to the porous nature of the cortex and the excellent vascularity of osteoporotic bone.

Subchondral resorption of bone, seen in some types of osteoporosis, leads to mechanical weakening and may conceivably be associated with epiphyseal collapse. This complication is typically seen in hyperparathyroidism and steroid-induced osteopenia but not in other varieties of osteoporosis.

b. Insufficiency Fractures. Insufficiency fractures are a type of stress fracture that result from usual or normal stresses applied to weakened or abnormal bones. These fractures may occur in osteoporotic patients at typical sites, including the symphysis pubis and pubic rami (112,113), sacrum (114–117), supra-acetabular region (118,119), other regions of the pelvis (114,119), femoral neck (120), tibia (121,122), and sternum (117,123,124) (Fig. 14). Potential contributing factors include rheumatoid arthritis and corticosteroid or radiation therapy. Progressive thoracic kyphosis in osteoporotic patients has been implicated as a cause of sternal insufficiency fractures (117,124). The presence of osteoporosis makes accurate radiologic diagnosis difficult. Subtle patchy osteosclerosis is often the only subtle radiographic sign of insufficiency fractures. Scintigraphy is a useful initial screening examination and should be supplemented with conventional or computed tomography when necessary (27) (Fig. 15).

The radiographic and scintigraphic appearance of certain insufficiency fractures is unique. Insufficiency fractures of the pubic rami often exhibit considerable osteolysis and bone fragmentation, simulating a malignant tumor. Sacral insufficiency fractures produce a characteristic scintigraphic appearance in which verti-

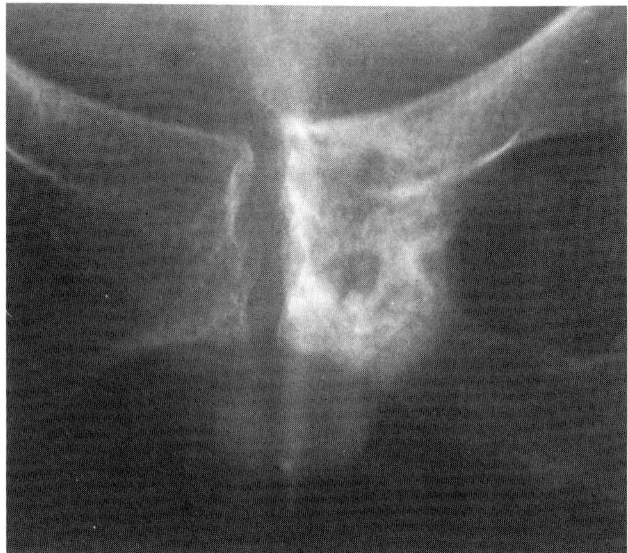

Figure 14 Osteoporosis: insufficiency fracture—symphysis pubis. The radiographic appearance of such fractures includes irregular osteolysis and osteosclerosis simulating a malignant neoplasm. (From Ref. 27. Courtesy of V. Vint, MD, San Diego, Calif.)

cal and horizontal regions of uptake of the bone-seeking radiopharmaceutical agent produce a configuration referred to as the "H" pattern (125). Although radionuclide imaging is the most sensitive study in detecting sacral insufficiency fractures, radiography can reveal subtle areas of increased density (125). Iliac insufficiency fractures are characterized radiographically by poorly defined zones of increased density of variable size affecting the supra-acetabular region, near the sciatic notch, and adjacent to the sacroiliac joint (118,119). Although these sacral and iliac fractures can occur in isolation, they are often seen in combination. Similar fractures of the tibial plateau resemble osteoarthritis or spontaneous osteonecrosis, whereas those of the sternum are caused by progressive kyphosis owing to vertebral collapse in the osteoporotic thoracic spine.

c. Reinforcement Lines (Bone Bars)

In patients with chronic osteopenia, usually related to osteoporosis associated with disuse, physical trauma, surgical amputation, or debilitating illness, radiographs of the tubular bones, particularly the femur and tibia, commonly reveal strands of horizontal trabeculae of variable thickness, extending partially or completely across the marrow cavity. They frequently branch and are oriented at right angles

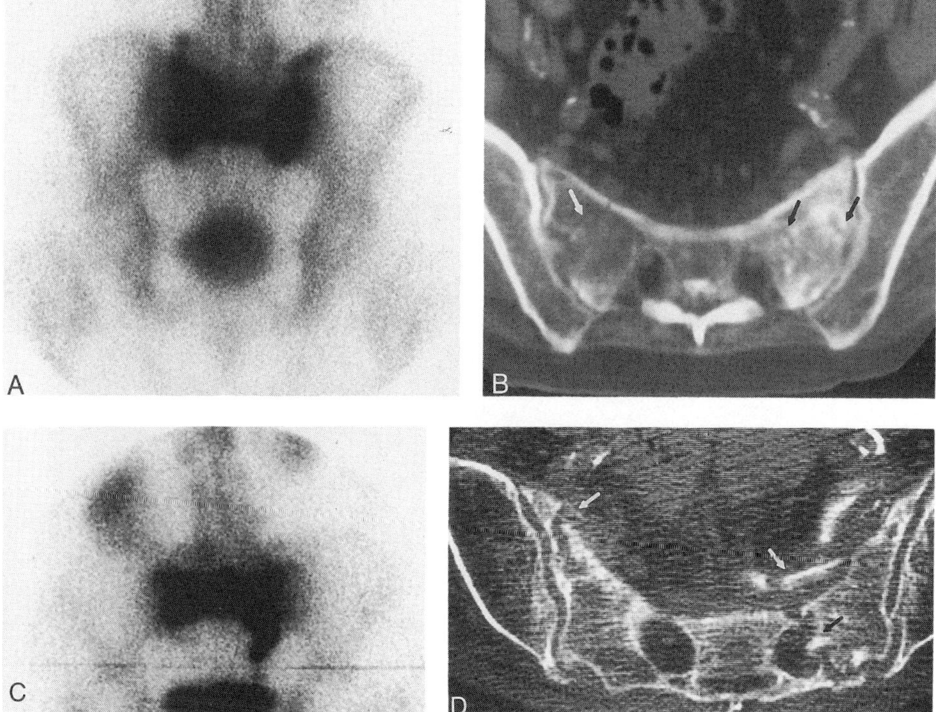

Figure 15 Osteoporosis: insufficiency fracture—sacrum. (A,B) In an 80-year-old woman with osteoporosis, the spontaneous onset of low-back pain occurred. Routine radiographs were interpreted as normal. The bone scan (A) reveals intense accumulation of radiopharmaceutical agent in the sacrum. Computed tomography (B) shows sacral fractures (arrows) and bone sclerosis. The sacral foramen on the left is involved. (C,D) In a 74-year-old woman in a nursing home, a similar history was obtained. Accumulation of the bone-seeking radionuclide (C) is evident in the sacrum. Computed tomography (D) documents fractures with extensive fragmentation (arrows). Note disruption of the sacral foramen. (From Ref. 27. Courtesy of T. Georgen, MD, San Diego, Calif.)

to the cortex in the diaphysis and at an oblique angle in the metaphysis. These "reinforcement lines" or "bone bars" are seen in both adults and children (Fig. 16). When viewed *en face*, they are linear; when viewed in profile, they appear as punctate or short linear dense foci, often simulating a bone infarction or cartilaginous tumor. Histologically, mature lamellar bone without evidence of recent bone deposition is observed.

Several hypotheses have been advanced to explain the pathogenesis of bone

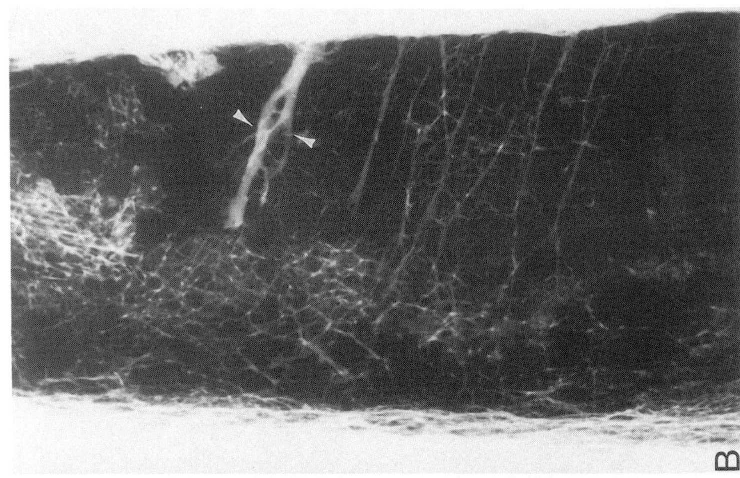
B

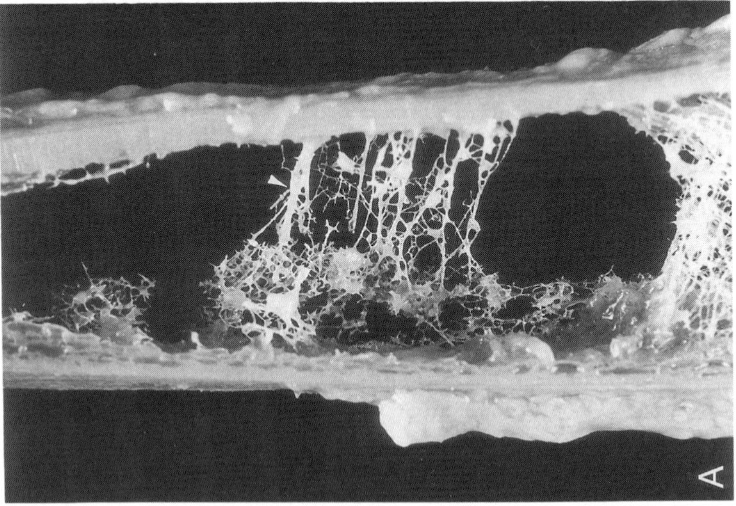
A

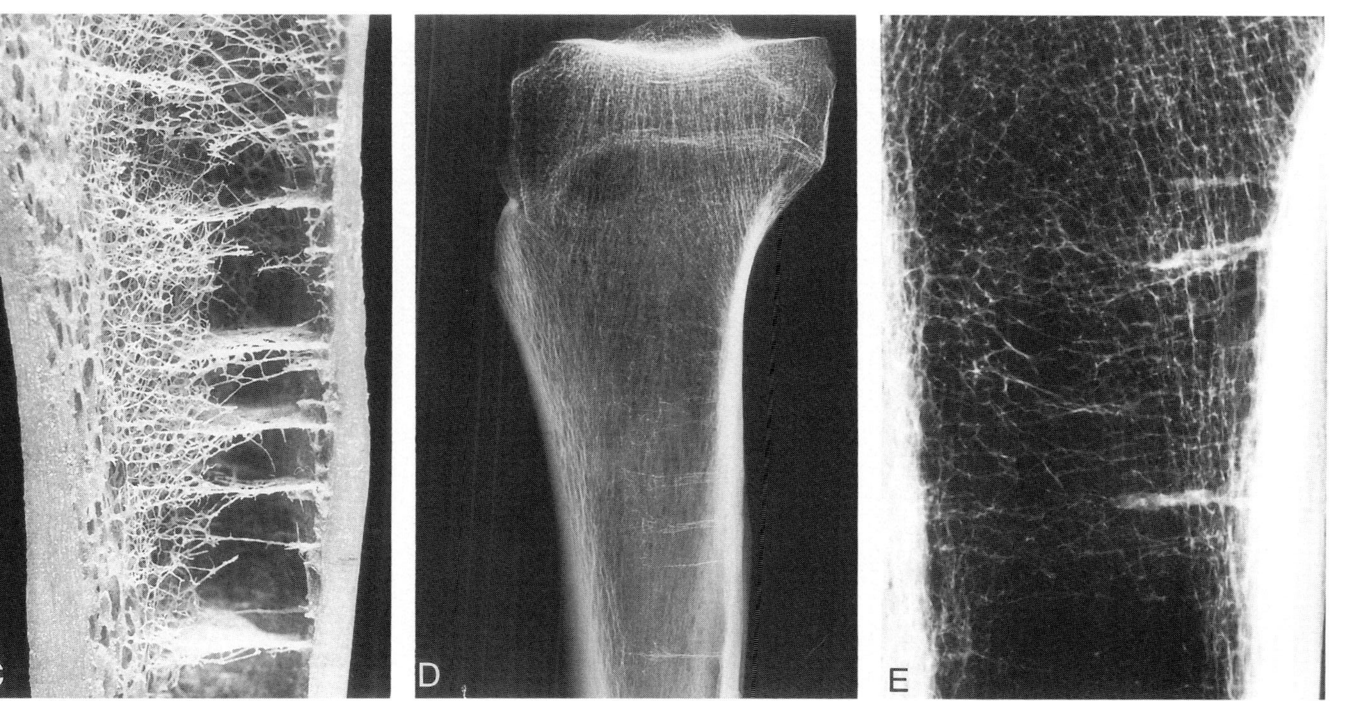

Figure 16 Reinforcement lines (bone bars): radiographic-pathologic correlation. (A,B) A photograph and magnification radiograph of a macerated midsagittal section of the femur show a branching bone bar (arrowheads) extending incompletely across the distal portion of the diaphysis. It is oriented at approximately 75° to the cortex. Numerous similar but thinner bars are evident distally, some extending across the entire medullary canal. (C,D) In this tibia, which has been sectioned in the sagittal plane, numerous parallel bars arise from the posterior surface of the bone. They are oriented at approximately 90° to the cortex and extend almost entirely across the medullary canal. (E) In another tibial specimen, observe several broad bone bars which are oriented in precisely the same fashion as the neighboring trabeculae. They terminate by branching into small trabeculae. (From Ref. 27.)

bars. One suggestion is that these are normal variations in the trabecular pattern of bone. This hypothesis is feasible in regions such as the humerus or femoral neck, where prominent trabeculae are commonly present, but it does not explain the presence of bone bars in regions such as the distal portion of the femur and proximal portion of the tibia, where prominent trabeculae are normally not encountered. Another suggestion has been that bone bars form normally during skeletal growth, remain hidden in the normal skeleton, and are unmasked by osseous resorption. A third explanation is that bone bars are initially formed in the osteoporotic skeleton in response to biomechanical stress.

B. Regional Osteoporosis

"Regional osteoporosis" is a term used to describe osteoporosis confined to a region or segment of the body, usually in the appendicular skeleton. The three classic forms of regional osteoporosis are transient regional osteoporosis, reflex sympathetic dystrophy, and osteoporosis of disuse and immobilization (Table 5).

1. Transient Regional Osteoporosis

Transient regional osteoporosis is a general term encompassing two separate (but probably related) conditions: transient osteoporosis of the hip, and regional migratory osteoporosis (126,127). These diseases are characterized by rapidly developing osteoporosis affecting periarticular bone. Both conditions occur in the absence of obvious inciting events such as trauma or immobilization, and both are self-limited and reversible. They also share similar clinical, radiologic, and pathologic features.

a. Transient Osteoporosis of the Hip. Transient osteoporosis of the hip was first described in 1959 (128). Initially, it was thought to occur most frequently in women during late pregnancy. It now is known that this condition is typically seen in young and middle-aged adults, particularly men. The patient complains of hip pain, antalgic limp, and limitation of joint motion with no history of antecedent trauma or infection. The clinical course is usually self-limited, full recovery occurring in 2–6 months (129–135).

Table 5 Major Causes of Regional Osteoporosis

Transient regional osteoporosis
Transient osteoporosis of the hip
Regional migratory osteoporosis
Reflex sympathetic dystrophy
Immobilization and disuse

Radiographic findings include progressive and marked osteoporosis of the femoral head beginning several weeks after the onset of clinical abnormalities. The femoral neck and acetabulum are usually involved less extensively than the femoral head. The femoral subchondral bone plate is thin but otherwise intact. The joint space is preserved. Femoral neck fractures may occur (136). In children, osseous enlargement may be seen (137). Radionuclide studies using bone-seeking agents reveal abnormal accumulation of isotope before osteoporosis becomes demonstrable radiographically (133,138–140). CT shows osteoporosis with cortical thinning (141), and MR imaging may reveal decreased signal intensity on T1-weighted images and increased signal intensity on T2-weighted images of affected sites (140,142–145) (Fig. 17). Joint effusions usually are seen on T2-weighted images (144,145). Restoration of normal radiographic bone density and MR imaging signal intensity occurs rapidly—within approximately 1 year (142).

Pathologically, bone biopsy reveals necrosis and an increase in resorption and new bone surface (146). Joint fluid may be increased in quantity, and synovial biopsy either yields normal results or shows mild chronic inflammatory changes (126).

The cause of transient osteoporosis of the hip is unknown. Self-limited osteonecrosis of bone (147) and neurogenic factors (27) have been proposed as possible etiologic factors. Findings from MR imaging and scintigraphy suggest that this condition is actually a transient bone marrow edema (140). Transient osteoporosis of the hip is occasionally bilateral, with either simultaneous or successive involvement of the two sides, suggesting a relationship with regional migratory osteoporosis (127,148–150).

b. Regional Migratory Osteoporosis. The second form of transient osteoporosis is migratory in nature and most commonly affects the knee, ankle, and foot (150–154). Regional migratory osteoporosis is also referred to as "transient painful osteoporosis of the lower extremity" (149,155–158). More common in men than in women, this condition usually becomes evident in the fourth and fifth decades of life (Fig. 18).

The disease is characterized by the rapid development of local pain and swelling of the lower extremity. The symptoms last up to 9 months and then diminish and disappear. Subsequent involvement may occur in other regions of the same or opposite extremity. Several recurrences can occur successively within 2 years or be separated by 2 years or longer (126).

Evidence of osteoporosis appears within weeks or months of the onset of clinical findings. The osteoporosis also appears rapidly, diminishes subsequently, and appears at other sites. Periarticular osteoporosis can extend for a considerable distance from the joint. The joint space typically remains normal; however, marked subchondral bone thinning can occur to an extent that the joint space is difficult to define. Erosions do not occur in this disorder. Bone scintigraphy

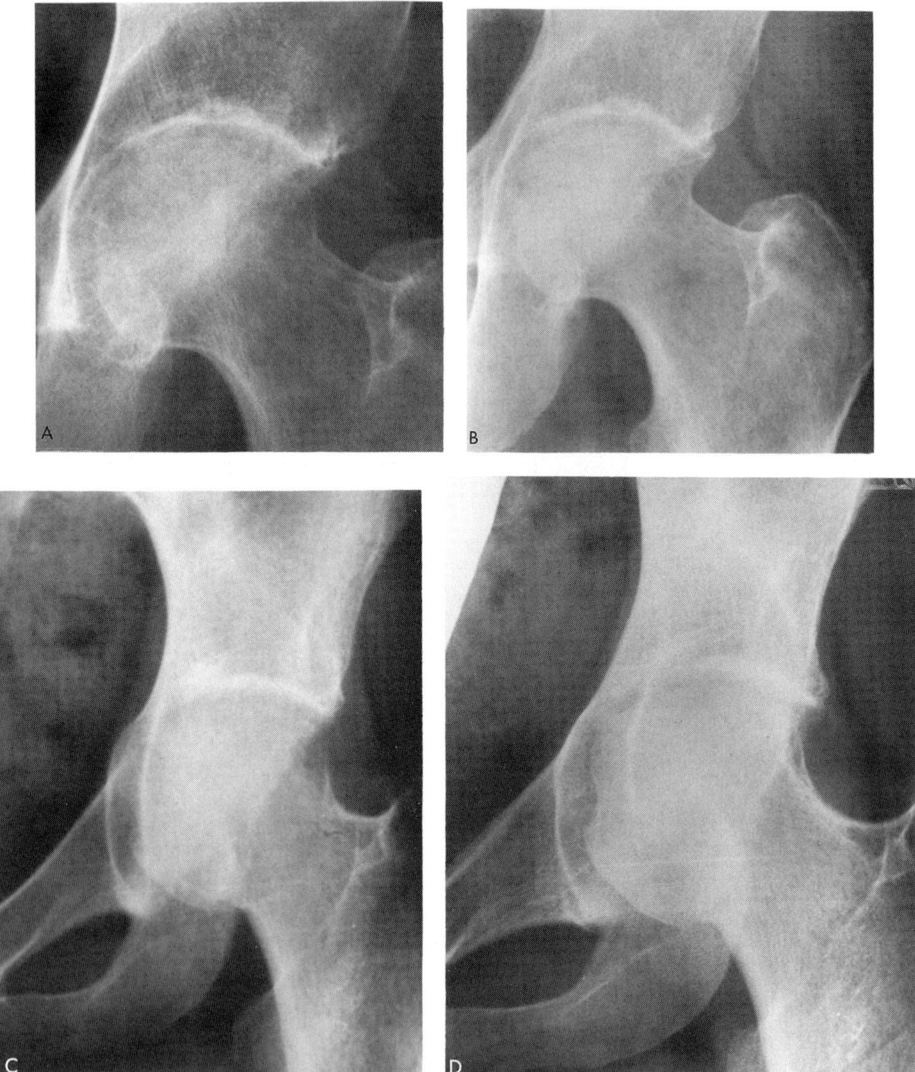

Figure 17 Transient osteoporosis of the hip. (A,B) A 49-year-old male complained of progressive hip pain. Joint aspiration was unrewarding. The initial radiograph (A) shows periarticular osteoporosis, particularly of the femoral head, with thinning and obscuration of the subchondral bone plate. The articular space is relatively normal, and there is no osseous collapse. Two months later (B), without institution of specific therapy, the osteoporosis is less striking. The joint space is well maintained. (C,D) A 23-year-old woman developed the rapid onset of hip pain. Laboratory values were unremarkable with the exception of mild elevation of the erythrocyte sedimentation rate. Aspiration of the hip

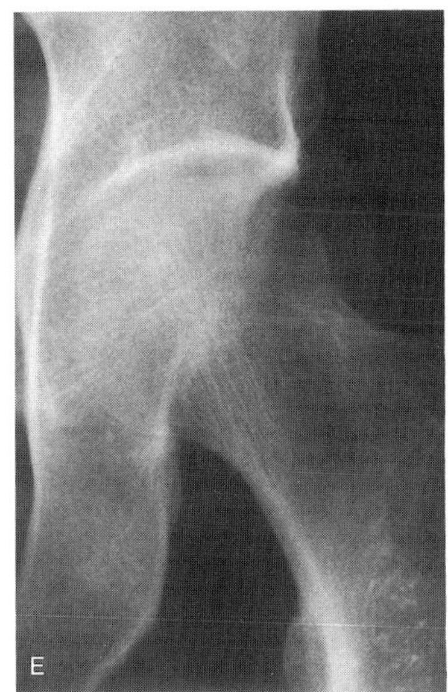

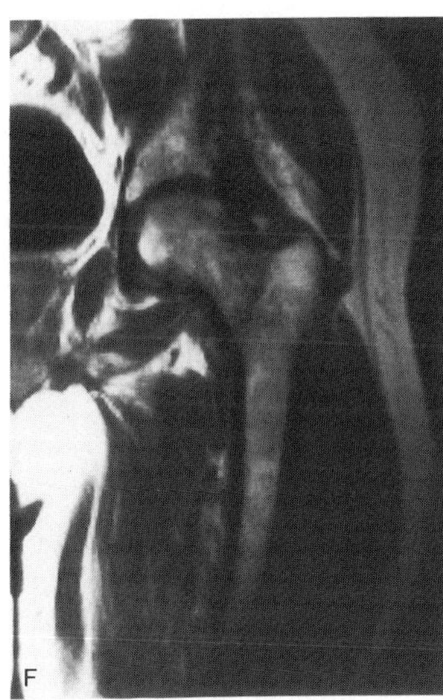

demonstrated no growth of organisms following appropriate culture. On the initial radiograph (C), there is marked osteopenia of the femoral head with loss of definition of the subchondral bone plate. The joint space is relatively preserved. Acetabular protrusion was evident bilaterally. Ten weeks later (D), without specific therapy, osteoporosis has largely disappeared. (E,F) In this 60-year-old man, the radiograph (E) shows subtle osteopenia in the femoral head. The coronal spin-echo magnetic resonance image (TR, 0.9 s, TE, 26 ms) (F) reveals a decreased signal intensity in the femur. (From Ref. 27. C,D, Courtesy of R. Richley, MD, San Diego, Calif.)

reveals increased activity (159–161) in involved areas, and radiographs can reveal a wavy periosteal bone formation along the shaft of tubular bones (151).

Laboratory analysis may reveal increased urinary excretion of calcium, hydroxyproline, and fluoride (158). Elevated alkaline phosphatase activity and hypophosphatemia have also been observed in this condition (162).

The migratory nature of this disease is the major feature differentiating it from transient osteoporosis of the hip. Usually the joint nearest the diseased articulation is the next to be involved successively. Also, several joints can be involved simultaneously (150,151). A variant of this condition, termed partial transient osteoporosis, has been described in which a portion of a joint is involved (163). In this variant form, only one digit of a foot or hand, or one femoral condyle, can be affected.

Histologic examination in regional migratory osteoporosis reveals thickened synovium with chronic inflammatory cellular reaction (154). The bone itself is osteoporotic, with increased numbers of osteoblasts and osteoclasts (151).

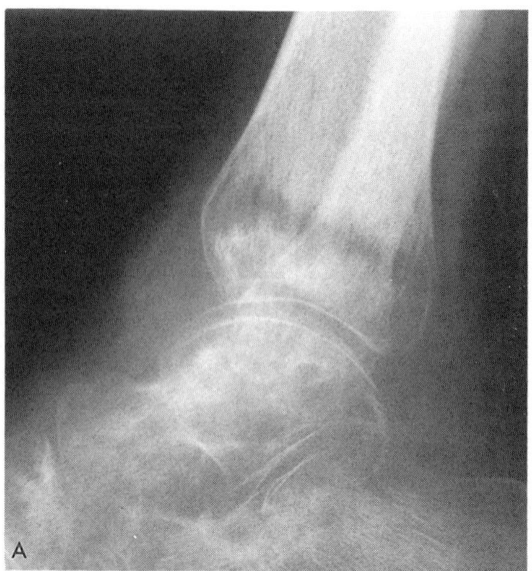

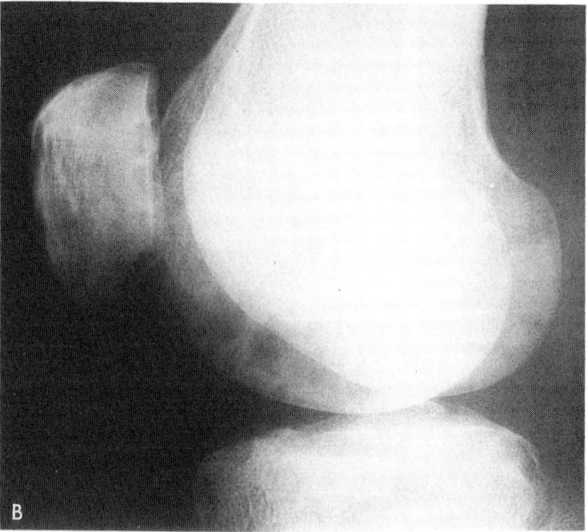

Figure 18 Regional migratory osteoporosis. (A,B) Typical in this condition are transient pain and swelling of one articulation associated with periarticular osteoporosis, followed by spontaneous improvement and involvement of an adjacent articulation. Observe the soft-tissue swelling and bandlike osteopenia of the tibia and talus (A) and the spotty osteoporosis of the distal femur and patella. (From Ref. 27.)

The pathogenesis of regional migratory osteoporosis is unknown, but it has been linked to reflex sympathetic dystrophy, transient osteoporosis of the hip, and denervation from a local inflammatory reaction of the nerve endings or from radiculopathy (153).

2. *Reflex Sympathetic Dystrophy*

Reflex sympathetic dystrophy (RSD) was first described in 1864 (164). Several terms have been applied to RSD, including causalgia (165), acute bone atrophy (166), Sudeck's atrophy (167), posttraumatic osteoporosis (168), and the shoulder-hand syndrome (169). RSD remains the most appropriate name for this entity (170–172,187).

Several neurally related visceral, musculoskeletal, neurologic, or vascular conditions are potential precipitators of RSD. Occasionally, an incipient cause for RSD is not identifiable. Reported associated conditions include myocardial infarction, cerebrovascular disorders, degenerative cervical spine disease, disk herniation (173), polymyalgia rheumatica (174), posttraumatic, postsurgical, and postinfectious states, calcific tendinitis, vasculitis, and neoplasm (175–177). RSD is more common in adults than children. When it occurs in children, it usually follows physical injury, is self-limited and benign, and results in no clinical residua (178,179).

The pathogenesis of RSD is unclear. The most widely held theory focuses on the internuncial pool (180), in which an injury or lesion is assumed to produce painful impulses that travel via afferent pathways to the spinal cord, where a series of reflexes are initiated that spread by way of the interconnecting pool of neurons. These latter reflexes stimulate the lateral and anterior tracts, provoking efferent impulses in pathways that travel to the peripheral nerves, producing the local findings of RSD (180). Another theory holds that the causalgic pain in this syndrome results from activation of sensory fibers by sympathetic impulses (181). This sympathetic nervous system theory is supported by evidence that increased blood flow and venous oxygen saturation occur in the affected extremity (182–185). Further evidence supporting the existence of sympathetic involvement is the presence of nerve fibers in the periosteum that are sympathetic in origin and that contain vasoactive intestinal peptide, a substance that dramatically stimulates bone resorption (186). This condition can involve the knee after meniscectomy (187,188).

The clinical presentation is highly variable. The disease most commonly affects the shoulder and hand. Men and women are affected equally, with onset usually occurring after the age of 50 years. Initially, stiffness, pain, tenderness, and weakness may be associated with swelling, vasomotor changes, hyperesthesia, and disability. The duration of RSD varies, and in some cases findings persist for years, becoming irreversible (189).

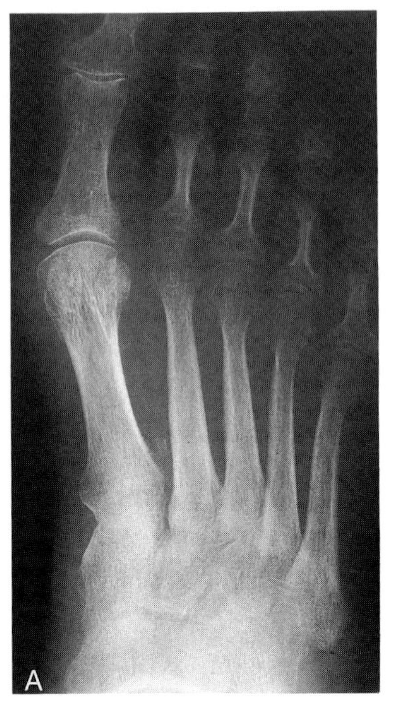
A

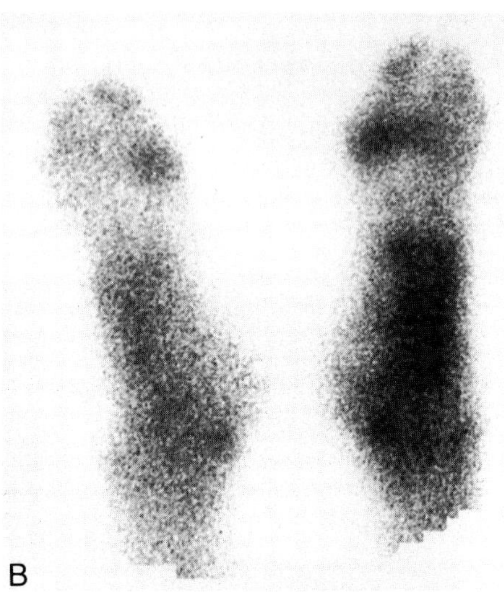
B

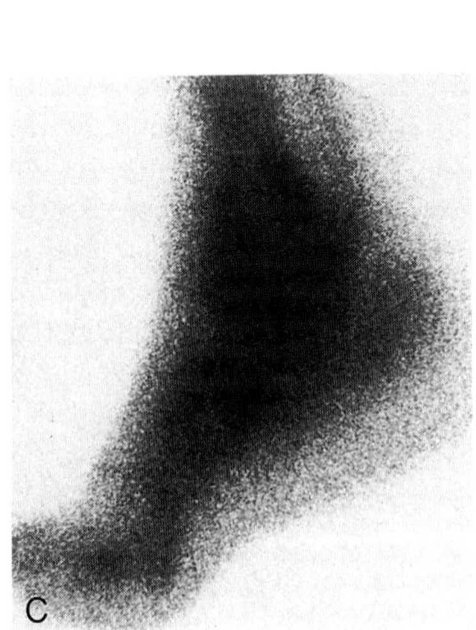
C

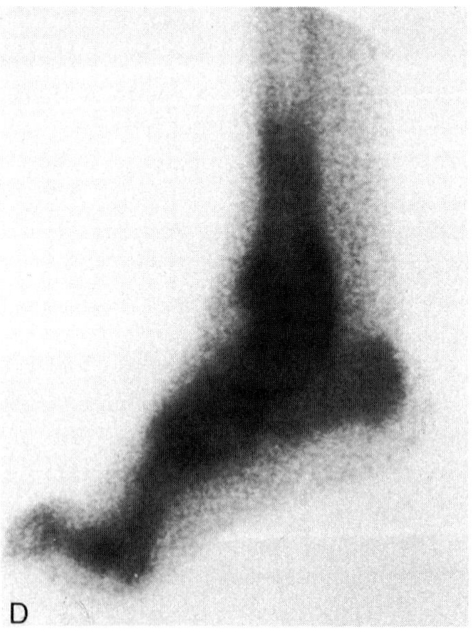
D

Radiographic evaluation is important in the diagnosis of RSD (126) (Fig. 19). Soft-tissue swelling and regional osteoporosis are the most important radiographic findings. High-resolution radiography reveals five types of bone resorption: 1. resorption of cancellous or trabecular bone in the metaphyseal region, most prominent in children, with bandlike, patchy, or periarticular osteoporosis; 2. subperiosteal bone resorption; 3. intracortical bone resorption with striation and tunneling of cortices; 4. endosteal bone resorption; 5. Subchondral and juxta-articular erosion.

These changes collectively can resemble the osteopenia seen in hyperparathyroidism. Because of the widespread nature and severity of bone resorption in RSD, radiography often reveals severe and rapid osteopenia, particularly in a periarticular distribution simulating the appearance of primary articular disorders (190). The absence of intra-articular erosions and joint space loss allows differentiation from arthritic processes and the regional distribution allows differentiation from hyperparathyroidism.

Bone and joint scintigraphy also reveals characteristic abnormalities that often precede both clinical and radiographic changes (170–173,191,192). Joint scintigraphy reveals radionuclide accumulation of ^{99m}Tc-pertechnetate in involved joints, presumably from increased vascularity of synovial membranes. This same pattern is also seen in articular disorders characterized by synovial inflammation and hyperemia (193). Similar uptake of radionuclide is seen in involved bones of RSD patients with bone scintigraphy, also presumed to result from increased blood flow (194). Occasionally, especially in children, decreased or normal uptake of radionuclide is observed on bone scans (195,196). The consensus, made on the basis of radiographic, scintigraphic, and quantitative bone mineral analyses, is that RSD is a bilateral process in at least 25–50% of cases but that its distribution is almost universally asymmetric (170,172,191,197).

Pathologically, several abnormalities have been identified. Synovial biopsies in symptomatic joints reveal edema, proliferation, and disarray of synovial lining cells, capillary proliferative changes, fibrosis of the subsynovium, and slight

---

Figure 19 Reflex sympathetic dystrophy syndrome: scintigraphic abnormalities. (A,B) In this 55-year-old woman who developed symptoms and signs of the reflex sympathetic dystrophy syndrome following a burn, a radiograph (A) reveals diffuse and periarticular osteopenia. A delayed image during a bone scan (B) shows abnormal uptake of the radionuclide in the midfoot and forefoot on the left side with similar but mild changes in the opposite foot. (C,D) In a 34-year-old woman who also was burned (in areas other than the foot and ankle), an early (blood pool or tissue phase) image (lateral view of ankle and foot) during a bone scan (C) demonstrates diffuse radionuclide activity. The delayed image (D) documents the intense radionuclide accumulation in the bones about the ankle and the midfoot and forefoot. (From Ref. 27.)

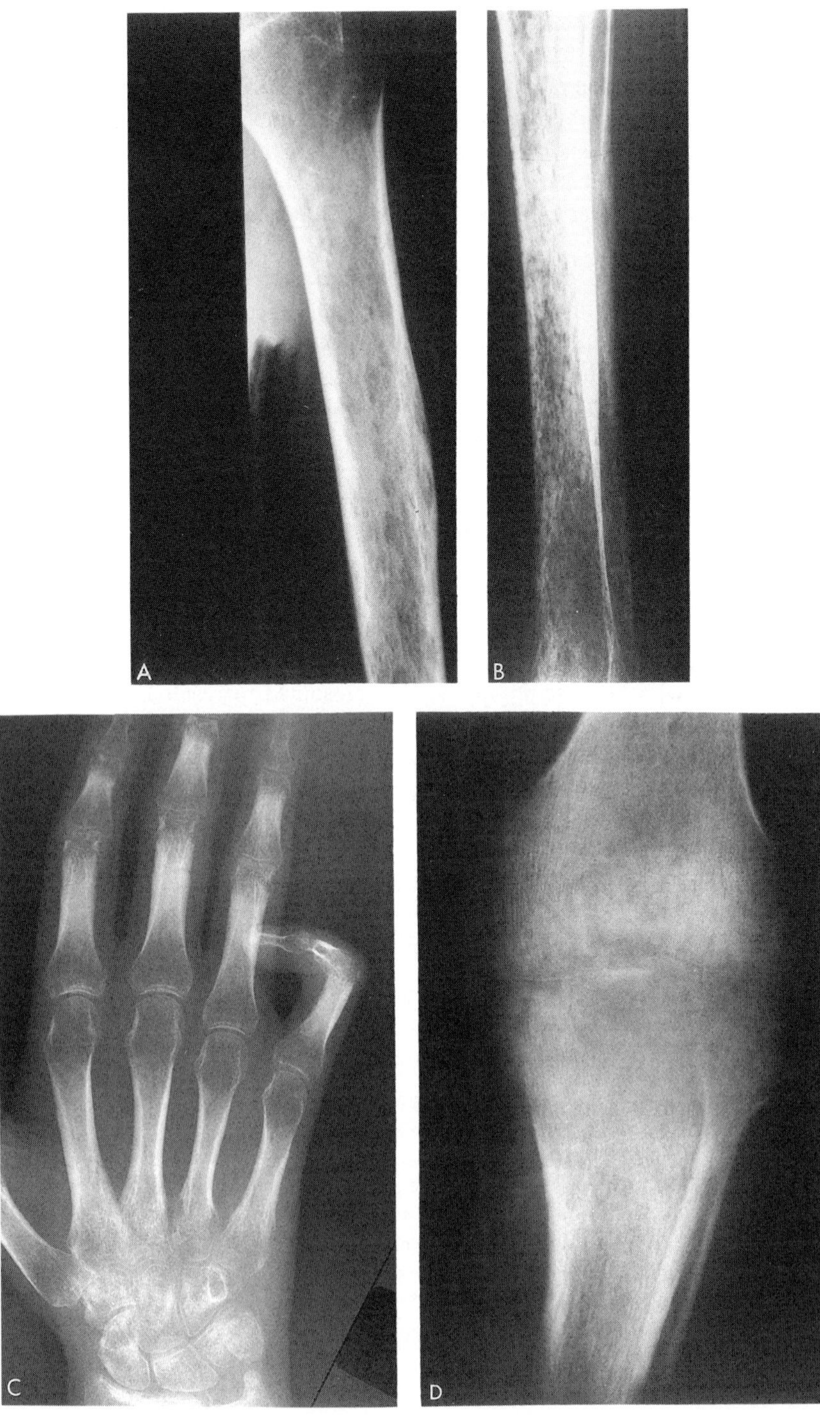
A
B
C
D

perivascular infiltration with chronic inflammatory cells (170). Fibrosis of superficial articular cartilage of the knee has been observed (198). The skin and subcutaneous tissues typically appear histologically normal. Bone reveals increased vascularity, prominent osteoclastic activity, and osteocytic degeneration (166,167,183,184,199).

The prominent pathogenetic role of local hyperemia in RSD explains the severe and rapid regional osteoporosis with periarticular accentuation that characterizes this condition (94).

3. Osteoporosis of Disuse and Immobilization

A unique type of osteoporosis occurs in areas of the skeleton that have been immobilized in patients with fractures, motor paralysis from central nervous system disease or trauma, and bone and joint inflammation (200). Disuse osteoporosis is associated with increased urinary and fecal calcium excretion with a subsequent negative calcium balance during the period of immobilization. The radiographic appearance of disuse osteoporosis depends on the age of the patient and the extent and duration of the negative calcium balance. Osteoporosis appears sooner after immobilization in younger persons and is more severe when calcium loss is more prominent (27). Osteoporosis generally appears within 2 or 3 months after paralysis has developed (126), and initially affects the appendicular skeleton. Although the pelvis is often involved, changes in the spine are not prominent. The changes seen after immobilization are similar to those in paralysis (201). Significant osteoporosis is more common after 8 weeks of immobilization, although it can be present before this, especially in persons younger than 20 years or older than 50 (202) (Fig. 20).

Most commonly, a uniform pattern of regional osteopenia is seen in disuse osteoporosis. Speckled or spotty osteopenia characterized by small, spherical, lucent regions also may be observed, particularly in periarticular locations and in the carpal and tarsal bones. Two other patterns characteristic of disuse osteoporosis are bandlike subchondral or metaphyseal osteopenia and cortical lamellation or scalloping of long bones (126,201). The radiographic appearance of these

---

Figure 20 Osteoporosis of immobilization and disuse. (A–C) Neurologic injuries. As a result of disease due to neurologic abnormality, variable patterns of bone resorption can be observed, which may appear very aggressive in nature. In the upper humeral shaft (A), scalloping of the endosteal surface of the cortex simulates the findings of plasma cell myeloma. Intracortical lucent areas also are observed. In the tibia and fibula in a different patient (B), a permeative pattern of bone destruction simulates the appearance of neoplasm or infection. In the hand in a third patient (C), periarticular osteoporosis is striking. A contracture is obvious. (D) Amputation. Following a below-the-knee amputation for osteomyelitis in this diabetic patient, patchy or spotty osteoporosis is evident, particularly in periarticular areas. The joint space is poorly evaluated because of knee flexion. (From Ref. 27.)

types of disuse osteoporosis can simulate those of malignancy (202). A double cortical line in the acetabular roof has been described as a reliable sign of disuse osteoporosis and appears to result from severe intracortical bone loss (203).

The typical distribution of disuse osteoporosis is regional. Occasionally, a generalized or scattered pattern of osteoporosis develops in quadriplegic persons; a similar appearance is observed in astronauts as a result of weightlessness due to lack of gravitational forces (204,205).

Laboratory abnormalities include hypercalcemia, hypercalciuria, and hyperphosphoremia (206). The pathogenesis of disuse osteoporosis is that of a high-turnover osteoporosis resulting from both increased bone resorption (1,126,207) and reduced bone formation (207,208). Although the process is self-limited and somewhat reversible (209,210), the period of recovery is several times longer than the period of bone loss, and the degree of recovery shows wide individual variation (211). Vascular stasis, neurologic factors, and humoral factors may all play a role in the development of disuse osteoporosis (212,213).

REFERENCES

1. Harris WH, Heaney RP. Skeletal renewal and metabolic bone disease. N Engl J Med 1969; 280:193–202.
2. Lutwak L, Whedon GD. Osteoporosis. DM 1963; April:1.
3. Griffiths HJ, Simmerman RE, The clinical application of bone mineral analysis. Skel Radiol 1978; 3:1.
4. Peppler WW, Mazess RB. Total body bone mineral and lean body mass by dual photon absorptiometry. I. Theory and measurement procedure. Calcif Tissue Int 1981; 33:353–363.
5. Drolner B, Nielsen PS. Measurement of bone mineral content (BMC) of the lumbar spine. I. Theory and application of a new two-dimensional dual-photon attenuation method. Scand J Clin Lab Invest 1980; 40:485–490.
6. Cameron JR, Mazess RB, Sorenson JA. Precision and accuracy of bone mineral determination by direct photon absorptiometry. Invest Radiol 1968; 3:141–150.
7. Genant HK, Boyd D. Quantitative bone mineral analysis using dual energy computed tomography. Invest Radiol 1977; 12:545–551.
8. Reich NE, Seidelmann FE, Tubbs RR, MacIntyre WJ, Meaney TF, Alfidi RJ, Pepe RG. Determination of bone mineral content using CT scanning. AJR 1976; 127: 593–594.
9. Posner, I, Griffiths HJ. Comparison of CT scanning with photon absorptiometric measurement of bone mineral content in the appendicular skeleton. Invest Radiol 1977; 12:542–544.
10. Ruegsegger P, Elsasser U, Anliker M, Gnehm H, Kind H, Prader A. Quantification of bone mineralization using computed tomography. Radiology 1976; 121:93–97.
11. Bradley JG, Huang HK, Ledley RS. Evaluation of calcium concentration in bones from CT scans. Radiology 197; 128:103–107.

12. Jensen PS, Orphanoudakis SC, Rauschkolb EN, Baron R, Lang R, Rasmussen H. Assessment of bone mass in the radius by computed tomography. AJR 1980; 134: 285–292.
13. Elsasser U, Ruegsegger P, Anliker M, Exner GU, Prader A. Loss and recovery of trabecular bone in the distal radius following fracture-immobilization of the upper limb in children. Klin Wochenschr 1979; 57:763.
14. Cann CE, Genant HK, Young DR. Comparison of vertebral and peripheral mineral losses in disuse osteoporosis in monkeys. Radiology 1980; 134:525–529.
15. Sartoris DJ, Andre M, Resnik C, Resnick D. Trabecular bone density in the proximal femur: quantitative CT assessment. Radiology 1986; 160:707–712.
16. Smith RW, Keiper DA. Dynamic measurement of the viscoelastic properties of bone. Am J Med Electron 1965; 4:156–160.
17. Selle WA, Jurist JM. Acoustical detection of senile osteoporosis. Proc Soc Exp Biol Med 1966; 121:150–152.
18. Sartoris DJ, Sommer FG, Marcus R, Madvig P. Bone mineral density in the femoral neck: quantitative assessment using dual-energy projection radiography. AJR 1985; 144:605–611.
19. Hangartner TN. Review: the radiologic measurement of bone. J Can Assoc Radiol 1986; 37:143–152.
20. Chesnut CH. The imaging and quantitation of bone by radiographic and scanning methodologies. In: Coe FL, Favus MJ, eds. Disorders of Bone and Mineral Metabolism. New York: Raven Press; 1992:443–454.
21. Lang FJ. Arthritis deformans und spondylitis deformans. In: Lubararsch O, Henke F, eds. Handbuch der Spezieller Pathologischen Anatomie und Histologie. Berlin: Springer-Verlag, 1934.
22. Trueta J. Studies of the Development and Decay of the Human Frame. Philadelphia: WB Saunders; 1968:316.
23. Lukert BP. Osteoporosis—a review and update. Arch Phys Med Rehabil 1982; 63: 480–487.
24. Michel BA, Lane NE, Jones HH, Fries JF, Bloch DA. Plain radiographs can be useful in estimating lumbar bone density. J Rheumatol 1990; 17:528–531.
25. Epstein DM, Dalinka MK, Kaplan FS, Aronchick JM, Marinelli DL, Kundel HL. Observer variation in the detection of osteopenia. Skel Radiol 1986; 15:347–349.
26. Finsen V, Anda S. Accuracy of visually estimated bone mineralization in routine radiographs of the lower extremity. Skel Radiol 1988; 17:270–275.
27. Resnick D, Niwayama G. Osteoporosis. In: Resnick D, Niwayama G, eds. Diagnosis of Bone and Joint Disorders, 2nd ed. Philadelphia: WB Saunders; 1988:2023–2083.
28. Mayo-Smith W, Rosenthal DL. Radiographic appearance of osteopenia. Radiol Clin North Am 1991; 29:37–47.
29. Reynolds WA, Karo JJ. Radiologic diagnosis of metabolic bone disease. Orthop Clin North Am 1972; 3:521–543.
30. Steinbach HL. The roentgen appearance of osteoporosis. Radiol Clin North Am 1964; 2:191–207.
31. Singh M, Nagrath AR, Maini PS. Changes in trabecular pattern of the upper end of the femur as an index of osteoporosis. J Bone Joint Surg [Am] 1970; 52:457–467.

32. Kerr R, Resnick D, Sartoris DJ, Kursunoglu S, Pineda C, Haghighi P, Greenway G, Guerra J Jr. Computed tomography of proximal femoral trabecular patterns. J Orthop Res 1986; 4:45–56.
33. Kerr R, Resnick D, Pineda C. CT analysis of proximal femoral trabecular pattern simulating skeletal pathology. J Comput Assist Tomogr 1988; 12:227–230.
34. Siffert RS. Trabecular patterns in bone. AJR 1967; 99:746–755.
35. Singh M, Riggs B, Beabout JW, Jowsey J. Femoral trabecular pattern index for evaluation of spinal osteoporosis. Ann Intern Med 1972; 77:63–67.
36. Dequeker J, Gautama K, Roh YS. Femoral trabecular patterns in asymptomatic spinal osteoporosis and femoral neck fracture. Clin Radiol 1974; 25:243–246.
37. Roh YS, Dequeker J, Mulier JC. Trabecular pattern of the upper end of the femur in primary osteoarthrosis and in symptomatic osteoporosis. J Belge Radiol 1974; 57: 89–94.
38. Osborne D, Effmann E. Disturbances of trabecular architecture in the upper end of the femur in childhood. Skel Radiol 1981; 6:165–173.
39. Horsman A, Nordin BE, Simpson M, Speed R. Cortical and trabecular bone status in elderly women with femoral neck fracture. Clin Orthop 1982; 166:143–151.
40. Seror P, Sebert JL, Rouleau L, Blotman F, Simon L. L'indice femoral de Singh dans l'osteoporose vertebrale. Sem Hop Paris 1982; 58:2315–2317.
41. Wicks M, Garrett R, Vernon-Roberts B, Fazzalari N. Absence of metabolic bone disease in the proximal femur in patients with fracture of the femoral neck. J Bone Joint Surg [Br] 1982; 64:319–322.
42. Kovarik J, Kuster W, Seidl G, Linkesch W, Dorda W, Willvonseder R, Kotscher E. Clinical relevance of radiologic examination of the skeleton and bone density measurements in osteoporosis of old age. Skel Radiol 1981; 7:37–41.
43. Cooper C, Barker DJP, Hall AJ. Evaluation of the Singh index and femoral calcar width as epidemiological methods for measuring bone mass in the femoral neck. Clin Radiol 1986; 37:123–125.
44. Parfitt AM, Duncan H. Metabolic bone disease affecting the spine. In: Rothman RH, Simeone FA, eds. The Spine. Philadelphia: WB Saunders; 1975:599.
45. Kranendonk DH, Jurist JM, Lee HG. Femoral trabecular patterns and bone mineral content. J Bone Joint Surg [Am] 1972; 54:1472–1478.
46. Khairi MR, Cronin JH, Robb JA, Smith DM, Yu PL, Johnston CC Jr. Femoral trabecular pattern index and bone mineral content measurement by photon absorption in senile osteoporosis. J Bone Joint Surg [Am] 1976; 58:221–226.
47. Wilson CR. Bone-mineral content of the femoral neck and spine versus the radius or ulna. J Bone Joint Surg [Am] 1977; 59:665–669.
48. Griffiths HJ, Virtama P. Cortical thickness and trabecular pattern of the femoral neck as a measure of osteopenia. Invest Radiol 1990; 10:1116–1119.
49. Disen A, Frey HM, Langholm R, Vagslid T. Appearance of trabecular bone in the femoral neck (Singh index). Acta Radiol Diagn 1979; 20:372–378.
50. Pogrund H, Rigal WM, Makin M, Robin G, Menczel J, Steinberg R. Determination of osteoporosis in patients with fractured femoral necks using Singh index. Jerusalem study. Clin Orthop 1985; 156:189–195.
51. Robertson A. Singh and metacarpal cortical indices. Australas Radiol 1978; 12:257–261.

52. Kawashima T, Uhthoff HK. Pattern of bone loss of the proximal femur: a radiologic, densitometric, and histomorphometric study. J Orthop Res 1991; 9:634–640.
53. Hansson T, Roos B. Microcalluses of the trabeculae in lumbar vertebrae and their relation to the bone mineral content. Spine 1981; 6:375–380.
54. Hurxthal LM. Measurement of anterior vertebral compressions and biconcave vertebrae. AJR 1968; 103:635–644.
55. Adami S, Gatti D, Rossini M, Adamoli A, James G, Girardello S, Zamberlan N. The radiological assessment of vertebral osteoporosis. Bone 1992; 13(suppl): S33–S36.
56. Brandner ME. Normal values of the vertebral body and intervertebral disk index in adults. AJR 1972; 114:411–414.
57. Resnick DL. Fish vertebrae. Arthritis Rheum 1982; 25:1073–1077.
58. Barnett E, Nordin BEC. The radiologic diagnosis of osteoporosis: a new approach. Clin Radiol 1960; 11:166.
59. Resnick D, Niwayama G. Intravertebral disk herniations: cartilaginous (Schmorl's) nodes. Radiology 1978; 126:57–65.
60. Geist ES. The intervertebral disc. JAMA 1931; 96:1696.
61. Hansson T, Roos B. The amount of bone mineral and Schmorl's nodes in lumbar vertebrae. Spine 1983; 8:266–271.
62. Coventry MB, Ghormley RK, Kernohan JW. Intervertebral disc: its microscopic anatomy and pathology. Changes in the intervertebral disc concomitant with age. J Bone Joint Surg 1945; 27:233–245.
63. Hassler O. The human intervertebral disc. A microangiographical study on its vascular supply at various stages. Acta Orthop Scand 1970; 40:765–777.
64. Coventry MB, Ghormley RK, Kernohan JW. Intervertebral disc; its microscopic anatomy and pathology; pathological changes in the intervertebral disc. J Bone Joint Surg 1945; 27:460–474.
65. Schmorl G, Junghanns H. The Human Spine in Health and Disease, 2nd ed. New York: Grune & Stratton; 1971:158.
66. Pogrund H, Bloom RA, Weinberg H. Relationship of psoas width to osteoporosis. Acta Orthop Scand 1986; 57:208–210.
67. Steiger P, Block JE, Friedlander A, Genant HK. Precise determination of para spinous musculature by quantitative CT. J Comput Assist Tomogr 1988; 12:616–620.
68. Hordon LD, Francis RM, Marshall DH, Smith AH, Peacock M. Are scintigrams of the spine useful in vertebral osteoporosis? Clin Radiol 1986; 37:487–489.
69. Garn SM, Poznanski AK, Nagy JM. Bone measurement in the differential diagnosis of osteopenia and osteoporosis. Radiology 1971; 100:509–518.
70. Evans RA, McDonnell GD, Schieb M. Metacarpal cortical area as an index of bone mass. Br J Radiol 1978; 51:428–431.
71. Dequeker J. Quantitative radiology: radiogrammetry of cortical bone. Br J Radiol 1976; 49:912–920.
72. Robertson A. A look at bone. Australas Radiol 1976; 20:346–366.
73. Meema HE. Radiology of osteoporosis. Ther Umsch 1977; 34:628–633.
74. Meema HE. Recognition of cortical bone resorption in metabolic bone disease in vivo. Skel Radiol 1977; 2:11.

75. Meema HE, Meema S. Comparison of microradioscopic and morphometric findings in the hand bones with densitometric findings in the proximal radius in thyrotoxicosis and in renal osteodystrophy. Invest Radiol 1972; 7:88–96.
76. Meema HE, Meema S. Improved roentgenologic diagnosis of osteomalacia by microradioscopy of hand bones. AJR 1975; 125:925–935.
77. The osteoporoses in the late 1980's: a field in flux. IM 1982; 3:65.
78. Courpron P. Bone tissue mechanisms underlying osteoporoses. Orthop Clin North Am 1981; 12:513–545.
79. Meema HE. Radiologic study of endosteal, intracortical, and periosteal surfaces of hand bones in metabolic bone diseases. Hand Clin 1991; 7:37–51.
80. Frost HM. Bone Remodelling and its Relationship to Metabolic Bone Diseases. Springfield, Ill: Charles C. Thomas, 1973.
81. Villaneuva AR, Ilnicki L, Duncan J, Frost HM. Bone and cell dynamics in the osteoporoses: a review of measurements by tetracycline bone labeling. Clin Orthop 1966; 49:135–150.
82. Wilson JS, Genant HK. In vivo assessment of bone metabolism using the cortical striation index. Invest Radiol 1979; 14:131–136.
83. Bloom RA, Pogrund H, Libson E. Radiogrammetry of the metacarpal: a critical reappraisal. Skel Radiol 1983; 10:5–9.
84. Forrester DM, Kirkpatrick J. Periostitis and pseudoperiostitis. Radiology 1976; 118: 597–601.
85. Dequecker J. Bone Loss in Normal and Pathological Conditions. Leuven, Belgium: University Press, 1972.
86. Garn SM. Earlier Gain and Later Loss of Cortical Bone. Springfield, Ill: Charles C. Thomas, 1970.
87. Bloom RA, Pogrund H. Humeral cortical thickness in female Bantu—its relationship to the incidence of femoral neck fracture. Skel Radiol 1982; 8:59–62.
88. Hermanutz KD, Ehlenz P, Verburg B. Morphometrie und Bestimmung kortikodiaphyser Indizes Klavikula im konventionellen Thoraxrontgenbild bei Gesunden und Knockenerkrankungen. ROFO 1982; 137:281–286.
89. Bras J, Van Ooij CP, Abraham-Inpijn L, Kusen GJ, Wilmink JM. Radiographic interpretation of the mandibular angular cortex: a diagnostic tool in metabolic bone loss. Part I. Normal state. Oral Surg 1982; 53:541–545.
90. Bras J, Van Ooij CP, Abraham-Inpijn L, Wilmink JM, Kusen GJ. Radiographic interpretation of the mandibular angular cortex: a diagnostic tool in metabolic bone loss. Part II. Renal osteodystrophy. Oral Surg 1982; 53:647–650.
91. Lusted LB, Keats TE. Atlas of Roentgenographic Measurement, 3rd ed. Chicago: Year Book Medical Publishers; 1972:138.
92. Steinbach JL, Gold RH, Preger L. Roentgen Appearance of the Hand in Diffuse Disease. Chicago: Year Book Medical Publishers; 1975:32.
93. Schworer I, Schmidtkunz U. Die bandformige Osteoporose. ROFO 1978; 128: 264–267.
94. Jaworski ZF, Lok E. The rate of osteosclerosis bone erosion in haversian remodelling sites of adult dog's rib. Calcif Tissue Res 1972; 10:103.

95. Joyce JM, Keats TE. Disuse osteoporosis: mimic of neoplastic disease. Skel Radiol 1986; 15:129–132.
96. Brower AC, Allman RM. Vascular influence on patterns of deossification. Arthritis Rheum 1982; 25:333–338.
97. Genant H. Osteoporosis. Bone Disease (Third Series) Syllabus. Chicago: American College of Radiology, 1980.
98. Mohajery M, Brooks SL. Oral radiographs in the detection of early signs of osteoporosis. Oral Surg Oral Med Oral Pathol 1992; 73:112–117.
99. Mitchell DC. Fractures in brittle bone diseases. Orthop Clin North Am 1972; 3: 787–792.
100. Cooper C, Atkinson EJ, O'Fallon WM, Melton LJ. Incidence of clinically diagnosed vertebral fractures: a population-based study in Rochester, Minnesota, 1985–1989. J Bone Miner Res 1992; 7:221–227.
101. Dias JJ, Wray CC, Jones JM. Osteoporosis and Colles' fractures in the elderly. J Hand Surg [Br] 1987; 12:57–59.
102. Harma M, Karjalainen P. Trabecular osteopenia in Colles' fracture. Acta Orthop Scand 1986; 57:38–40.
103. Parfitt AM. Trabecular bone architecture in the pathogenesis and prevention of fracture. Am J Med 1987; 82(suppl 1B):68–72.
104. Firooznia H, Rafii M, Golimbu C, Schwartz MS, Ort P. Trabecular mineral content of the spine in women with hip fracture: CT measurement. Radiology 1986; 159: 737–740.
105. Hoiseth A, Alho A, Husby T, Engh V. Are patients with fractures of the femoral neck more osteoporotic? Eur J Radiol 1991; 13:2–5.
106. Cummings SR. Are patients with hip fractures more osteoporotic? Am J Med 1985; 78:487–494.
107. Evans RA, Ashwell JR, Dunstan CR. Lack of metabolic bone disease in patients with fracture of the femoral neck. Aust NZ J Med 1981; 11:158–161.
108. Dalen N, Jacobsson B. Rarefied femoral neck trabecular patterns, fracture displacement, and femoral head vitality in femoral neck fractures. Clin Orthop 1986; 217: 97–98.
109. Patel U, Skingle S, Campbell GA, Crisp AJ, Boyle IT. Clinical profile of acute vertebral compression fractures in osteoporosis. Br J Rheumatol 1991; 30:418–421.
110. De Smet AA, Robinson RG, Johnson BE, Lukert BP. Spinal compression fractures in osteoporotic women: patterns and relationship to hyperkyphosis. Radiology 1988; 166:497–500.
111. Salomon C, Chopin D, Benoist M. Spinal cord compression: an exceptional complication of spinal osteoporosis. Spine 1988; 13:222–224.
112. De Smet AA, Neff JR. Pubic and sacral insufficiency fractures: clinical course and radiologic findings. AJR 1985; 145:601–606.
113. Casey D, Mirra J, Staple TW. Parasymphyseal insufficiency fractures of the os pubis. AJR 1984; 142:581–586.
114. Cooper KL, Beabout JW, Swee RG. Insufficiency fractures of the sacrum. Radiology 1985; 156:15–20.

115. Lourie H. Spontaneous osteoporotic fracture of the sacrum. An unrecognized syndrome of the elderly. JAMA 1982; 248:715–717.
116. Schneider R, Yacovone J, Ghelman B. Unsuspected sacral fractures: detection by radionuclide bone scanning. AJR 1985; 144:337–341.
117. Cooper KL. Insufficiency fractures of the sternum: a consequence of thoracic kyphosis? Radiology 1988; 167:471–472.
118. Cooper KL, Beabout JW, McLeod RA. Supraacetabular insufficiency fractures. Radiology 1985; 157:15–17.
119. Davies AM, Bradley SA. Iliac insufficiency fractures. Br J Radiol 1991; 64:305–309.
120. Dorne HL, Lander PH. Spontaneous stress fracture of the femoral neck. AJR 1985; 144:343–347.
121. Bauer G, Gustafsson M, Mortensson W, Norman O. Insufficiency fractures in the tibial condyles in elderly individuals. Acta Radiol (Diagn) 1981; 22:619–622.
122. Manco LG, Schneider R, Pavlov H. Insufficiency fractures of the tibial plateau. AJR 1983; 140:1211–1215.
123. Itani M, Evans GA, Park WM. Spontaneous sternal collapse. J Bone Joint Surg [Br] 1982; 64:432–434.
124. Sapherson DA, Mitchell SCM. Atraumatic sternal fractures secondary to osteoporosis. Clin Radiol 1990; 42:250–251.
125. Rawlings CE, Wilkins RH, Martinez S, Wilkinson RH. Osteoporotic sacral fractures: a clinical study. Neurosurgery 1988; 22:72–76.
126. Arnstein AR. Regional osteoporosis. Orthop Clin North Am 1972; 3:585–600.
127. Naides S, Resnick D, Zvaifler N. Idiopathic regional osteoporosis. J Rheumatol 1985; 12:763–768.
128. Curtiss PH Jr, Kincaid WE. Transitory demineralization of the hip in pregnancy. J Bone Joint Surg [Am] 1959; 41:1327–1333.
129. Pantazopoulos T, Exarchou E, Hartofilikidis-Garofalidis G. Idiopathic transient osteoporosis of the hip. J Bone Joint Surg 1973; 55:315–320.
130. DeMarchi E, Sancroce A, Solarino GB. Su Di una peculiare artoatia rarefacente dell'anca. Arch Putti Chir Organi Mov 1966; 21:62–66.
131. Lequesne M. L'algodystrophie de la hanche. Presse Med 1968; 76:793–802.
132. Lequesne M. Transient osteoporosis of the hip. A nontraumatic variety of Sudeck's atrophy. Ann Rheum Dis 1968; 27:463–472.
133. Valenzuela F, Aris H, Jacobelli S. Transient osteoporosis of the hip. J Rheumatol 1977; 4:59–64.
134. Lequesne M, Mauger M. 100 cases of transient osteoporosis of the hip in 74 patients. Rev Rhum Mal Osteoartic 1983; 50:401–410.
135. Kaplan SS, Stegman CJ. Transient osteoporosis of the hip: a case report and review of the literature. J Bone Joint Surg [Am] 1985; 67:490–493.
136. Karasick D, Edeiken J. Case report 19. Skel Radiol 1977; 1:181.
137. Nicol RO, Williams PF, Hill DJ. Transient osteopaenia of the hip in children. J Pediatr Orthop 1984; 4:590–592.
138. Gaucher A, Colomb J-N, Naoun AR, Faure G, Netter P. The diagnostic value of ^{99m}Tc-diphosphonate bone imaging in transient osteoporosis of the hip. J Rheumatol 1979; 6:574–583.

139. Bray ST, Partain L, Teates CD, Guilford WB, Williamson BRJ, McLaughlin RC. The value of the bone scan in idiopathic regional migratory osteoporosis. J Nucl Med 1979; 139:1268–1271.
140. Wilson AJ, Murphy WA, Hardy DC, Totty WG. Transient osteoporosis: transient bone marrow edema? Radiology 1988; 167:757–760.
141. Dihlmann W, Thomas W. Diagnostischer Algorithmus fur die transitorische Huftosteoporose—unter Einbeziehung der Computertomographie. ROFO 1983; 138: 214–219.
142. Hauzeur DP, Hanquinet S, Gevenois P-A, Appelboom T, Bentin J, Perlmutter N. Study of magnetic resonance imaging in transient osteoporosis of the hip. J Rheumatol 1991; 18:1211–1217.
143. Urbanski SR, de Lange E, Eschenroeder HC. Magnetic resonance imaging of transient osteoporosis of the hip. J Bone Joint Surg [Am] 1991; 73:451–455.
144. Takatori Y, Kokubo T, Ninomiya S, Nakamura T, Okutsu I, Kamogawa M. Transient osteoporosis of the hip: magnetic resonance imaging. Clin Orthop 1991; 271:190–194.
145. Bloem JL. Transient osteoporosis of the hip: MR imaging. Radiology 1988; 167: 753–755.
146. Hunder GG, Kelly PJ. Roentgenologic transient osteoporosis of the hip. A clinical syndrome? Ann Intern Med 1968; 68:539–552.
147. Dihlmann W, Delling G. Ist die transitorische Huftosteoporose eine transitorische Osteonekrose? Z Rheumatol 1985; 44:82–86.
148. Rosen RA. Transitory demineralization of the femoral head. Radiology 1970; 94:509–512.
149. Swezey RL. Transient osteoporosis of the hip, foot and knee. Arthritis Rheum 1970; 13:858–868.
150. Duncan H, Frame B, Frost H, Arnstein AR. Regional migratory osteoporosis. South Med J 1969; 62:41–44.
151. Steiner RM, McKeever C. Regional migratory osteoporosis. J Can Assoc Radiol 1973; 24:70–75.
152. Gupta RC, Popovtzer MM, Huffer WE, Smyth CJ. Regional migratory osteoporosis. Arthritis Rheum 1973; 16:363–368.
153. McCord WC, Nies KM, Campion DS, Louie JS. Regional migratory osteoporosis: a denervation disease. Arthritis Rheum 1978; 21:834–838.
154. Byrd JW, Ricciardi JM, Jung BI. Regional migratory osteoporosis and tarsal tunnel syndrome. Clin Orthop 1981; 157:164–169.
155. Langloh ND, Hunder GG, Riggs BL, Kelly PJ. Transient painful osteoporosis of the lower extremities. J Bone Joint Surg [Am] 1973; 55:1188–1196.
156. Durivage J, Levesque H-P. L'osteoporose douloureuse transitoire. Union Med Can 1976; 105:562–569.
157. Levy D, Hinterbuckner C. Transient or migratory osteoporosis of lower extremity. NY State J Med 1976; 76:739–742.
158. Jacox RF, Waterhouse C, Taves DR. Transient painful osteolysis—a metabolic study. J Rheumatol 1982; 9:279–283.
159. O'Mara RE, Pinals RS. Bone scanning in regional migratory osteoporosis. Case report. Radiology 1970; 97:579–581.

160. Strashun A, Chayes Z. Migratory osteolysis. J Nucl Med 1979; 20:129.
161. Tannenbaum H, Esdaile J, Rosenthall L. Joint imaging in regional migratory osteoporosis. J Rheumatol 1980; 7:237.
162. Gerster J-C, Jaeger P, Gobelet C, Boivin G. Adult sporadic hypophosphatemic osteomalacia presenting as regional migratory osteoporosis. Arthritis Rheum 1986; 29:688–692.
163. Lequesne M, Kerboull M, Bensasson M, Perez C, Dreiser R, Forest A. Partial transient osteoporosis. Skel Radiol 1977; 2:1.
164. Mitchell SW, Morehouse GR, Keen WW. Gunshot Wounds and Other Injuries of Nerves. Philadelphia: JB Lippincott, 1864.
165. Mitchell SW. Injuries of Nerves and Their Consequences. Philadelphia: JB Lippincott, 1872.
166. Sudeck P. Uber die akute (reflectorische) Knochenatrophie nach Entzundungen and Verletzungen an den Extremitaten und ihre Klinische Erscheinungen. Fortschr Geb Roengenstr Nuklearmed 1901–1902; 5:277.
167. Lenggenhager K. Sudeck's osteodystrophy: its pathogenesis, prophylaxis and therapy. Minn Med 1971; 54:967–972.
168. Fontaine R, Herrmann L. Post-traumatic painful osteoporosis. Ann Surg 1933; 97: 26–61.
169. Steinbrocker O. The shoulder-hand syndrome. Am J Med 1947; 3:402–407.
170. Kozin F, McCarty DJ, Sims J, Genant H. The reflex sympathetic dystrophy syndrome. I. Clinical and histologic studies: evidence for bilaterality, response to corticosteroids and articular involvement. Am J Med 1976; 60:321–331.
171. Kozin F, Genant H, Bekerman C, McCarty DJ. The reflex sympathetic dystrophy syndrome. II. Roentgenographic and scintigraphic evidence for bilaterality and of periarticular accentuation. Am J Med 1976; 60:332–338.
172. Genant HK, Kozin F, Bekerman C, McCarty DJ, Sims J. The reflex sympathetic dystrophy syndrome. A comprehensive analysis using fine-detail radiography, photon absorptiometry, and bone and joint scintigraphy. Radiology 1975; 117:21–32.
173. Bernini PM, Simeone FA. Reflex sympathetic dystrophy associated with low lumbar disc herniation. Spine 1981; 6:180–184.
174. Wysenbeek AJ, Calabrese L, Scherbel AL. Reflex sympathetic dystrophy syndrome complicating polymyalgia rheumatica. Arthritis Rheum 1981; 24:863–864.
175. Michaels RM, Sorber JA. Reflex sympathetic dystrophy as a probable paraneoplastic syndrome: case report and literature review. Arthritis Rheum 1984; 27:1183–1185.
176. Taggart AJ, Iveson JMI, Wright V. Shoulder-hand syndrome and symmetrical arthralgia in patients with tubo-ovarian carcinoma. Ann Rheum Dis 1984; 43:391–393.
177. Medsger TA Jr, Dixon JA, Garwood VF. Palmar fasciitis and polyarthritis associated with ovarian carcinoma. Ann Intern Med 1982; 96:424–431.
178. Ruggeri SB, Athreya BH, Doughty R, Gregg JR, Das MM. Reflex sympathetic dystrophy in children. Clin Orthop 1982; 163:225–230.
179. Rush PJ, Wilmot D, Saunders N, Fladman D, Shore A. Severe reflex neurovascular dystrophy in childhood. Arthritis Rheum 1985; 28:952–956.
180. Lorente de No R. Analysis of the activity of chains of internuncial neurons. J Neurophysiol 1938; 1:207–244.

181. Doupe J, Cullen CH, Chance GQ. Post-traumatic pain and causalgic syndrome. J Neurol Neurosurg Psychiatry 1944; 7:33–48.
182. Lehman EP. Traumatic vasospasm: a study of 4 cases of vasospasm in the upper extremity. Arch Surg 1934; 29:92–107.
183. DeTakats G. Reflex dystrophy of the extremities. Arch Surg 1937; 34:939–956.
184. Miller DS, DeTakats G. Post-traumatic dystrophy of the extremities: Sudeck's atrophy. Surg Gynecol Obstet 1942; 75:558–582.
185. Stolte BH, Stolte JB, Leyten JF. De pathofysiologie van het schouderhandsyndroom. Ned Tijdschr Geneeskd 1970; 114:1208–1209.
186. Hohmann EL, Elde RP, Rysavy JA, Einzig S, Gebhard RL. Innervation of periosteum and bone by sympathetic vasoactive intestinal peptide-containing nerve fibers. Science 1986; 232:868–871.
187. Kim HJ, Kozin F, Johnson RP, Hines R. Reflex sympathetic dystrophy syndrome of the knee following meniscectomy. Report of three cases. Arthritis Rheum 1979; 22: 177–181.
188. Martin VM. Reflex sympathetic dystrophy syndrome of the knee after meniscectomy. Arthritis Rheum 1980; 23:780.
189. Steinbrocker O. The painful shoulder. In: Hollander JL, McCarty DJ Jr, eds. Arthritis and Allied Conditions, 8th ed. Philadelphia: Lea & Febiger; 1942:1461.
190. Doherty M, Watt I, Dieppe P. Apparent bone erosions in painful regional osteoporosis. Rheumatol Rehabil 1980; 5:95–96.
191. Kutzner J, Hahn K, Grimm W, Brod KH. Skelettszintigraphische Untersuchungen bei der Sudeckschen Knochendystrophie. ROFO 1974; 121:361–369.
192. Ryan LM, Carrera GF, Soin JS, Kozin F. Radiographic and scintigraphic changes in patients with the reflex sympathetic dystrophy syndrome. Arthritis Rheum 1980; 23: 741 (abstract).
193. McCarty DJ, Polcyn RE, Collins PA, Gottschalk A. ^{99m}Technetium scintiophotography in arthritis. I. Technic and interpretation. Arthritis Rheum 1970; 13:11–20.
194. Genant HK, Bautovich GJ, Singh M, Lathrop KA, Harper PV. Bone-seeking radionuclides: an in vivo study of factors affecting skeletal uptake. Radiology 1974; 113: 373–382.
195. Laxer RM, Allen RC, Malleson PN, Morrison RT, Petty RE. Technetium-99m methylene diphosphonate bone scans in children with reflex neurovascular dystrophy. J Pediatr 1985; 106:437–440.
196. Doury P, Granier R, Pattin S, Metges PJ. Algodystrophie avec hypofixation a la scintigraphic osseuse par les pyrophosphates de technetium-99m. Sem Hop Paris 1981; 57:1325–1327.
197. Steinbrocker O, Spitzer N, Friedman H. The shoulder-hand syndrome in reflex dystrophy of the upper extremity. Ann Intern Med 1948; 29:22–52.
198. Arlet J, Ficat P, Durroux R, de Gercourt RG. Histopathology of bone and cartilaginous lesions in reflex sympathetic dystrophy (RSD) of the knee: sixteen cases. Rev Rhum Mal Osteoartic 1981; 48:315–321.
199. Basle MF, Rebel A, Renier JC. Bone tissue in reflex sympathetic dystrophy syndrome—Sudeck's atrophy: structural and ultrastructural studies. Metab Bone Dis Relat Res 1983; 4:305–311.

200. Wronski TJ, Morey ER. Inhibition of cortical and trabecular bone formation in the long bones of immobilized monkeys. Clin Orthop 1983; 181:269–276.
201. Jones G. Radiological appearances of disuse osteoporosis. Clin Radiol 1969; 20: 345–353.
202. Keats TE, Harrison RB. A pattern of post-traumatic demineralization of bone simulating permeative neoplastic replacement: a potential source of misinterpretation. Skel Radiol 1978; 3:113.
203. Yagan R, Radivoyevitch M, Khan MA. Double cortical line in the acetabular roof: a sign of disuse osteoporosis. Radiology 1987; 171–175.
204. Mack PB, LaChance PA, Vose GP, Vogt FB. Bone demineralization of foot and hand of Gemini-Titan IV, V, and VII astronauts during orbital flight. AJR 1967; 100: 503–511.
205. Vose GP. Review of roentgenographic bone demineralization studies of the Gemini space flights. AJR 1974; 121:1–4.
206. Bunts RC. Management of urologic complications in 1000 paraplegics. J Urol 1958; 79:733–741.
207. Heaney RP. Radiocalcium metabolism in disuse osteoporosis in man. Am J Med 1962; 33:188–200.
208. Jowsey J. Quantitative microradiography: a new approach in the evaluation of metabolic bone disease. Am J Med 1966; 40:485–491.
209. Mattsson S. The reversibility of disuse osteoporosis: experimental studies in the adult rat. Acta Orthop Scan Suppl 1972; 144:11–12.
210. Jaworski ZF, Liskova-Kiar M, Uhthoff HK. Effect of long-term immobilisation on the pattern of bone loss in older dogs. J Bone Joint Surg [Br] 1980; 62:104–110.
211. Mazess RB, Whedon GD. Immobilization and bone. Calcif Tissue Int 1983; 35: 265–267.
212. Dunning MF, Plum F. Hypercalciuria following poliomyelitis: its relationship to site and degree of paralysis. Arch Intern Med 1957; 99:716–731.
213. Geiser M, Trueta J. Muscle action, bone rarefaction and bone formation. J Bone Joint Surg [Br] 1958; 40:282–290.
214. Vigorita VJ. Osteoporosis: a diagnosable disorder? Pathol Annu 1988; 23:185–212.

7

Noninvasive Methods for Assessment of Bone Density, Architecture, and Biomechanical Properties: Fundamental Concepts

DEXTER M. WONG

University of California, San Diego, Medical Center
San Diego, California

DAVID J. SARTORIS

University of California, San Diego, School of Medicine, and University of California, San Diego, Medical Center
San Diego, California

Osteoporosis is the most common disease of bone and affects millions of people. Osteopenia is any bone condition in which a loss of bone mineral compromises bone strength. Osteoporosis is a subcategory of osteopenia specific to certain populations. Osteoporosis affects all bones in the skeleton, but is particularly likely to induce fractures in the wrist, hip, and spine (1). There are three types of osteoporosis: type I volutional; type II volutional; and secondary osteoporosis (2). Post- and periomenopausal women are a major target population that is susceptible to osteoporosis. Women suffering from periomenopausal, or type I volutional, osteoporosis are likely to suffer from fractures in bone highly composed of trabecular bone such as the wrist and vertebrae (2). Numerous studies have shown that women who have experienced menopause have accelerated bone loss for 5–15 years following the onset of menopause (3). The estimated increased risk of fracture in females over the age of 50 years is +16% for the hip and + 32% for the spine (4). Peak bone mass in humans is reached between the ages of 20 and 30. Bone mineral density after approximately 30 years of age begins to decrease due to a greater relative rate of bone resorption versus bone formation (5). Health problems due to senile, or type II volutional, osteoporosis are evident and clinically significant, especially among populations of people aged 70–80 years (6). Senile osteoporosis affects both cortical and trabecular bone. Thus, fracture frequently occurs in the hip, pelvis, and humerus (2). Secondary osteoporosis is a rarer disease which can be caused by poor health such as hormonal irregularities or improper steroid use (2). In general, the normal populations at greatest risk of osteoporosis are elderly, white, postmenopausal and female (7). Other factors that may be important in the pathogenesis of osteoporosis are low body weight and poor health maintenance such as smoking, alcoholism, and lack of exercise (1).

Osteoporosis and risk of fracture are most commonly evaluated by measuring the bone mineral density (BMD) or bone mineral content (BMC) of the patient (Figure 1). BMD is strongly associated with the strength of bone (8). Thus as BMD decreases, the risk of fracture increases (4). BMD is equal to BMC divided

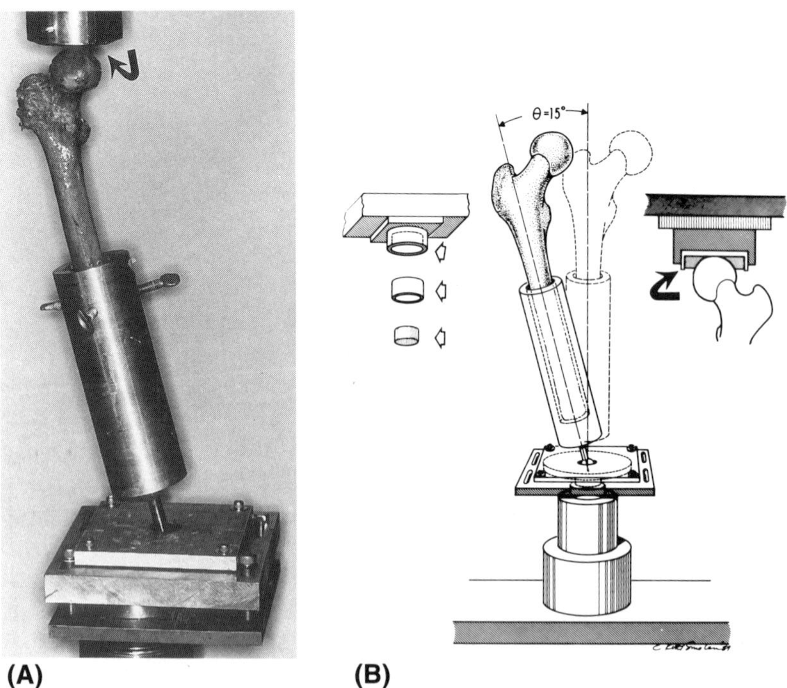

Figure 1 Bone mineral density (BMD) is currently the most measurable, but by no means the only, determinant of bone strength and fracture risk. Strength can be estimated from BMD based on the results of correlative studies involving biomechanical testing of cadaveric specimens: an example is shown of an experimental apparatus designed to simulate hip fracture (A and B; arrows = support components for femoral head). Fracture risk can be estimated from BMD based on the results of long-term longitudinal population studies.

by the projected area or volume of the bone being studied; and is an attempt to normalize for size differences. It is not entirely agreed upon that either measurement is superior over the other in evaluating osteoporosis (9). Numerous studies have shown that a well-defined threshold of bone density separates patients with little risk of osteoporotic fracture and those likely to incur this complication of the disease (7). Thus, as bone density diminishes below the estimated density threshold, the risk of osteoporotic fracture increases significantly (in some studies exponentially).

The cost of osteoporosis is tremendous in terms of morbidity and dollars spent on treatment and prevention. In the United States, there are approximately 1.5 million fractures per year due to osteoporosis. There are an estimated 25 million Americans affected by the condition, 85% of whom are women. Approximately $10 billion per year is spent on the treatment of osteoporosis and management of fractures, with a projected cost of $60 billion by the year 2000 (10).

Preventive measures for combating osteoporosis could ultimately lead to reduced morbidity and lower health care costs. A significant component of a comprehensive prevention program is the detection of osteoporosis at the earliest possible age (Figure 2). In the last 50 years many techniques for bone mass measurement have been developed and refined, enabling the clinician to more effectively diagnose and monitor the treatment of osteoporosis. Specifically, methods for measuring bone density have evolved from in vivo bone biopsies to broad-band ultrasound attenuation and magnetic resonance inferometry. The numerous methods have been extensively compared and tested in controlled prospective experiments and reviewed in epidemiological studies. It is the focus of this chapter to succinctly review the theory and methodology, as well as the advantages and disadvantages, of existing and developing bone densitometric techniques.

In vivo bone biopsies were among the first methods used to measure bone mineral density and trabecular histomorphometry. Bone biopsies are seldom performed in vivo except in patients with undiagnosed forms of metabolic bone disease. Bone biopsies are performed on cadavers when evaluating other bone densitometry techniques in research studies focusing on the accuracy of noninvasive methods. In vivo bone biopsies are too invasive and time-consuming the patient; they also require sophisticated histopathological analysis of the core specimen that is not widely available (4).

Noninvasive techniques are thus used almost exclusively in clinical practice at the present time (Figure 3). The most common and established methods are radiogrammetry (R), radiographic absorptiometry (RA), single-photon absorptiometry (SPA), dual-photon absorptiometry (DPA), single-energy x-ray absorptiometry (SXA), dual-energy x-ray absorptiometry (DXA), quantitative computed tomography (QCT), and ultrasonography (speed of sound [SOS] and broad-band ultrasound attenuation [BUA]). Magnetic resonance (MR) inferometry has been proposed as a possible method for the measurement of bone mass and trabecular

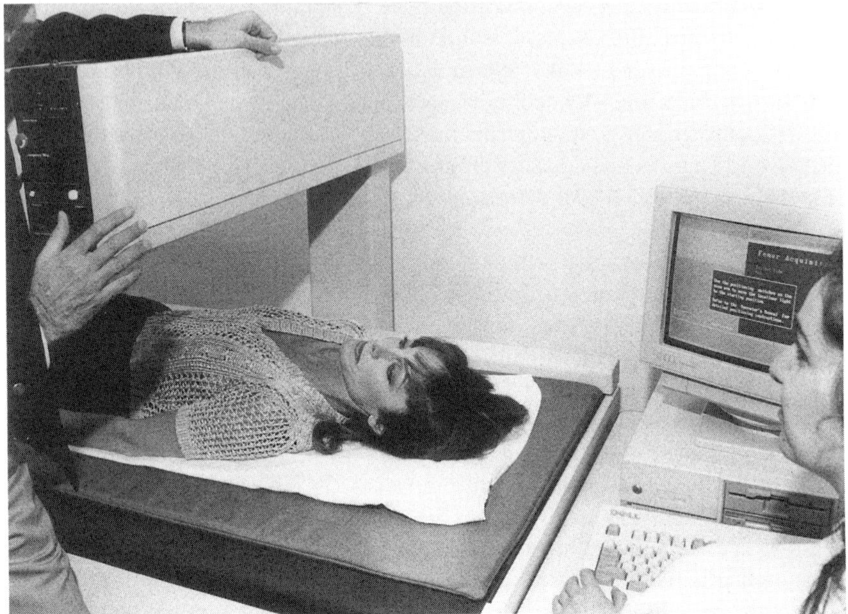

Figure 2 Bone densitometry is an extremely powerful tool for patient education and compliance with lifestyle modification as well as pharmacologic intervention. Communication and explanation of results by the physician are thus essential components of a comprehensive bone mass measurement program. The patient shown has undergone DXA of the proximal femur on a Lunar DPX system.

bone architecture; however, its use remains in the research and development phase.

I. RADIOGRAMMETRY

Radiogrammetry is a noninvasive densitometric method that utilizes roentgenograms of the hand for measuring cortical thickness of the metacarpals (Figure 4). Metacarpal thickness is used to project risk of hip fracture based on estimated extrapolations. Test results of radiogrammetry are poor to controversial (12). The reported inaccuracy is largely due to the irregularities in the shape of the metacarpal cortical regions and intracortical resorption (2).

II. RADIOGRAPHIC ABSORPTIOMETRY

RA was among the first noninvasive techniques for measuring bone density (13). Paired radiographs of the hands provide the necessary information for determining the BMD of the phalanges (7). However, RA has several important shortcomings; the method was initially an inherently labor-intensive, operator-dependent test (14). As a result, the accuracy of RA was poor early in its development. Researchers were also concerned about the low sensitivity of RA since certain studies demonstrated that up to 40% of bone mass may be lost before RA could detect it (11).

Recent improvements in RA, however, may increase the utility of the technique in measuring BMD. Initially, radiographs could be misinterpreted due to film quality, exposure time, and voltage differences (14). Operator variability and error also contributed to the poor reliability and error of RA. A recent review of RA by Yates et al. (14), however, has emphasized the merits of RA. Error in the method can be significantly reduced by careful standardization. By using a standardized aluminum wedge as a calibration phantom placed next to the phalanges during the radiograph, as well as digitized radiographic images and computer analysis, error can be significantly reduced. After exposure the radiographs are sent to a central processing site where this analysis can be performed. At the processing center, a microdensitometer scans the radiograph and computes BMD by averaging the results from the phalanges (15) (Figure 5). One such establishment is the Osteogram company based in Manhattan Beach, California (56). In an investigation, Yang et al. measured a short term in vivo precision of 0.6% for the phalanges (56).

The new developments in RA render it a promising diagnostic tool for selected patients. RA measures primarily appendicular bone, specifically the middle phalanges. There are valid concerns that measurement of BMD in the appendicular skeleton may not accurately predict bone mineral content of the axial skeleton (7). Presently, RA is at best a simple, low-cost, low-risk screening tool for osteoporosis (15). Improvements and extensive studies of RA will perhaps increase its utility in diagnosing and monitoring osteoporosis.

III. SINGLE-PHOTON ABSORPTIOMETRY

SPA was first introduced in 1963 by Cameron and Sorenson (16). SPA measures the BMD of the appendicular skeleton. Osteoporosis of the appendicular skeleton can be detected directly from such BMD measurements, and used to estimate bone mass in other portions of the skeleton such as the vertebrae and hip. SPA is best employed in areas where soft-tissue thickness is constant. Some studies have shown that BMD of the radius or calcaneus is useful for prediction of fracture risk in other parts of the skeleton, particularly the vertebral column (17). In fact, bone mass determination at any site in the skeleton can predict fracture risk locations (18), although not as well as site-specific measurements.

SPA is most useful when employed at the distal third of the radius, which is approximately 95% cortical bone and 5% trabecular bone. The relatively higher cancellous bone content of the distal radius as compared to more proximal sites renders it the best region for BMD measurement (7). SPA utilizes a single-photon

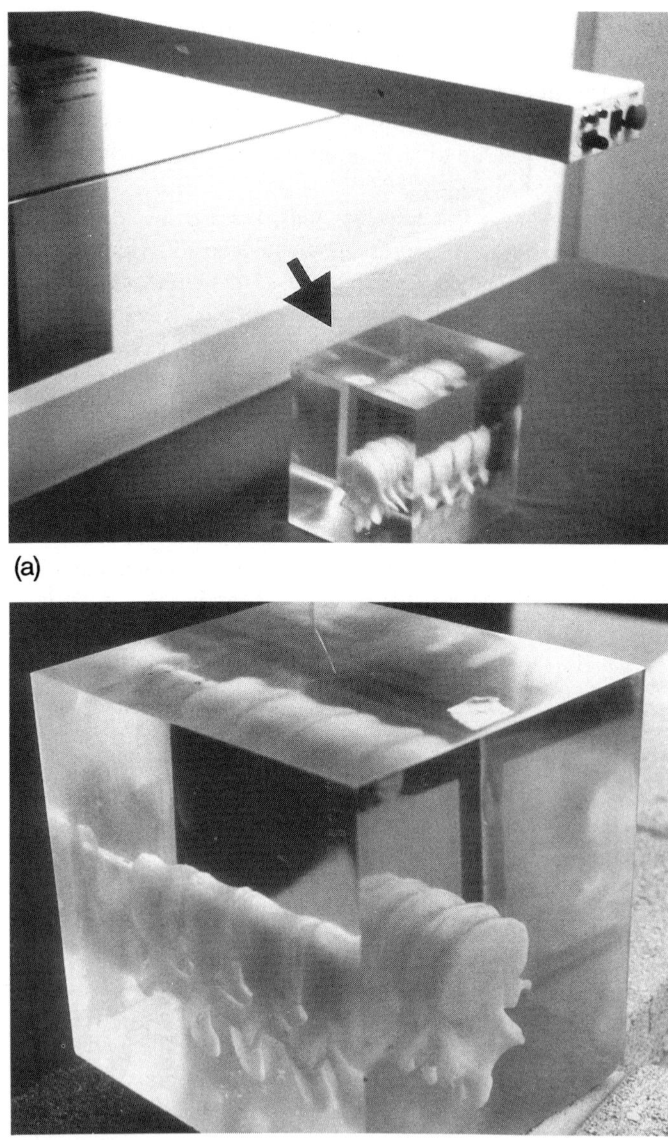

(a)

(b)

Figure 3 (a) Daily calibration scans of a bone- and tissue-equivalent phantom (arrow) are essential to ensure acceptable system accuracy and precision, particularly with dedicated densitometric methods such as DXA (a Hologic QDR-1000 system is shown). (b, c) The Hologic anthropomorphic spine phantom contains 58.0 ± 0.3 g calcium hydroxyapatite excluding the transverse processes (which add −2%) and was the first calibration phantom developed specifically for DXA. It remains widely utilized for both clinical and research applications.

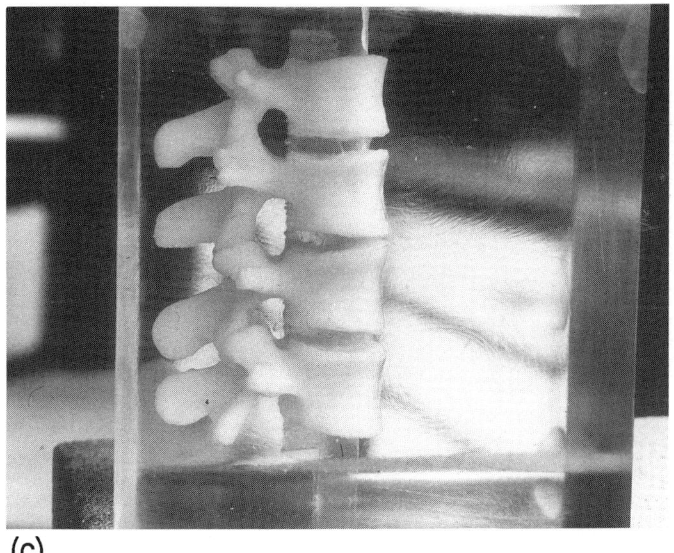

(c)

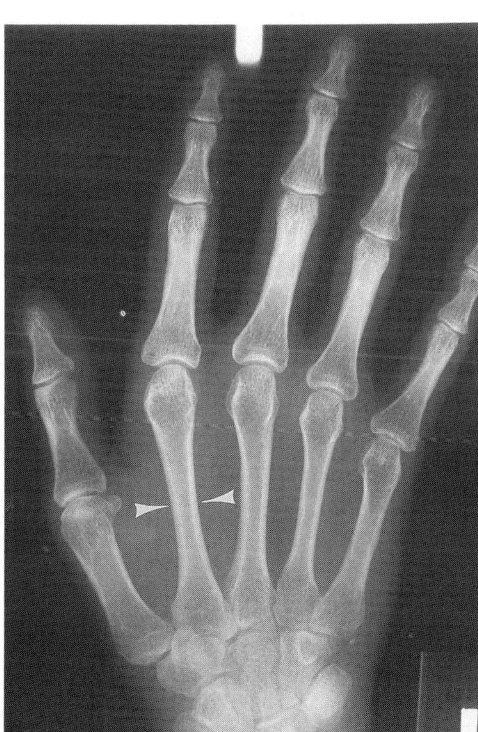

Figure 4 Radiogrammetry. Cortical thickness measurements of the middiaphysis of the second metacarpal bone (arrowheads) are corrected for bone width and compared to normative standards available in the literature.

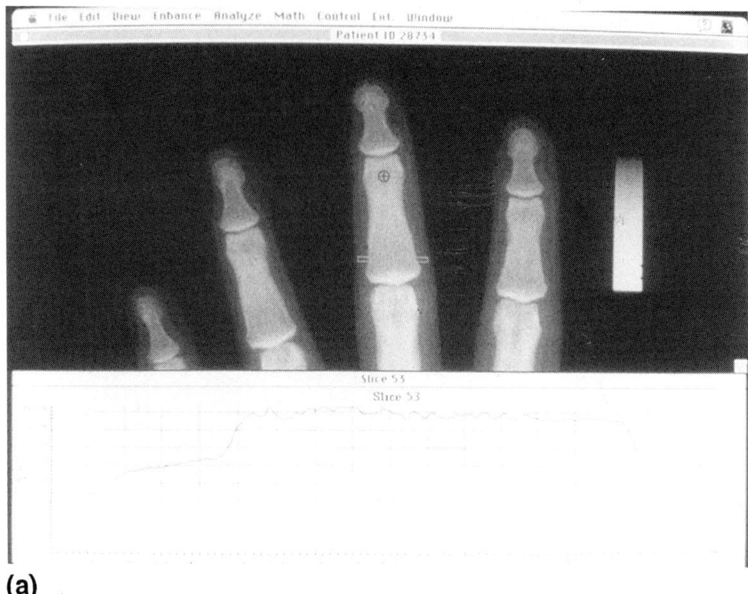

(a)

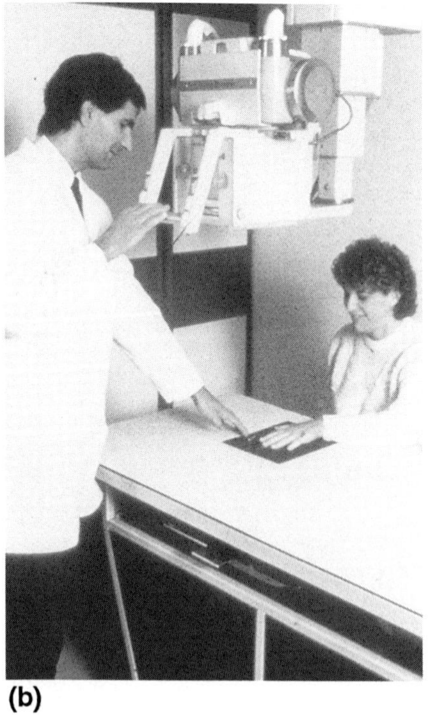

(b)

Figure 5 Radiographic absorptiometry. Computerized density analysis of the second through fourth middle phalanges (a) is performed on paired conventional radiographs using different technical factors (b). (Courtesy of Compumed Corporation, Manhattan Beach, CA.)

source of either ^{125}I or ^{241}Am (19). ^{125}I and ^{241}Am have photon energies of 28 keV and 60 keV, respectively (7). Measurement of BMD by SPA requires that the patient immerse the forearm in a water bath or use tissue-equivalent bracelets to compensate for variations in soft-tissue thickness (skin, muscle, fatty tissue, etc.) (20,21). A narrow beam of photons of approximately 1–3 mm in diameter is projected through the water bath or tissue-equivalent material surrounding the forearm. The transmitted radiation is then collected by a sodium iodide crystal radiation detector (22). Attenuation of photons results in a highly reproducible BMC measurement (11,16). The in vitro precision error of the method has been determined to be as low as 0.1–0.3% (20,21).

SPA is a useful and clinically proven tool for BMD measurement. The procedure is relatively easy to perform and has acceptable in vivo reproducibility. The scan times are usually 10 minutes or less and the method exposes the patient to less than 0.1 mrem total dose (4). Bone densitometry of the distal radius provides a useful technique for predicting risk of forearm fracture (23). The BMD of the distal radius can be used by the clinician to estimate the extent of osteoporosis in other parts of the skeleton, such as the hip, vertebrae, and other appendicular sites (4). Although the technique has been time-tested as a reliable diagnostic tool, SPA is not without significant drawbacks.

SPA requires the use of a water bath or other tissue-equivalent material to provide reliable measurements. A water bath is cumbersome and may introduce significant error in the BMC measurement. Because SPA is confined to sites where soft-tissue thickness is low and bone is relatively homogeneous, measurements are usually performed on the calcaneus or distal radius. These determinations are used to infer fracture risk in other parts of the skeleton. There is significant controversy over the accuracy of predicting fracture in other parts of the skeleton from measurements at these sites. However, SPA is relatively inexpensive as compared to other recently developed methods for bone densitometry. SPA requires costly biannual replacement of the ^{125}I photon source (17). This problem has recently been overcome by the development of single-energy x-ray absorptiometry, which utilizes similar technical principles but replaces the radionuclide source with an x-ray tube. The x-ray source is more reliable, more durable, and less costly than the photon source (24). Though SXA is a relatively new tool with few prospective studies completed, BMD measurements should be comparable to or better than SPA (24).

IV. DUAL-PHOTON ABSORPTIOMETRY; SINGLE-ENERGY X-RAY ABSORPTIOMETRY

The evolution of SPA led to the implementation of a dual-photon source in the technique known as dual-photon absorptiometry, or DPA, which is capable of measuring BMD at axial skeletal sites SXA. As of 1989, DPA was used in over 1,000 health care systems and clinics for bone density measurements (25). The radioactive source for DPA is usually ^{153}Gd, which simultaneously emits photon energies of 44 keV and 100 keV (7). DPA is a more versatile densitometric method than SPA, in that it can be used to measure predominantly trabecular bone of the lumbar spine and proximal femur (26). Direct measurement of the spine and hip was an improvement over SPA, which estimates axial skeletal bone mass from appendicular BMD measurements. Dual-photon energies allow for selective tissue subtraction and eliminate the need for a water bath or tissue-equivalent material when measuring BMD. In DPA, attenuation of the photon beams by bone is significantly greater than by soft tissue. Attenuation due to soft tissue can be subtracted using a mathematical equation based on differences in energy-dependent absorption between bone and soft tissue, leaving attenuation values due exclusively to bone (4).

Although DPA has proven its utility in clinical settings, the method also has significant drawbacks. The scanning time required for the spine or proximal femur is approximately 15–30 minutes, exposing the patient to 0.5 mrem. Comparatively, SPA of the calcaneus exposes the patient to less than 0.1 mrem, and the procedure takes from 5 to 10 minutes (4). Longer scan times are more uncomfortable for the patient, and there is more chance that the subject may move during the procedure, compromising precision and accuracy. There is also concern over the ability of DPA to measure bone mineral changes in patients over an acceptable period of time, owing to its relatively high precision error. Furthermore, integration of cancellous and compact bone by DPA is not as desirable as selective assessment of high-turnover trabecular bone as afforded by quantitative computed tomography (QCT).

The effectiveness of DPA is particularly compromised in elderly and severely osteoporotic populations (7). Extraosseous calcification in the arteries and degenerative deformities or fractures in the vertebrae can reduce the reproducibility and accuracy of DPA (27). Some of the shortcomings of DPA have been overcome by the development of dual-energy x-ray absorptiometry, or DXA.

V. DUAL-ENERGY X-RAY ABSORPTIOMETRY

DXA became commercially available in 1987 (7) (Figure 6). DXA uses a radiographic source as opposed to the radionuclides used in SPA and DPA (4). Selective energy switching or a k-edge filter produces a dual-energy incident x-ray, analogous to the output of ^{153}Gd in DPA (22) (Figure 7). There are approximately 2,500 DXA systems currently being utilized in hospitals and clinics worldwide (4). DXA is capable of determining BMD in the lumbar spine (both frontal and lateral projections) (Figure 8), proximal femur, total body (Figure 9), and any appendicular site (4) (Figures 10, 11).

DXA is more versatile than SPA and is better in many respects than DPA. Firstly, DXA measurements compensate for variable soft-tissue thickness in a manner analogous to DPA (4). Secondly, DXA can measure varying amounts of both cancellous and cortical bone in the axial skeleton, whereas SPA is limited to measuring primarily appendicular sites where cortical bone generally predominates (4). Thirdly, the cost to operate DXA is lower than that of SPA and DPA as repeated radioisotope source replacements are unnecessary (28). Studies have shown that DXA has a significantly lower precision error at all sites than DPA, and is hence better for monitoring changes in bone mass over shorter periods of time (7) (Figure 12).

DXA also requires a shorter scan time for the patient, which helps to provide better accuracy. Also, the radiation exposure for a DXA scan is significantly lower than that of DPA. For example, a typical DXA scan of the proximal femur takes approximately 5–10 minutes and exposes the patient to 0.1 mrem (Figure 13), whereas a DPA scan of the same site requires up to 30 minutes while exposing the patient to 0.3–0.5 mrem (4). In general, DXA exposes patients to relatively low levels of radiation, equivalent to $<1\%$ of the average natural background radiation that humans experience (29). Overall, the resolution of the DXA image is better than that of DPA and approaches that of a radiograph with the latest systems (30) (Figure 14). Its diagnostic sensitivity is comparable to that of DPA for lumbar spine measurements (31) and highly correlated ($r = .97$) with BMD measurements obtained by SPA (28). DXA is perhaps the best absorptiometric tool of those currently available on the market, and is rapidly replacing the use of DPA worldwide. However, SPA and SXA remain useful tools, particularly for measuring BMD of the distal radius and predicting risk of forearm fracture.

DXA is thus an effective and accurate tool for noninvasive bone mass measurement. However, the DXA machine is relatively expensive and cumbersome, and the technique is inherently unable to selectively measure high-turnover cancellous bone owing to its projectional nature (32). Lack of portability and high equipment cost may inhibit certain clinics and private practices from implementing DXA on a larger scale.

VI. QUANTITATIVE COMPUTED TOMOGRAPHY

Noninvasive, cross-sectional methods have also been developed and used by clinicians and researchers worldwide. Quantitative computed tomography (QCT) is an effective cross-sectional bone densitometric method that is used mainly for measuring BMD of the thoracolumbar spine. Vertebral trabecular bone is measured because of its high turnover rate; cancellous bone is more sensitive to the effects of aging, treatment, and disease than cortical bone owing to its approximately eightfold greater surface area for cellular activity (33). Therefore, QCT can effectively monitor changes in bone density over time due to the positive influences of treatment and/or exercise, or the deleterious effects of aging, menopause, and disease. QCT has become a more popular bone densitometric technique over the past 15 years, and was developed at the University of California, San Francisco (7). It utilizes an imaging CT scanner, a single- or dual-energy source, and mineral phantoms for calibration of the scan (7). Cann and Genant

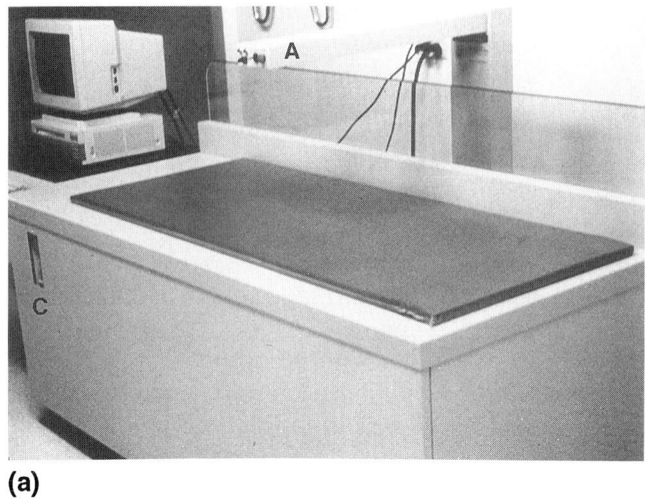

(a)

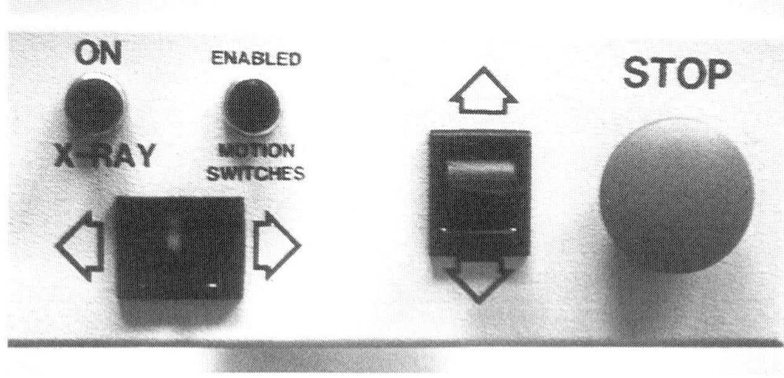

(b)

Figure 6 (a) The Hologic QDR-1000 device was the first commercially available DXA system, introduced in 1987 (A = detector arm; C = computer diskette drive for scan archiving). (b, c) Close-up views of detector arm positioning controls and computer monitor, printer, and keyboard. (d) Frontal lumbar spine scan and data from one of the earliest clinical studies performed on the system, as part of multicenter establishment of normative data for this emerging technology.

(34) introduced a simultaneous calibration system. In this approach the patient lies on a surface containing mineral samples of known densities which are perpendicular to the plane of the axial CT slices; the phantom consists of bone, fat, and water equivalents. The phantom bone material is usually dipotassium hydrogen phosphate (K_2HPO_4), which closely approximates the attenuation characteristics of calcium hydroxyapatite ($Ca_{10}(PO_4)_6(OH)_2$) in mineralized bone (7). The phantom facilitates accurate measurement of bone density via a linear regression and

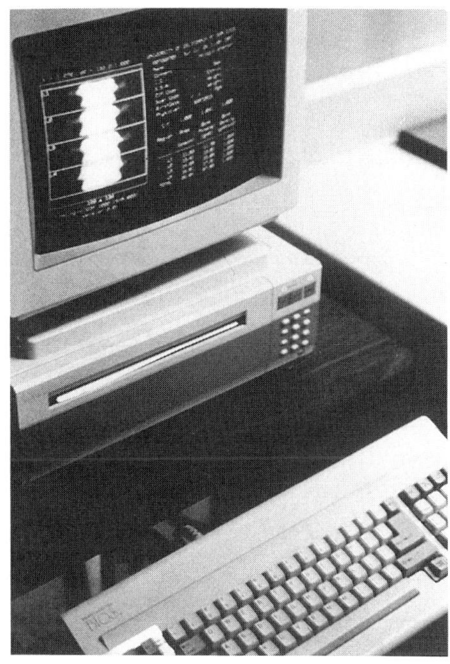

(c)

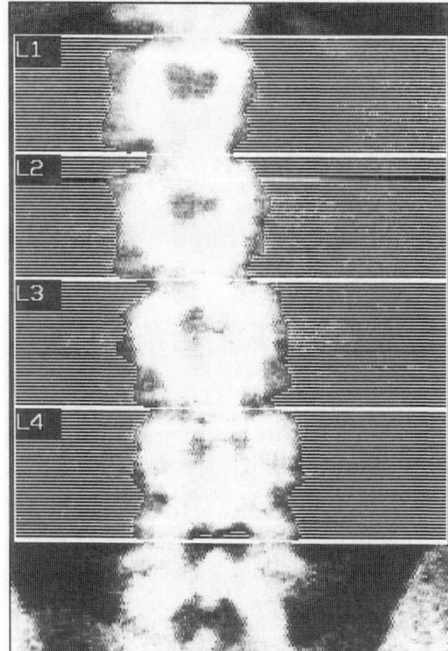

UNIVERSITY OF CALIFORNIA AT SAN DIEGO
A0806870C Thu Aug 06 16:06 1987
Name:
Comment: volunteer
I.D.: Sex: F
S.S.#: 548-72-5812 Ethnic: W
ZIP Code: 92105 Height:5'5 "
Scan Code: Weight: 132
BirthDate: 07/22/48 Age: 39
Physician: DR. SARTOIS

C.F. 1.000 1.041 1.000

Region	Area (cmxcm)	Bone Mineral (gHA)	Bone Density (gHA/cm2)
L1	12.92	13.11	1.015
L2	14.11	15.72	1.114
L3	15.75	18.31	1.162
L4	16.89	18.70	1.107
TOTAL	59.68	65.84	1.103

(d)

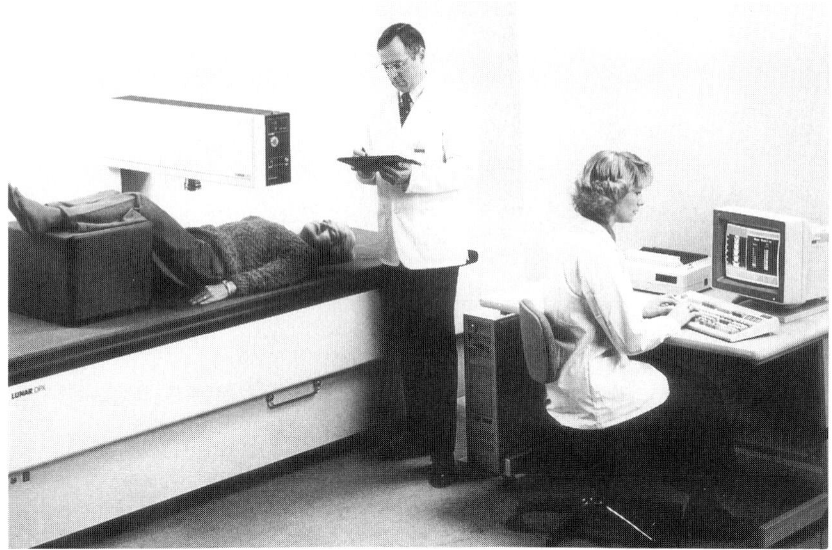

Figure 7 Selective K-edge filtration-type dual-energy x-ray absorptiometer. The patient is undergoing a lumbar spine density measurement on a Lunar DPX system.

interpolation. A tissue-equivalent material is placed between the patient and the phantom to negate the influence of air on the calculated CT densities (7). The examination takes approximately 20 minutes excluding analysis time. Attenuation values for the region of interest (ROI) are corrected, averaged, and plotted against normative data for age, gender, and ethnicity (4).

There are several advantages of QCT over projectional techniques for measuring BMD. QCT independently measures trabecular BMD and can also selectively evaluate cortical bone, unlike DXA (Figure 15). Three-dimensional histograms can also be generated from QCT images, allowing the radiologist to study osseous architecture (4). In addition to bone density, osseous architecture is an important determinant of bone strength. SPA, DPA, and DXA cannot optimally evaluate three-dimensional structure of a bone.

Several investigations demonstrated an apparent superiority of QCT over SPA and DPA. The three most common bone densitometry techniques used for assessment of osteoporosis are SPA, QCT, and DPA. Vertebral osteoporosis has recently been targeted in a comparative study by Heuck et al. (35). Testing was performed on 68 postmenopausal women with varying degrees of vertebral compression fracture. Extensive testing and statistical analysis revealed that QCT was the best discriminator in separating subjects with mild deformity from true fracture pa-

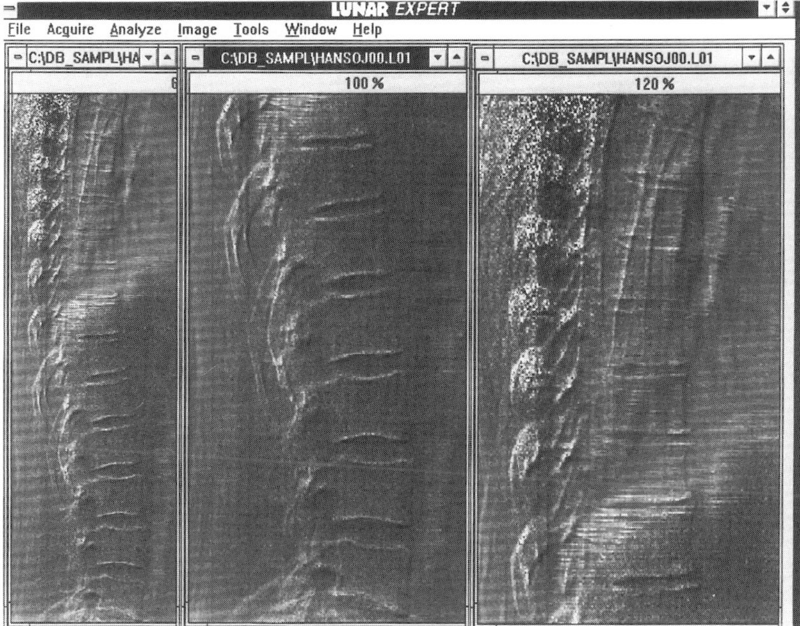

(a)

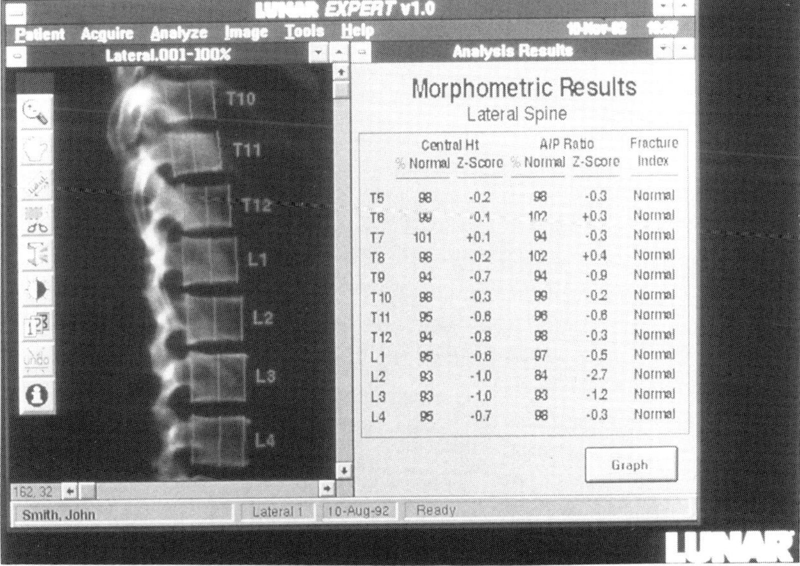

(b)

Figure 8 (a) Lateral DXA of the thoracolumbar spine using a Lunar Expert system (*EXPERT* 12-minute acquisition, 84-kg, 44-year-old male). Such images not only afford bone mineral density measurement but can also be combined with morphometric analysis (b) as an index of vertebral body deformation secondary to metabolic bone disease.

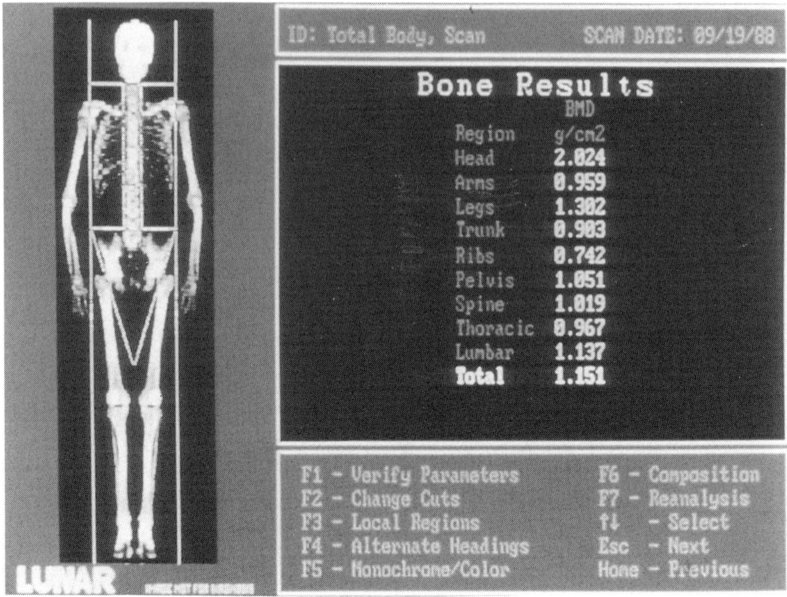

Figure 9 DXA image and data from a total body scan, obtained using a Lunar DPX system. Body fat and lean body mass can be measured from the same scan data, thus providing a comprehensive assessment of body tissue composition.

tients. SPA was deemed statistically insignificant in predicting vertebral fracture (35). An additional study has proven the efficacy of QCT; in this study of 45 bone samples, BMD measurements obtained by this method incurred only a 1.4% accuracy error (36).

QCT is a powerful tool for measuring bone mineral density changes since it directly measures trabecular bone, which has a higher turnover rate than cortical bone (36). Cancellous bone will reflect rapid and subtle variations due to osteoporosis and other diseases, aging, and treatment. QCT measurements also exclude calcium deposits in body tissue, such as aortic calcification (7). Projectional methods, on the other hand, do not compensate for extraneous ossification related to degenerative disease, which can compromise the accuracy of BMD measurements (Figure 16). Overall, QCT provides an excellent measurement of BMD in the spine. (37)

However, QCT exposes the patient to the highest dose of radiation of all densitometric methods. A single- or dual-energy scan can expose the patient to several dozen millirems, whereas a typical lateral spine DXA measurement involves a dose of only 0.3 mrem. The typical QCT scan times are 20–25 minutes, considerably longer than most current absorptiometric scan times (4). Although QCT is accurate in measuring trabecular bone of the thoracolumbar spine, Hayes

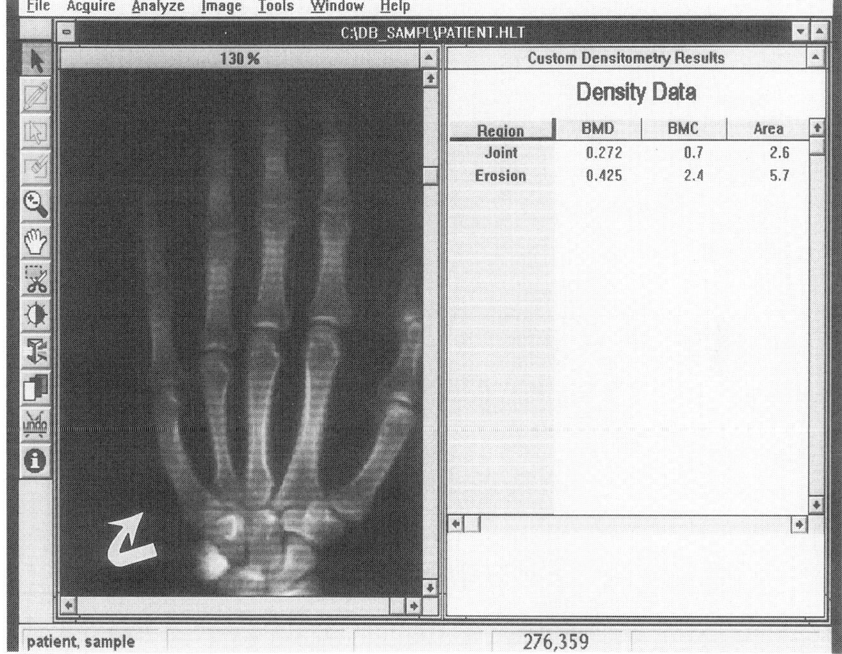

Figure 10 A recent experimental application of DXA and other techniques involves the measurement of periarticular bone density alterations secondary to erosive disease and hyperemia among patients with inflammatory articular disorders such as rheumatoid arthritis. A frontal image of the hand and wrist is shown (arrow), obtained on a Lunar Expert system (*EXPERT* 20-second acquisition, 86-kg, 44-year-old white male).

et al. have reported that determinations of cortical bone density by QCT are inaccurate (37).

QCT is an established and clinically proven method for measuring BMD despite high radiation exposure, relatively inferior precision and accuracy, and inability to study extraspinal sites without a dedicated system. Future modifications and improvements should render QCT more efficacious in the diagnosis and management of osteoporosis.

Peripheral QCT (pQCT) is one of the newer techniques developed to assess bone density. Peripheral QCT measures bone density of the appendicular skeleton, such as the radius and the tibia. PQCT systems measure trabecular and cortical bone density independently (38) (Figure 17). This offers a distinct advantage over SPA and SXA of the distal forearm, which are limited to evaluating chiefly cortical bone (39).

PQCT is performed in a manner similar to that of conventional QCT. The peripheral bone of interest is scanned in precise slices over a preestablished area using a thickness of several millimeters. The most commonly measured site is the

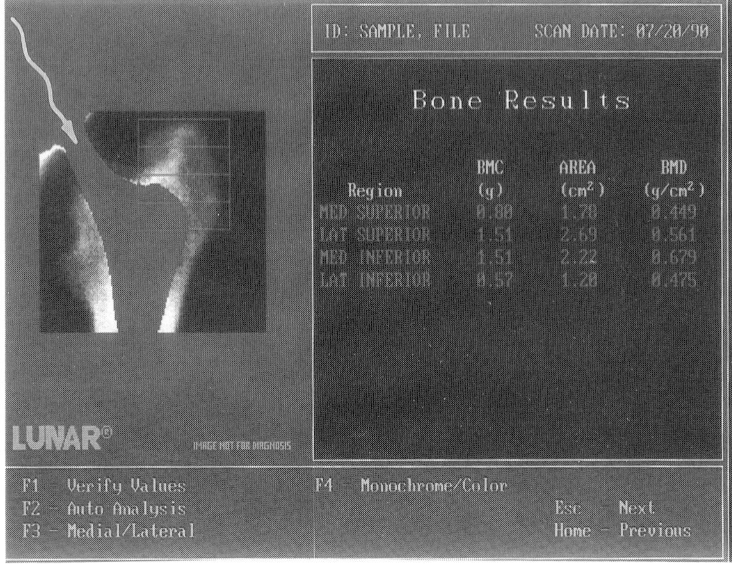

(a)

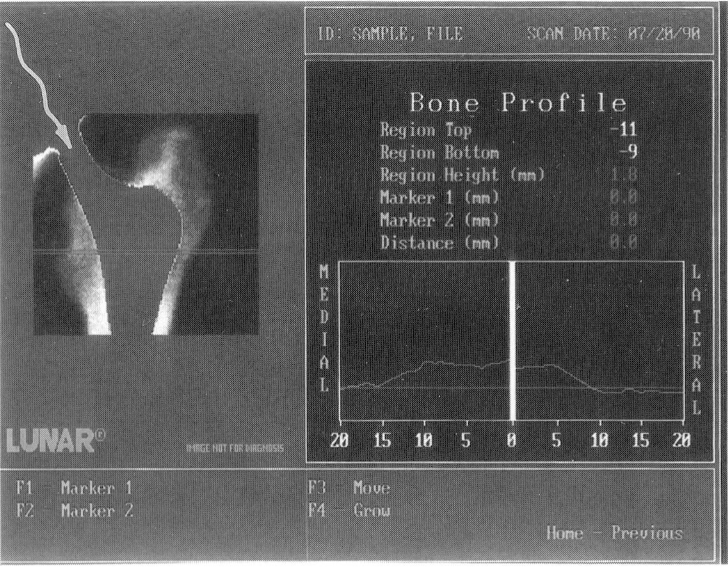

(b)

Figure 11 An important investigational application of DXA as a potential tool in orthopedic surgery is the evaluation of bone density changes related to internal fixation hardware. (a) Following total hip replacement (arrow), bone mineral density is measured in various regions-of-interest around the femoral component. (b) An alternative approach involves line-by-line analysis of bone density profiles across selected portions of the component (arrow). Either method can be used to gauge the extent of stress-shielding and possibly to predict early loosening or histiocytic reaction to the hardware and/or polymethylmethacrylate cement.

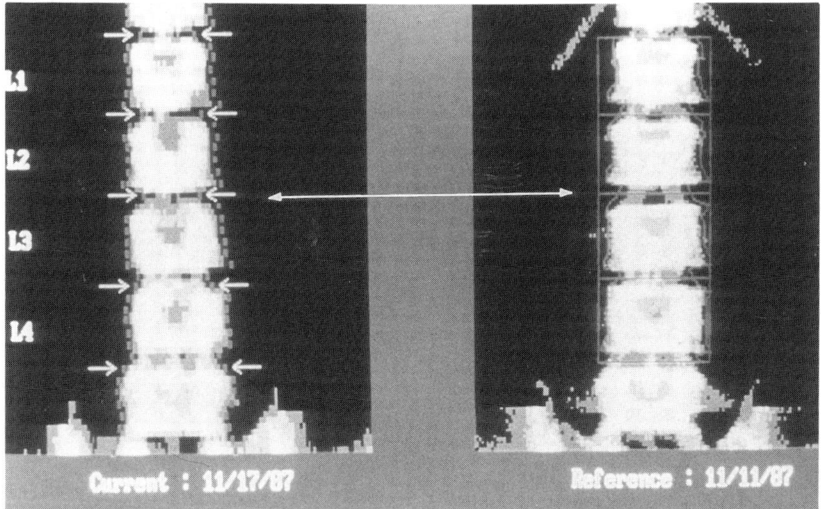

Figure 12 The software of most dedicated bone densitometry systems has a comparison function which affords reproducible placement of regions-of-interest (double-headed arrow), thus facilitating low precision error on longitudinal studies of a given patient. This allows confident detection of smaller incremental changes in bone density over time; frontal DXA scans of the lumbar spine are shown, derived from a Lunar DPX system.

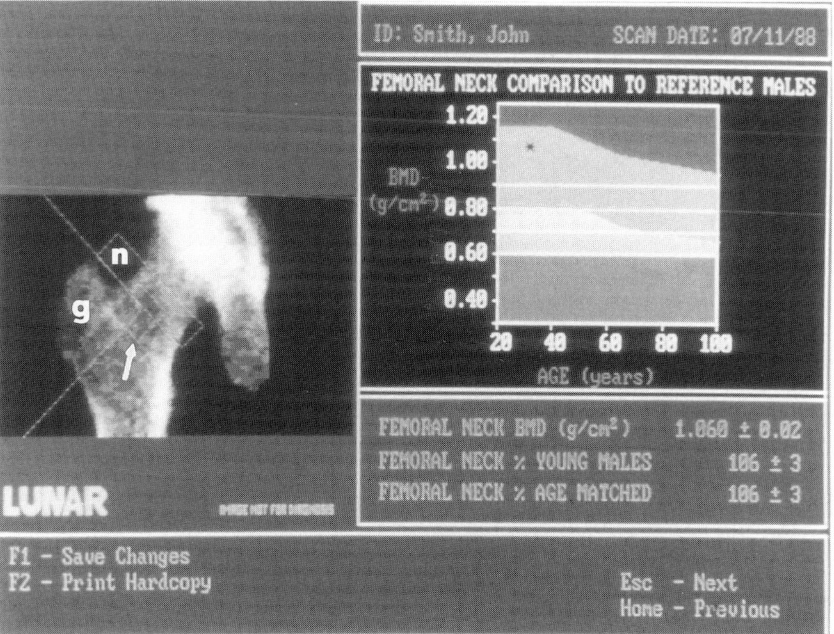

Figure 13 DXA image and data from a proximal femur scan obtained on a Lunar DPX system. Regions-of-interest studied by all commercially available DXA scanners include the femoral neck (n), Ward's triangle (arrow), and the greater trochanter (g.).

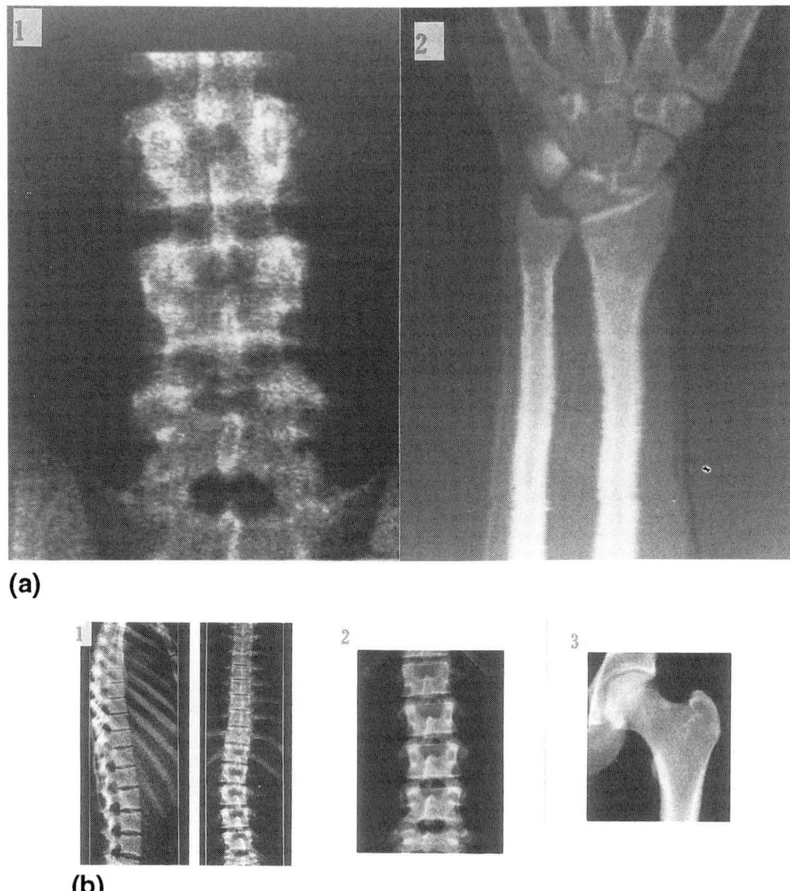

Figure 14 Image quality and spatial resolution have continued to improve with the evolution of DXA technology, approaching those of conventional radiography, without the distortion and soft-tissue interference inherent in the latter. (a) Frontal images of the lumbar spine (1) and forearm (2) generated by a Hologic QDR-1000 system. (b) A Hologic QDR-2000 Plus device was used to produce these lateral and frontal images of the thoracolumbar spine (1), frontal image of the lumbar spine (2) and frontal image of the proximal femur (3).

ultradistal portion of the forearm. This region of the forearm is the common site of Colles fracture (40), which frequently occurs in patients with low bone density and relatively minor trauma.

Calibration of the equipment is performed by scanning phantoms of known calcium hydroxyapatite content. In a recent study by Butz et al., in vivo precision error of the model XCT 900 pQCT machine was found to be extremely low (mean coefficient of variation of 1.08%) (38).

Relatively few studies involving pQCT have been performed to date, although results have been fairly promising. In the study by Butz et al., significant correlation was observed between pQCT of the radius and DXA of the femoral neck; in contrast, there were low coefficients of correlation (0.4% to 0.5%) between pQCT and DXA of the lumbar spine (41).

VII. ULTRASONOGRAPHY

There was no correlation between radial pQCT and BUA as determined by ultrasonography (38). Another study has indicated a good correlation between pQCT of the forearm and SPA of the distal radius. In another study, patients with Colles fracture had their distal forearms measured for BMD by SPA; results were between 3% and 12% lower in these patients than in age-matched control subjects (42). In a similar study of Colles fracture patients versus controls, QCT of the distal forearm in the fracture group was 9% lower for cortical MLS (mass per unit length), and 23% lower for trabecular TBD (trabecular bone density) (43). These studies illustrate a potential role for pQCT in assessing risk of Colles fracture.

The observed good correlation between pQCT of the forearm and DXA of the femoral neck indicates that it may be a useful tool for predicting hip fractures. Furthermore, in a study by Smith et al., TBD of the distal forearm by pQCT was found to be 36% lower in vertebral fracture patients than in age-matched control patients (42). Unfortunately, the accepted range of "normal" trabecular bone density is relatively large. In light of these arguments, the use of pQCT as a diagnostic tool is not recommended until further refinements are made. However, its use as a clinical method for monitoring large changes in BMD is well documented.

Ultrasound is another relatively new technique for measuring bone density. It was first introduced by Langton et al. in 1984 (44). There is a direct mathematical relationship among the velocity, intensity, and shape of a sound wave propagating through a medium and its stiffness and mass density (45); specifically, sound waves are affected by bone mass and bone architecture (46). These principles are the basis for broad-band ultrasound attenuation (BUA) in bone densitometry. An incident wave is projected through bone, and a resultant wave is recorded. Subtracting the incident wave from the resultant wave provides information that is used to derive bone density (45).

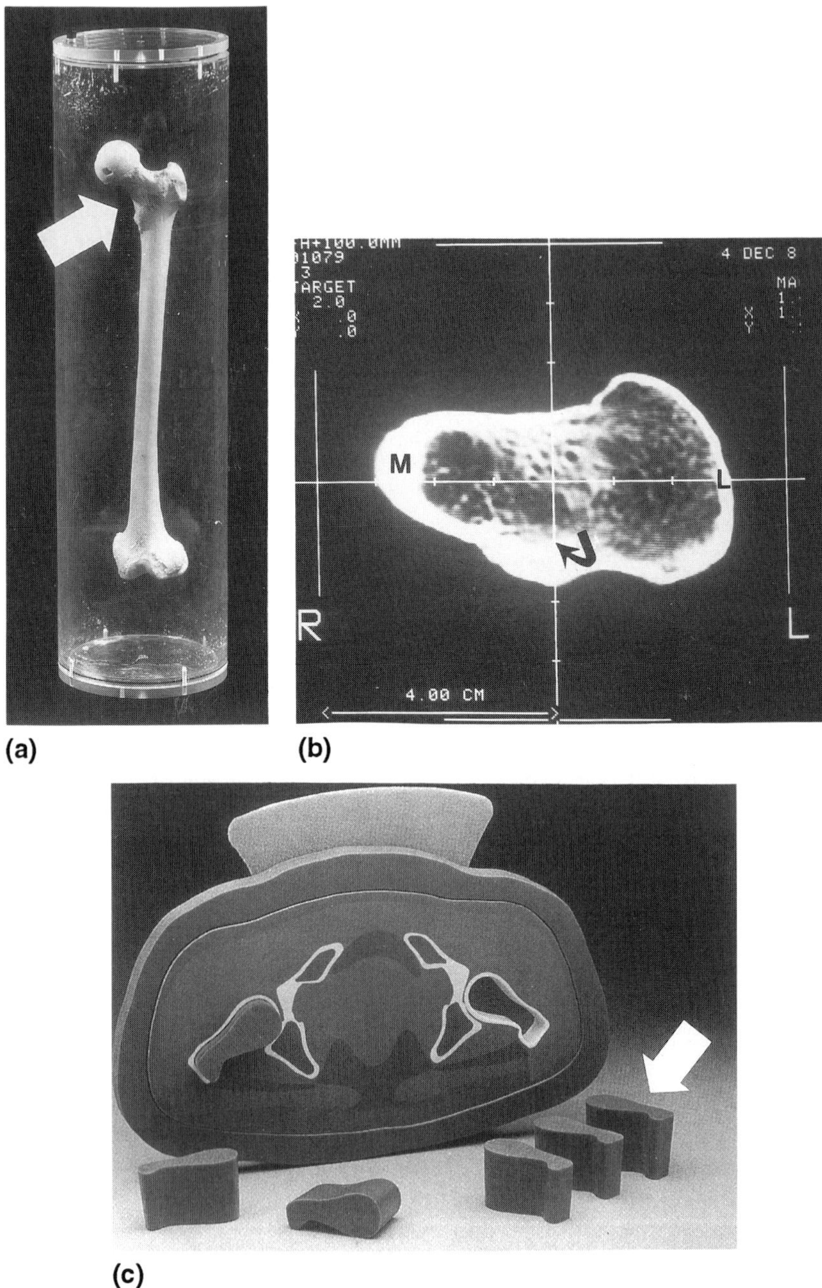

Figure 15 (a) Owing to its inherently complex architecture, the proximal femur (arrow) has always been more amenable to reproducible bone mass measurement using projectional as opposed to cross-sectional techniques. However, quantitative computed tomography has been performed at this site using CT scanners designed for imaging (b; M = medial cortex, L = lateral cortex, arrow = region of Ward's triangle) rather than dedicated bone densitometry, which is currently under development for this region. Correction for variations in

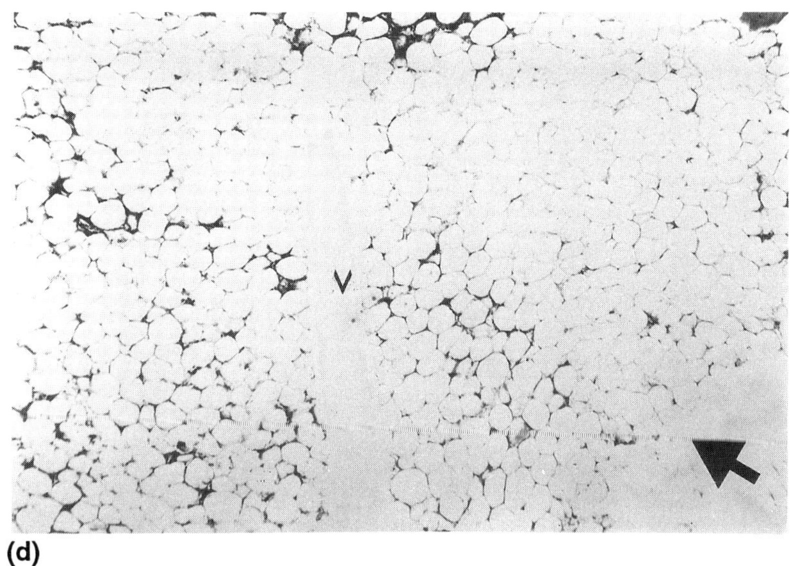

(d)

x-ray tube output over time is achieved by linear regression and interpolation analysis, after scanning either a body-torso or other calibration phantom (c) containing variable known quantities of a mineral equivalent material (such as dipotassium hydrogen phosphate or calcium hydroxyapatite [arrow]). (d) The major advantage of cross-sectional over projectional densitometric methods is their unique ability to selectively measure high-turnover trabecular bone (arrow), which has an approximately eightfold greater surface area for cellular activity as compared to cortical bone. (V = vascular channel in sectioned vertebral body).

The calcaneus or heel is often the site of BUA measurements (Figure 18). Although the calcaneus is not a common fracture site, it is comprised of approximately 90% cancellous bone (47). The high bone turnover rate at the heel renders it a theoretically useful area in which to estimate bone mass and response to treatment in other parts of the skeleton. BUA of the calcaneus is highly correlated to BMD of the spine and hip (48). To measure BMD by BUA, the heel is placed in a water bath between two ultrasound transducers after an initial baseline measurement in the empty water bath. To negate the effects of the dermis on the ultrasound measurements, the skin must initially be soaked in the water bath for about 4 minutes (4). Subsequently, an ultrasonic wave is projected through the water bath and heel (4). Attenuation results are then collected and processed into BMD values.

BUA is a relatively new and promising tool in bone densitometry. BUA does not expose the patient to ionizing radiation, unlike QCT and absorptiometric techniques. BUA also can evaluate the spatial architecture of the bone. Knowledge of the three-dimensional osseous structure is helpful in determining bone

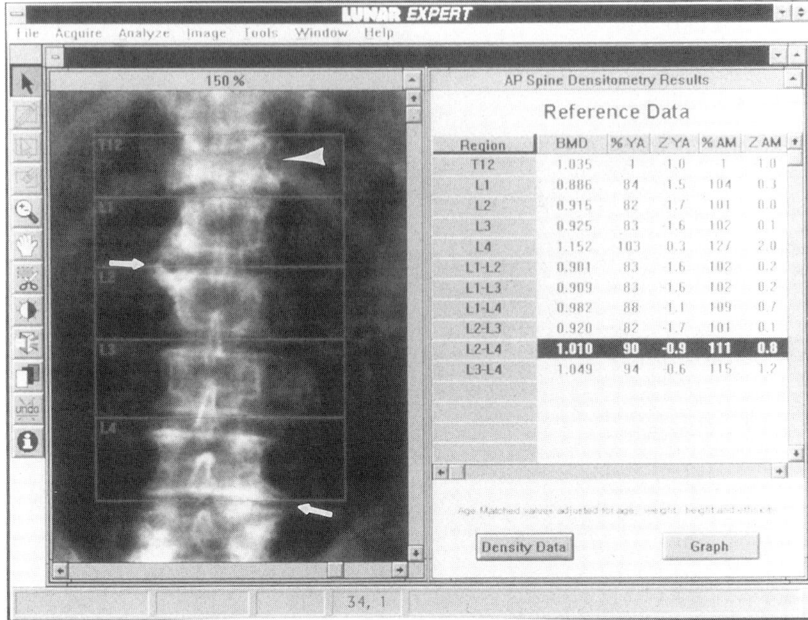

Figure 16 High-resolution DXA image and data from a lumbar spine scan in the frontal projection, obtained on a Lunar Expert system. False elevation of the measured BMD values at several levels is caused by spinal degenerative disease (arrows) and a compression fracture of T12 (arrowhead).

strength (47). BUA is also an inexpensive densitometric test (49), and preliminary testing has shown promising results. In investigations comparing BUA to other densitometric tests, the ultrasound method has performed comparably. In a recent study involving 87 healthy patients and 17 patients with osteoporosis, BUA of the calcaneus was compared to DXA of the femoral neck. It is well established that with age, bone density decreases; BUA correlated with increasing age at $r = -0.44$, while DXA of the femoral neck correlated with age at $r = -0.43$ (46). BUA is not, however, without limitations, since the variability in measurements is suspect (50). Also, the reproducibility of BUA measurements have been poor to average. Poor reproducibility may be due in part to water bath temperature variation and differences in foot positioning (49).

The consensus among researchers studying BUA is that this densitiometric method, though not yet perfected, is a promising tool for the diagnosis of osteoporosis. BUA is relatively inexpensive, emits no radiation, can detect both structure and bone density, and is relatively easy to use.

Magnetic resonance imaging (MRI) is another nonionizing bone densitometric

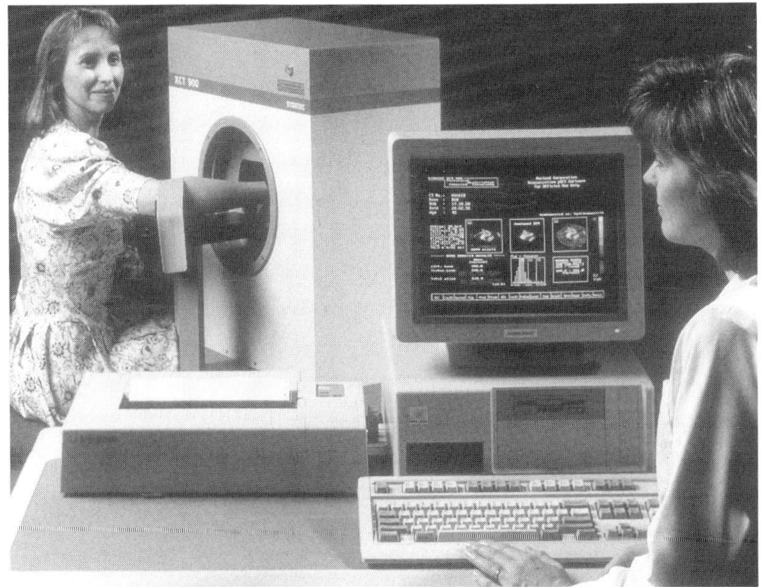

(a)

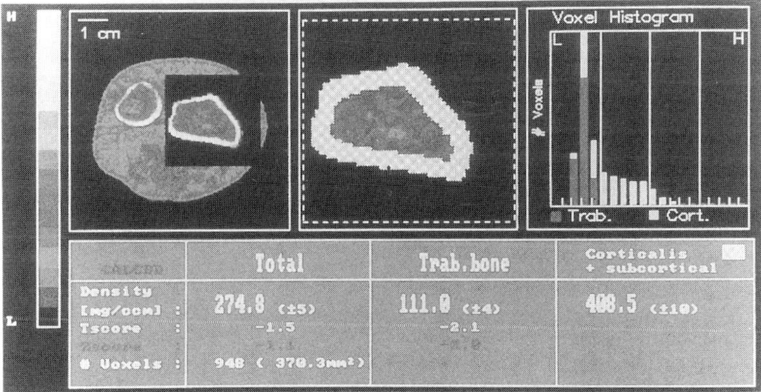

(b)

Figure 17 Peripheral quantitative CT. A dedicated XCT 900 Stratec scanner (a) affords cross-sectional analysis of bone density in the distal portion of the radius, including trabecular and cortical components (postmenopausal osteoporotic female) (b). (Courtesy of Norland Corporation, Ft. Atkinson, WI.)

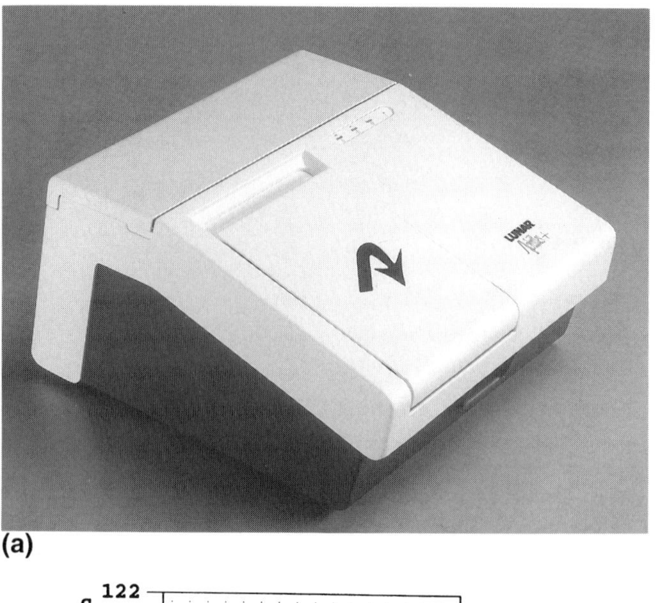

(a)

LUNAR

STIFFNESS

122

100

78

56

20 40 60 80 100

AGE (years)

Stiffness	105 ± 3
% Young Adult	105 ± 3
% Age Matched	159 ± 3

RIGHT HEEL

Age (Years)....................36	Weight (lbs)....................0	Ethnic...........................W
Sex..............................F	Height (in).....................0	System.......................1013
STIFFNESS.....................105	SOS (m/s)....................1575	BUA (dB/MHz)...................127

	Stiffness[1] %	Z
Young Adult	105	0.46
Age Matched	159	3.56

(b)

Figure 18 (a) The Lunar Achilles Plus is a dedicated system for ultrasonographic evaluation of bone in the calcaneus. The scan support device opens toward the patient (arrow), and measurements of speed of sound (SOS) and broad-band ultrasound attenuation (BUA) are performed. (b) The scan report from this instrument yields an estimate of bone stiffness, which is compared to normative data from young adult and age-matched control subjects.

technique. Use of MRI in densitometry is a relatively new strategy. MRI operates on the principle of magnetism and resonance frequency. Hydrogen is richly abundant in the human body, and the amount of hydrogen in specific portions of the marrow is correlated to its bone density. Due to its +1 charge, hydrogen has an associated magnetic moment (51), and magnetically, hydrogen can be treated as a proton. Protons placed in a magnetic field tend to orient in the direction of the field; when resonance frequency is applied to the protons, they reorient themselves. When the resonance frequency signal is turned off, the protons return to their original positions over time. The time required for this phenomenon is expressed in several parameters: T1 (spin-lattice relaxation time); T2 (spin-spin relaxation time); and T2* (magnetic field inhomogeneity induced relaxation time) (51). Generally, T1 refers to the time required for the protons to realign with the magnetic field. T2 refers to the time it takes for out-of-phase nuclei to negate the signal of neighboring protons (52). Relaxation times along with other data such as spin density, chemical shift, and diffusion effects are then mapped into an image through complex mathematics (51) (Figure 19).

T2 relaxation time is more pronounced in normal bone than in osteoporotic bone. Furthermore, cortical bone does not produce a significant signal in MRI due to short T2 relaxation times. However, the trabecular network containing bone marrow causes significant changes in the induced magnetic field (51). As the body ages, bone density decreases; trabeculae of cancellous bone become more rarefied, allowing fatty marrow to accumulate in the vacated spaces (7). The highly rarefied trabecular network produces significant T2 relaxation times, which are used in conjunction with other data to map an MR image.

Genant has reported that an in vitro study of MRI versus QCT found a correlation of r=0.94 in bone density measurements (53). The use of MRI as a diagnostic tool is controversial due to a lack of studies and widespread clinical use. However, MRI remains among the more promising and revolutionary techniques in bone densitometry, particularly since it provides additional information on trabecular architecture and connectivity.

Osteoporosis is a serious disease causing millions of fractures and thousands of deaths each year. Early diagnosis and preventive treatment will help to curtail some of the costs and suffering due to osteoporosis. Numerous methods have been developed to measure bone density and estimate bone strength. R is not a reliable tool for measuring bone density, and is antiquated by more recently developed densitometric tools. RA is one of the oldest methods, although recent improvements have rendered it a promising technique for BMD determination in selected patients. Until further testing is done, however, RA is at best considered a convenient, inexpensive alternative method that may be used to screen people at risk for osteoporosis. SPA and SXA are effective tools for measuring BMD; these techniques are of greatest value at the distal radius, where results are predictive of Colles fracture risk (54,55).

SXA offers slight cost and performance advantages over SPA. DXA allows direct measurements of the proximal femur, spine, other regional sites, and whole

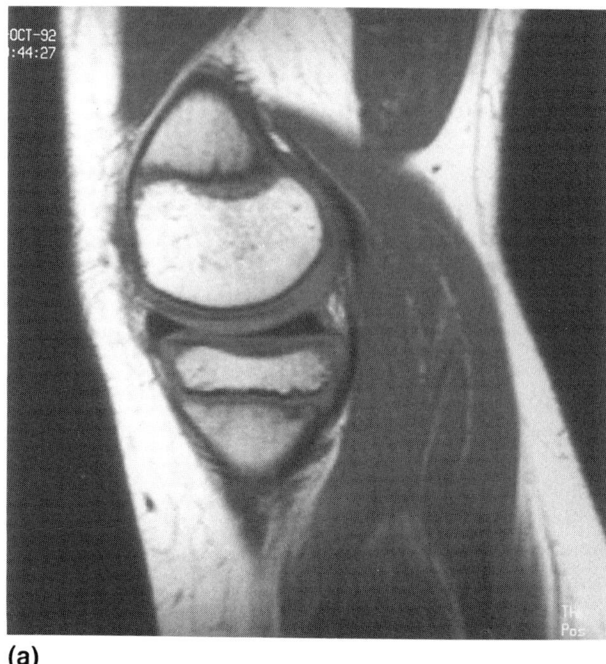

(a)

Figure 19 Spin-echo (a) and gradient-echo (b) magnetic resonance images of the knee joint of a normal volunteer in the sagittal plane. The bone marrow signal intensity on a gradient-echo sequence increases as one moves from the epiphysis through the metaphysis to the diaphysis of a bone (owing to progressively decreasing trabecular bone content), whereas the intensity on a spin-echo sequence remains constant for a given TR (repetition time) and TE (echo time). For this reason, T2* (provided by gradient-echo sequences) as opposed to T1 or T2 (provided by spin-echo sequences) relaxation times are used to indirectly measure trabecular bone density using a technique known as magnetic resonance inferometry.

body. Osteoporotic fractures of the hip and spine are often the most debilitating and potentially fatal; hence, direct measurement of these areas of the skeleton is preferred over SPA's estimation from measurements made at other sites. QCT BMD measurements offer two distinct advantages over projectional methods: they are not influenced by extraosseous mineralization, and they provide information concerning osseous architecture, which is a major determinant of bone strength. PQCT offers an alternative to SPA or SXA in predicting risk of Colles fracture, and has potential as a diagnostic tool. Ultrasonography is a promising new technique in bone densitometry; it is simple to use, relatively inexpensive, and radiation-free. More testing and improvements must be accomplished before BUA can become a clinically valuable method for densitometry.

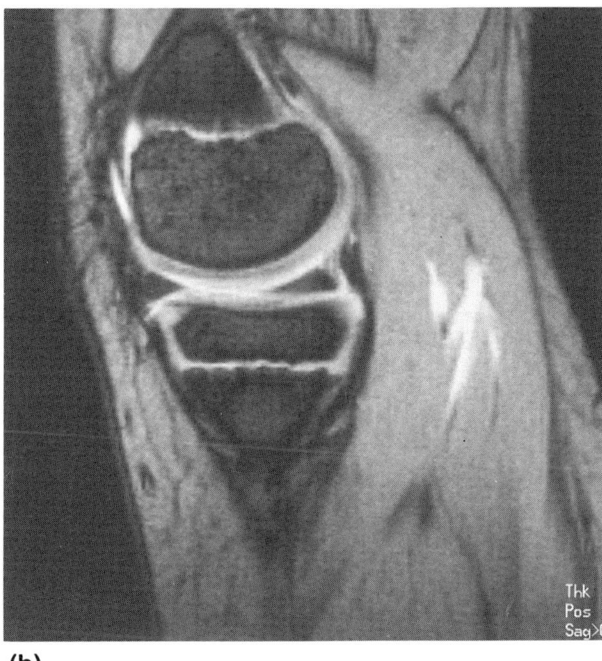

(b)

Finally, MRI is another radiation-free technique for bone densitometry; at this time it is not widely used for this purpose, but it also provides architectural information. Overall, the currently available tools for measuring and monitoring BMD are accurate and effective, but none of them is ideal. As osteoporosis becomes a larger problem worldwide, the anticipated improvements in both bone densitometry and osteoporosis therapy will most certainly abate present-day projections.

REFERENCES

1. Baran DT. Quantitative ultrasound: a technique to target women with low bone mass for preventive therapy. Am J Med 1995; 98(2A):37S–40S.
2. Hughes TH, Yu JS, Sartoris DJ. Imaging of osteoporosis. J South Orthop Assoc 1993; 2(3):173–184.
3. Nevitt MC. Epidemiology of osteoporosis. Rheum Dis Clin North Am 1994; 20(3): 535–559.
4. Hagiawara S, Yang S, Gluer C, Bendavid E, Genant HK. Non-invasive bone mineral density measurement in the evaluation of osteoporosis. Rheum Dis Clin North Am 1994; 20(3):651–669.

5. Parfitt AM. Implications of architecture for the pathogenesis and prevention of vertebral fractures. Bone 1992; 13(suppl 2):S41–S47.
6. Greenspan SL, Myers ER, Maitland LA, Resnick NM, Hayes WC. Fall severity and bone density as risk factors for hip fracture in ambulatory elderly. JAMA 94; 271(2): 128–133.
7. Lang P, Steiger P, Faulkner K, Gluer C, Genant HK. Osteoporosis. Current techniques and recent developments in quantitative bone densitometry. Radiol Clin North Am 1991; 29(1):49–76.
8. Hayes WC, Piazza ST, Zysett PK. Biomechanics of fracture risk prediction of the hip and spine by QCT. Radiol Clin North Am 1991; 29(1):1–18.
9. Cummings SR, Black DL. Bone mass measurements and risk of fracture in Caucasian women: a review of findings from prospective studies. Am J Med 1995; 98(2A): 24S–28S.
10. McBean LD, Forgac T, Finn SC. Osteoporosis: visions for care and prevention—a conference report. J Am Dietic Assoc 1994; 94(6):668–671.
11. Gupta S, Luna E, Belsky J, Gelfman N, Miller K, Davies T. Photon absorptiometry for non-invasive measurements of BMC. Clin Nucl Med 1984; 9(8):435–439.
12. Epstein RS, Lydick E, Suppapanya N, Ross PD, Yates AJ. Baseline measurement of bone mass from hand x-rays predicts hip fractures in a national sample of white women. Osteoporos Int. In press.
13. Garn SM. The earlier gain and later loss of cortical bone. In: Thomas CC, ed. Nutritional Perspective. Springfield, IL: Charles C. Thomas; 1970:146.
14. Yates AJ, Ross PD, Lydick E, Epstein RS. Radiographic absorptiometry in the diagnosis of osteoporosis. Am J Med 1995; 98(2A):41S–47S.
15. Cosman F, Herrington B, Himmelstein S, Lindsay R. Radiographic absorptiometry: a simple method for determination of bone mass. Osteoporos Int 1991; 2(1): 34–38.
16. Cameron JR, Sorenson J. Measurement of bone mineral in-vivo: an improved method. Science 1963; 142:230–232.
17. Leboff MS, Fuleihan GE, Angell JE, Chung S, Curtis K. Dual energy x-ray absorptiometry of the forearm: reproducibility and correlation with single-photon absorptiometry. J Bone Miner Res 1992; 7(7):841–846.
18. Kelley TL, Crane G, Baran DT. Single-x-ray absorptiometry of the forearm: precision, correlation and reference data. Calcif Tissue Int 1994; 54(3):212–218.
19. Markel MD, Wikenheiser MA, Morin RL, Lewallen DG, Chao EY. The determination of bone fracture properties by dual-energy x-ray absorptiometry and single-photon absorptiometry: a comparative study. Calcif Tissue Int 1991; 48(6):392–399.
20. Vogel JM, Anderson JT. Rectilinear transmission scanning of irregular bones for quantification of mineral content. J Nucl Med 1972; 13(1):13–18.
21. West RR, Reed GW. The measurement with bone mineral in-vivo by photon beam scanning. Br J Radiol 1980; 43:886.
22. DeLuca HF, Mazess R. Osteoporosis: Physiological Basis, Assessment and Treatment. New York: Elsevier Science, 1990.
23. Eastell R, Riggs BL, Wahner HW, O'Fallon WM, Amadio PC, Melton LJ III. Colles' fracture and bone density of the ultradistal radius. J Bone Miner Res 1989; 4(4):607–613.

24. Johnston CC Jr, Slemenda CW. Identification of patients with low bone mass by single-photon absorptiometry and single-energy-x-ray absorptiometry. Am J Med 1995; 98(2A):37S–40S.
25. Barden HS, Mazess RB. Bone densitometry of the appendicular skeleton. Top Geriatr Rehabil 1989; 4:1–12.
26. Wahner HW, Dunn WL, Riggs BL. Noninvasive bone mineral measurements. Semin Nucl Med 1983; 13(3):282–289.
27. Genant HK, Cann CE, Boyd DP, et al. Quantitative computed tomography for vertebral mineral determination. In: Frame B, Potts JT, eds. Clinical Disorders of Bone and Mineral Metabolism. Amsterdam: Excerpta Medica; 1983:40–47.
28. Nelson D, Feingold M, Mascha E, Kleerekoper M. Comparison of single-photon absorptiometry and dual-energy x-ray absorptiometry of the radius. Bone Miner 1992; 18(1):77–83.
29. Lewis MD, Blake GM, Fogelman I. Patient dose in dual x-ray absorptiometry. Osteoporos Int 1994; 4(1):11–15.
30. Johnson J, Dawson-Hughes B. Precision and stability of dual-energy x-ray absorptiometry measurements. Calcif Tissue Int 1991; 49(3):174–178.
31. Nuti R, Martini G, Richi G, Frediani B, Turchetti V. Comparison of total body measurements by dual-energy x-ray absorptiometry and dual-photon absorptiometry. J Bone Miner Res 1991; 6(7):681–687.
32. Lees B, Stevenson JC. Preliminary evaluation of a new ultrasound bone densitometer. Calcif Tissue Int 1993; 53(3):149–152.
33. Engelke K, Grampp S, Gluer CC, Jergas M, Yang SO, Genant HK. Significance of QCT bone mineral density and its standard deviation as parameters to evaluate osteoporosis. J QCT 1995; 19(1):111–116.
34. Cann CE, Genant HK. Precise measurement of vertebral mineral content using computed tomography. J Comput Assist Tomogr 1980; 4(4):493.
35. Heuck A, Block J, Gluer CC, Steiger P, Genant HK. Mild versus definite osteoporosis: comparison of bone densitometry techniques using different statistical models. J Bone Miner Res 1989; 4(6):891–900.
36. Reinbold W-D, Adler CP, Kalender WA, Lente R. Accuracy of vertebral mineral determination by dual-energy quantitative computed tomography. Skel Radiol 1991; 20(1):25–29.
37. Hayes WC, Piazza SJ, Zysset PK. Biomechanics of fracture risk prediction of the hip and spine by QCT. Radiol Clin North Am 1991; 29(1):1–18
38. Butz S, Wuster C, Scheidt-Nave C, Gotz M, Ziegler R. Forearm BMD as measured by peripheral quantitative computed tomography (pQCT) in a German reference population. Osteoporos Int 1994; 4(4):179–184.
39. Wahner HW, Eastell R, Riggs BL. Bone mineral density of the radius: where do we stand? J Nucl Med 1985; 26(11):1339–1341.
40. Eastell R, Wahner HW, O'Fallon WN, Amadio PC, Melton LJ III, Riggs BL. Unequal decrease in bone density of the lumbar spine and ultradistal radius in Colles and vertebral fracture syndromes. J Clin Invest 1989; 83(1):168–174.
41. Mazess RB, Harden HS. Interrelationships among bone densitometry sites in normal young women. Bone Miner 1990; 11(3):347–356.

42. Smith DA, Hosie CJ, Deacon AD, Hamblen DL. Quantitative gamma-ray computed tomography of the radius in normal subjects and osteoporotic patients. Br J Radiol 1990; 63(754):776–782.
43. Hesp R, Dore C, Page L, Summers R. Normal values for trabecular and cortical bone in the radius measured by computed tomography. Clinic Phys Physiol Meas 1985; 6(4):303–310.
44. Langton CM, Palmer SB, Porter RW. The measurement of broadband ultrasonic attenuation in cancellous bone. Eng Med 1984; 13(2):89–91.
45. Brandenberger GH. Clinical determination of bone quality: is ultrasound an answer. Calcif Tissue Int 1993; 53(suppl 1):S151–S156.
46. Poet JL, Tonolli-Serabian I, Camboulives H, Dufour M, Roux H. BUA of the os calcis: preliminary study. Clin Rheumatol 1994; 13(2):234–238.
47. Resh H, Pietchmann P, Bernecker P, Krexner E, Willvonsender R. Broadband ultrasound attenuation: a new diagnostic method in osteoporosis. AJR 1990; 155(4): 825–828.
48. Stewart A, Reid DM, Porter RW. Broadband ultrasound attenuation and dual-energy x-ray absorptiometry in patients with hip fractures: which technique discriminates fracture risk. Calcif Tissue Int 1994; 54(6):466–469.
49. Funke M, Kopka L, Vosshenrich R, Fischer U, Ueberschaer A, Oestmann J, Grabbe E. Broadband ultrasound attenuation in the diagnosis of osteoporosis: correlation with osteodensitometry and fracture. Radiology 1995; 194(1):77–81.
50. Zagzebski JA, Rossman PJ, Messina C, Mazess RB, Madsen EL. Ultrasound transmission measurements through the os calcis. Calcif Tissue Int 1991; 49(2):107–111.
51. Majumdar S, Genant HK. A review of the recent advances in magnetic resonance imaging in the assessment of osteoporosis. Osteoporos Int 1995; 5(2):79–82.
52. Easton EJ Jr, Powers JA. Musculoskeletal Magnetic Resonance Imaging. New Jersey: Slack Inc; 1986:6.
53. Majumdar S, Genant HK. Quantitation of susceptibility effects in trabecular bone and their correlation with bone density. In: Printed Program Supplement 22 of the 8th Annual Meeting of Society for Magnetic Resonance Imaging, 1990.
54. Wasnich RD, Ross PD, Davis JW, Vogel JM. A comparison of single and multi-site BMC measurements for assessment of spine fracture possibility. J Nucl Med 1989; 30(7):1166–1171.
55. Vogel JM, Wasnich JM, Ross PD. The clinical relevance of calcaneus bone mineral measurements: a review. Bone Miner 1988; 5(1):35–58.
56. Yang SO, Hagiwara S, Engelke K, et al. Radiographic absorptiometry for bone mineral measurement of the phalanges: precision and accuracy study. Radiology 1994; 192(3):857–859.

8

Quantitative Assessment of Osteoporosis: Current and Future Status

STEPHAN GRAMPP, MICHAEL JERGAS, PHILIPP LANG, and HARRY K. GENANT

University of California, San Francisco
San Francisco, California

CLAUS C. GLÜER

University of Kiel
Kiel, Germany

I. INTRODUCTION

Osteoporosis is defined as a decrease in bone mass accompanied by structural changes leading to an increase in fracture propensity. In cancellous bone the density and integrity of the trabecular network are reduced. In cortical bone, increased endosteal and intracortical resorption causes thinning and porosity of the bone tissue. All of these mechanisms lead to a reduction in bone strength. Bone strength itself depends on several factors such as bone mineral density (BMD), bone structure and size, material properties of the bone matrix, and the ability to heal microfractures. Studies suggest, however, that BMD is the most important determinant of bone fragility (1–5). The incidence of fractures has increased in the last decades due to the increased expectation of life (6–9). Early diagnosis of osteoporosis, fracture risk prediction, and assessment of therapy efficacy are therefore of great clinical and scientific interest.

Over the past several decades there has been considerable progress in the development and application of noninvasive methods of bone mass measurements, and a number of techniques are available for measuring bone mass at multiple sites of the skeleton (10–18). This chapter reviews methodology and developments in bone densitometry including the early approaches like radio-

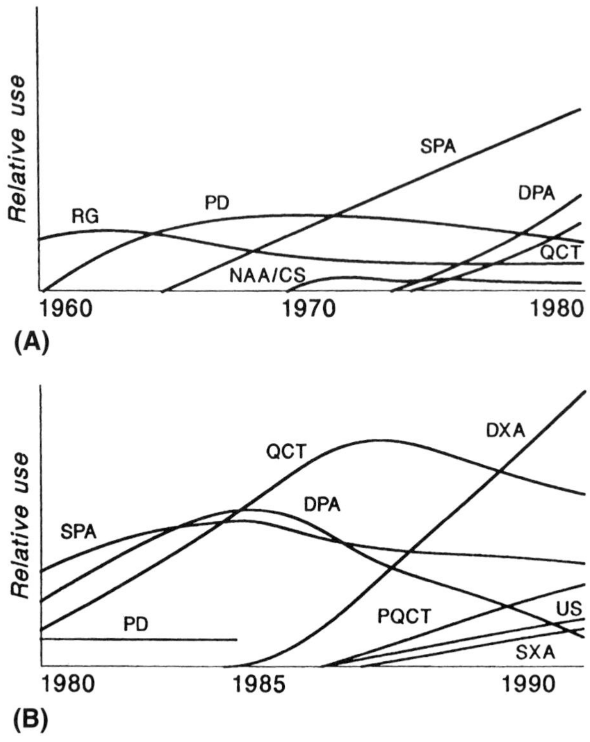

Figure 1 Relative use of equipment for bone density measurement from (A) 1960 to 1980; (B) 1980 to 1990. Abbreviations: RG = radiogrammetry; PD = photodensitometry; NAA/CS = neutron activation analysis and Compton scattering; SPA = single-photon absorptiometry; DPA = dual-photon absorptiometry; QCT = quantitative computed tomography; pQCT = peripheral quantitative computed tomography; DXA = dual x-ray absorptiometry; SXA = single x-ray absorptiometry; US = ultrasound.

grammetry, photo densitometry, neutron activation analysis, and Compton scattering techniques as well as the recent developments like quantitative ultrasound, magnetic resonance imaging, and finite element analysis. The development of the currently most widely used techniques, dual x-ray absorptiometry and quantitative computed tomography, is briefly reviewed. The relative use of most of these techniques is illustrated in Figure 1. The widespread clinical and scientific interest in bone densitometry will provide further impetus for improvement in the established methods as well as the development of newer techniques.

II. PAST METHODS

A. Techniques Based on Conventional X-rays

Indications of bone loss on radiographs are a reduction in density and changes in morphology such as thinning of the cortex, scalloping of the inner cortical surface, and intracortical tunneling. It has been estimated that in most cases early spinal osteoporosis (osteopenia) becomes detectable on conventional radiographs only after a loss of at least 30% of the skeletal calcium. The interobserver variances of this detection were considerable (probability of correct response = 0.53–0.95) (19) (Fig. 2). The method may not be adequate for the assessment of osteopenia, but it is an important part of the standard routine of a radiologist reading a radiograph. Semiquantitative grading techniques, like vertebral or femoral indices (Fig. 3), have not proven to be precise or sensitive enough to diagnose osteopenia at an early stage (20,21), but were employed successfully in epidemiological studies in the assessment of osteoporosis (22,23).

In radiogrammetry (RG), the ratio of cortical thickness to the overall thickness of tubular bones is calculated (20,24). This usually involves direct caliper measurements of inner and outer diameters of the cortex from which bone mass indices are finally calculated (Fig. 4) (25). The combined cortical thickness index is usually determined in the metacarpal bones due to their easy accessibility by x-ray imaging and the low radiation exposure to the patient. Though this method can detect endosteal and subperiosteal resorption, an assessment of intracortical porosity is not possible. Errors of this method occurred because of nonuniformity of the endosteal surface and variations in positioning of the hand (12,26). Like the semiquantitative methods, RG generally is regarded as inadequate for either diagnosing or for assessing the course of osteoporosis for individual patients; however, it appears to be adequate in epidemiological studies of large populations (27–29).

Another radiographic based approach is photo densitometry (PD), one of the first quantitative techniques developed to estimate BMD (30). Standardized radiographs of bones are obtained simultaneously with an aluminum step-wedge phantom. However, an x-ray beam, which passes through an absorbing tissue, is scattered according to composition and physical thickness of this tissue. Variations in the amount of soft tissue overlying the bone are not accounted for by PD. Therefore reasonable accuracy can only be ensured at appendicular bones, which are surrounded by a relatively negligible amount of soft tissue (e.g., calcaneus, metacarpals, or phalanxes).

The optical density of appendicular bone on the exposed film is determined by comparison with the defined density of the aluminum step-wedge using an optical densitometer (Fig. 5). The results are given in aluminum equivalent values. PD is a low-cost technique, which measures integral bone (trabecular and cortical). Re-

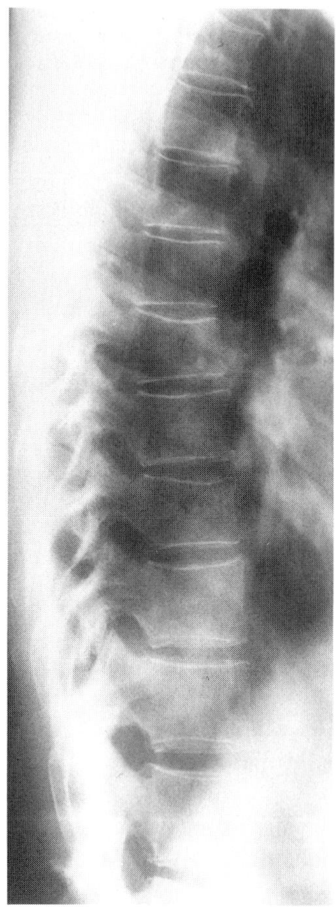

Figure 2 Conventional radiographs can be used for the visual estimation of BMD. Lateral radiograph at the thoracic spine: mild fractures at T7 and T9.

cent studies have shown that PD is significantly correlated with single-photon absorptiometry (SPA) and with spinal and femoral dual-photon absortiometry (DPA) (31). Yet numerous physical factors that influence the radiographic image also have an adverse effect on precision and accuracy with photo densitometry. Among these are inconsistencies in beam quality, instability of the x-ray source, film response, processing conditions, radiation scattering conditions, and variations resulting from a low-energy polychromatic beam transmitted through layers of soft tissue and bone of varying thickness and composition (i.e., beam hardening effects) (13). Beam hardening is caused by a loss of photons in the lower-energy

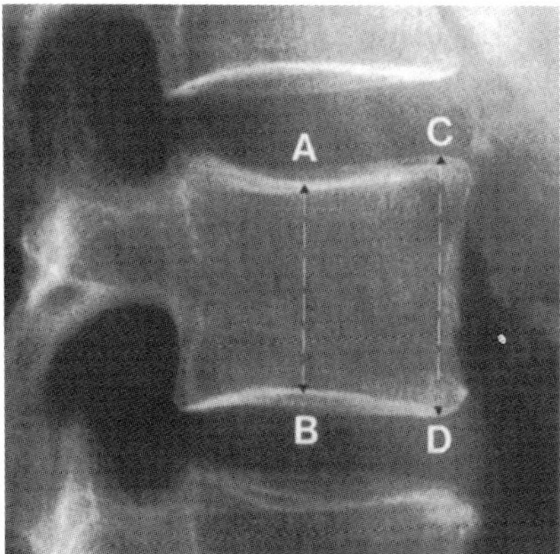

Figure 3 The Barnett-Nordin Index calculates the ratio of vertebral height in the middle of the vertebral body to the height at the anterior margin of the vertebral body: AB/CD.

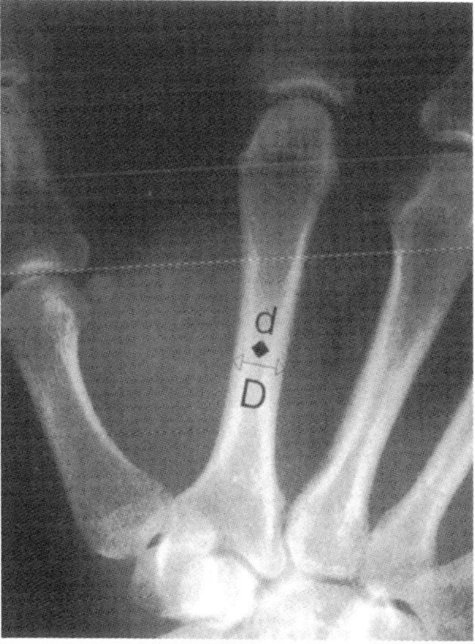

Figure 4 The Os Metacarpal II Index is calculated from the ratio of cortical thickness and bone diameter: D–d/D.

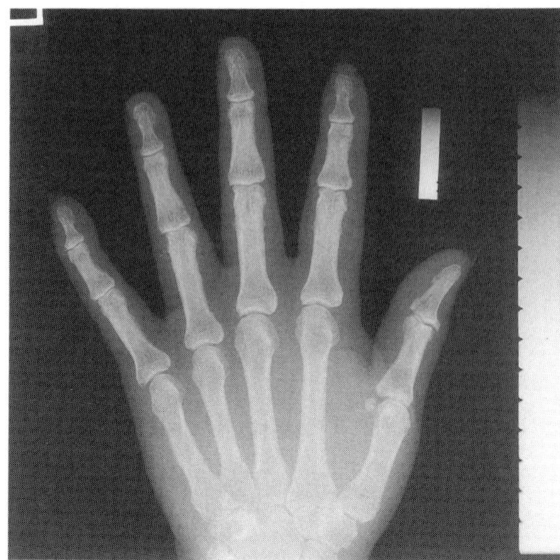

Figure 5 Standardized radiograph of the left hand together with two aluminum step wedges to compare metal and bone density by their amounts of x-ray absorption.

spectrum as the x-ray beam passes through tissue. These error sources are responsible for miscalculations of the BMD with a photodensitometer; however, newer calibration and analysis techniques have enhanced the suitability of the method (30–32).

B. Neutron Activation Analysis and Compton Scattering Techniques

Neutron activation analysis (NAA) of the total body or parts of the body, and Compton scattering techniques (CS) are among the earlier methods developed for quantitative bone analysis (33–37).

With neutron activation analysis, neutrons are used to bombard a small fraction of the total calcium-48 (^{48}Ca) or calcium-40 (^{40}Ca) contained in the human body, producing ^{49}Ca (with a half-life of 8.8 min). This process results in emission of gamma photons and can finally be counted and quantified with external detectors either directly at the point of neutron capture, or as the active nuclei decay. The delayed method of measuring the nuclear decay is more commonly used. After exposure to the neutron flux, the patient is transferred to a radiation counter to record the radiation, which is emitted as the nuclei decay. The neutrons (with energies of 1 to 5 MeV) are derived from accelerators, reactors, or alpha neutron sources. The technique provides an estimate of the bone mineral content because, at least in the skeleton, calcium makes up a constant fraction (0.395) of the mineralized tissue. Measurement sites can be either the total body or a selected body part (38). The sites are irradiated with neutrons in a standardized and reproducible fashion. The radiation dose for such measurements ranges from 200 to 3,000 mSv (39), depending on the neutron energy and the detector efficiency. Several studies suggested a precision and accuracy on the order of 2–5% (40).

The total body calcium measurement by NAA reflects primarily compact bone, which constitutes approximately 80% of the total skeletal mass and therefore correlates closely with other measurements of cortical bone. Total body calcium measurements obtained by NAA have been compared with results obtained by peripheral single-photon absorptiometry. Here correlation coefficients of approximately 0.9 were obtained (41–44). Processes occurring initially or predominantly in cancellous bone may not be detected as readily with this technique. For example, in osteoporotic patients, the correlation between peripheral measurements by photon absorptiometry and total body NAA was not high (45). Heterotopic calcification, such as vascular and osteochondral calcification, or heterotopic ossification, such as osteophytosis and myositis ossificans, can cause inaccuracies in the estimation of skeletal calcium by NAA.

In an attempt to measure predominantly cancellous bone, methods have been developed for partial body neutron activation in which areas of the trunk (e.g., pelvis, spine, and rib cage) are measured. Precision and dosages for these local measurements are comparable to those obtained with the total body activation techniques.

Compton scattering techniques have been used to estimate the density of selected volumes of bone (36,37,46–48). These methods make use of the information extracted primarily from the scattered beam, not from the transmitted beam. The electron density of a tissue volume is estimated by the extent of Compton scattering produced by incident radiation. Such radiation is generally of relatively high photon energy, on the order of 100–500 keV, emanating from a monoenergetic isotope source (49). A highly collimated gamma ray source and a highly collimated detector are positioned such that their "sensitive areas" project pathways that intersect perpendicular to each other within the object and that define the volume to be measured (Fig. 6). The technique measures a composite of all the medullar components producing the scatter, not simply the density of bone mineral. The detected scatter is proportional to the electron density, independent of the atomic number z. For this reason, the method is less sensitive to the calcium level than is single-photon absorptiometry applied at low energies. The precision of the method is 3–5%. Its accuracy is affected by photon attenuation in tissues outside the region of interest. The use of high photon energy diminishes these problems at the expense of an increased radiation dose (50–53). There is no reference on the effective dose equivalent of Compton scattering. When applied to the appendicular skeleton, however, the radiation dose should be relatively small.

A variant of the foregoing scattered photon technique is coherent scattering as proposed by Puumalainen and colleagues (54). With this method, both Compton-

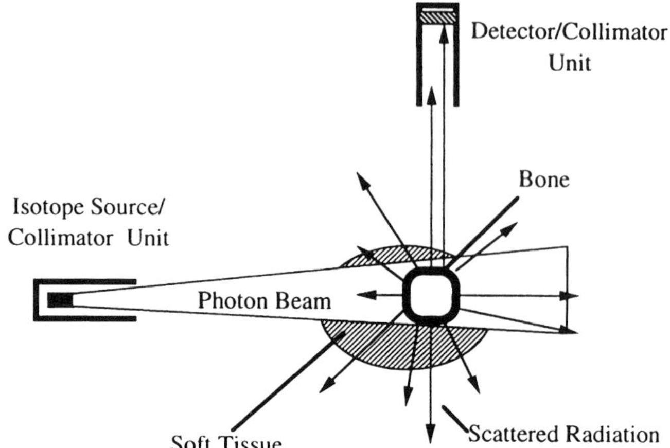

Figure 6 Principle of the instrumental layout used for the Compton scattering measurement. A highly collimated gamma ray source is positioned perpendicularly to a highly collimated detector, which counts photons scattered by the object in the beam path.

scattering and coherent scattering of photons are determined in a particular volume of tissue such as cancellous bone. This is made possible by the use of a solid-state detector, which provides good discrimination. Coherent scattering, like photoelectric absorption, depends on the cube of the atomic number (z^3); thus the ratio of coherent to Compton-scattered photons is a measure of the effective atomic number, independent of density. A decreased ratio may therefore be observed in osteopenic diseases. Likewise, the ratio is unaffected by scatter outside the region of interest, so complicated corrections for this potential inaccuracy are not necessary.

Only a few clinical studies have been performed with NAA or Compton scattering techniques (41,46,55–57). Their extreme technical requirements, the relatively high radiation dose for neutron activation analysis, and the development of competitive methods with comparable or better precision and easier use have all made these methods nearly obsolete in bone densitometry. Today neutron activation analysis and Compton scattering are regarded as investigational techniques with negligible clinical impact.

C. Single-Photon Absorptiometry

Single-photon absorptiometry (SPA), a quantitative method for measuring peripheral bone mineral density, was introduced in the 1960s (58–60). With this method a quantitative assessment of bone mineral content at a peripheral site of the skeleton (e.g., radius or calcaneus) is possible.

A highly collimated, monochromatic photon beam from a radionuclide source (usually ^{125}I) is used to measure photon attenuation. The extremity to be investigated is placed between the source and a scintillation detector and is scanned in a rectilinear fashion. The level of attenuation is then converted to bone mineral content (BMC) in grams (g) or areal bone mineral density (BMD) in grams per centimeters squared (g/cm^2) using a known standard. SPA overcomes errors, which may arise with the polychromatic, divergent x-ray beam of photodensitometry (i.e., beam hardening, source instability, and scattered radiation—film processing techniques) to a large extent. Variations in soft-tissue thickness may cause underestimation or overestimation of BMD. To keep the absorption of the soft tissue constant and to compensate for superimposition of layers of varying thickness, the extremity is placed in water, which fortunately has absorption properties similar to those of soft tissue (Fig. 7). Separate measurements of trabecular and cortical bone are not possible with SPA. Routine methods have been established for measuring the distal radius and the calcaneus. The commonly used site for bone densitometry by SPA is the distal third of the radial shaft, which is composed mostly of cortical bone (61–63). Measurements at this relatively homogeneous site of the distal radius demonstrate an accuracy of about 6% and a

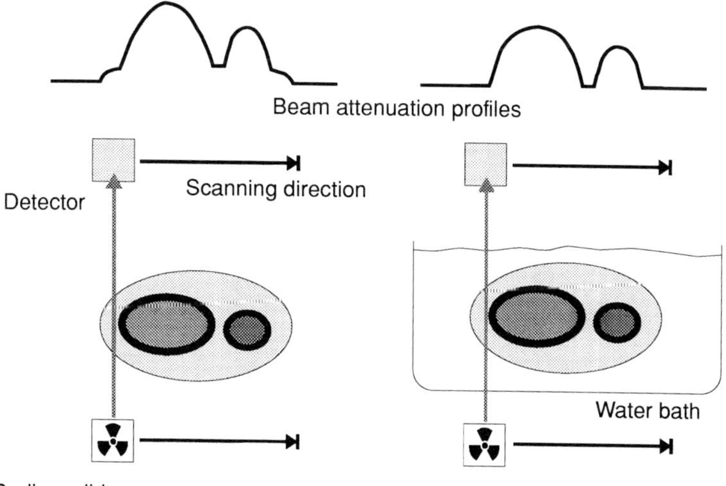

Figure 7 Principle of SPA. (Left) The beam intensity (demonstrated by the beam attenuation profiles) is demonstrated as a function of beam path through a simulated forearm. The soft tissue contributes critically to the amount of attenuation. (Right) Introduction of a water bath for immersing of the scanned extremity corrects for inconsistencies in the length of the path through soft tissue as it is expressed in the beam attenuation profile. The area under the beam attenuation profile is therefore proportional to the bone mineral content along the scan line.

reproducibility between 1% and 2% (relative precision as the coefficient of variation (CV) = standard deviation/mean × 100) (64,65). Metabolically more active trabecular bone is largely excluded by this approach. As a solution, measurements may be acquired at the ultradistal radius. This site yields a trabecular-to-cortical bone ratio of about 1, which is similar to the distribution ratio in the lumbar spine. The major problem in measuring BMD at the ultradistal radius is the great change in density values within a relatively small area. Anatomical definition of the ROI in this region could be problematic (64,66). Because of the complex and heterogeneous nature of the radius anatomy, measurements at this site were subject to positioning errors, but recently have been accomplished with rectilinear scanning devices (63). A computer-aided edge detection algorithm is necessary for this technique to facilitate exact location of the ROI and to ensure appropriate precision of the analysis (65).

The value of bone mineral measurements at the calcaneus has been somewhat controversial because of the potentially confounding relationship between BMD and body weight or exercise at this site (67,68). Nevertheless, recent studies have shown impressive results for the value of calcaneus measurements in predicting osteoporotic vertebral and femoral neck fractures (2,69–75).

SPA has proven to be a valuable tool in the diagnosis of osteoporosis, providing reasonable precision, low radiation dose (<1 μSv per measurement; see Table 1), and short examination times. The major disadvantage of the method is that the clinically important sites of the spine and the hip cannot be evaluated.

At present the technique is in use at approximately 250 clinical centers worldwide. Ongoing development of these systems is limited, however, although for some systems the radionuclide source has been replaced by an x-ray tube, resulting in improved precision and cost-effectiveness. This technique is referred to as single x-ray absorptiometry (SXA). Using an x-ray tube rather than a radionuclide source eliminates the need for replacing the source and thereby reduces radioactive waste. Furthermore, extensive quality control measures to compensate for radioactive decay do not apply. However, it may be necessary to correct for beam hardening due to the polychromatic spectrum of the x-ray source. BMD measurements of the appendicular skeleton have been adapted to dual-photon and dual x-ray absorptiometry based on the experiences made with SPA and SXA. Special software already exists for forearm measurements, which are widely used in clinical densitometry. There were also successful attempts to apply the method for BMD measurements at the calcaneus (76,77). The enormous versatility of dual x-ray absorptiometry that allows for an application of this technique at virtually any site contributes to the dwindling usage of SPA in bone densitometry.

D. Dual-Photon Absorptiometry

SPA measurements are not possible at sites with a variable soft-tissue thickness and composition (i.e., the axial skeleton, hip, or whole body). For these purposes

Table 1 Precision, Accuracy Error, and Radiation Dose of Techniques for Bone Mineral Measurement

Technique	Precision[a] (%)	Accuracy error (%)	Effective dose equivalent[b] (μSv)
Convent. radiographs and grading techniques	Kappa score: 0.39–0.92	Probability of correct response: 0.53–0.95	Lumbar spine lateral/AP 450/550
RG	1–2	4	1
PD	1–3.5	5–10	1
NAA	2–5	2–5	200–3,000
CS	>3		3,000
SPA	1–2	4–6	<1
DPA			
Lumbar spine	2–4	5–10	5
Proximal femur	3–5	5–10	3
DXA			
PA lumbar spine	1	4–8	1
Lateral lumbar spine	2–3	5–10	3
Proximal femur	1–2	4–8	1
Total body	1	1–2	3
QCT			
Single-energy QCT	2–4	5–15	50
Dual-energy QCT	4–6	3–10	100
Peripheral QCT	0.5–1	2–8	<2
Ultrasound[c]			
BUA (calcaneus)	1.6–3.8	NA	0
SOS (calcaneus)	0.3–1.9	NA	0
SOS (patella)	<2	NA	0
Magnetic resonance			
Radius	3.3–7	NA	0

[a]Kappa score and probability of correct response depend on study site and index employed.
[b]For perspective, the effective dose equivalent for an AP chest film is 50 μSv and annual background irradiation amounts to 2,400 μSv.
[c]Determining accuracy for ultrasound is difficult since the bone parameters assessed have not been fully defined.

where a constant path length of the beam cannot be maintained, dual-photon absorptiometry techniques (DPA) were developed and have been studied extensively to measure mineral content of the spine, hip, and whole body. The technique represents an extension of the principle of SPA. SPA requires a constant soft-tissue thickness for providing reliable data. At peripheral measuring sites an extremity can be assumed to be composed of bone, muscle, and other types of soft tissue, which can be simulated by immersion of this extremity in water. For the axial skeleton, however, this assumption is not valid. Considerable amounts of fat may lie in the path of the beam at these sites, and immersion of the whole body in water is hardly possible. To overcome these shortcomings of SPA, DPA uses a radionuclide source at two effective discrete energy levels.

When DPA was first employed, the radionuclide source consisted of radionuclide combinations such as ^{125}I and ^{241}Am. The dual emitter ^{153}Gd (with photons of predominantly 44 and 100 keV) was introduced in the early 1970s and became the standard radionuclide source for DPA (78). The principle of DPA and of the other dual-energy methods (dual x-ray absorptiometry = DXA and dual-energy quantitative computed tomography = DE-QCT) is based on the fact that radiation of distinct energies is attenuated by tissues to different extents (79). In both soft tissue and bone, a low-energy beam is attenuated to a greater degree than a high-energy beam. Because this attenuation occurs in bone to a much greater extent than in soft tissue, the contrast in attenuation between bone and soft tissue is greater for the low-energy beam than for the high-energy beam. DPA is based on this contrast difference. Entering both attenuation profiles into a mathematical equation system, the bony components can ideally be calculated. This is done by multiplying the high-energy curve by an appropriate factor (K); the soft-tissue portion of the intensity profile can be transformed to match that of the low-energy curve. When the rescaled high-energy profile is subtracted from the low-energy profile, the soft-tissue contribution is eliminated, resulting in only the bone contribution. The application of this technique eliminates the need for a constant path length. As in SPA, a scintillation detector is used and the scan is performed in a rectilinear fashion. A bone edge detection algorithm is used to outline bone structures and specific regions within the spine (usually L1–L4) and within the proximal femur (femoral neck, trochanter, Ward's triangle) and defines them automatically. The results are expressed in bone mineral density (g/cm^2).

Advantages of the method are the relatively low radiation dose (3–5 μSv) and a clinically sufficient accuracy (Table 1) (76,80,81). The possibility of measuring parts of the axial skeleton and the total body is clinically important, because of possible variations in BMD, which may be regionally presented (82). A shortcoming of DPA is the long scanning times, between 20 and 45 minutes. The precision errors (CVs) for short-term investigations were between 1.1% and 2.3% (76,81, 83–86) and for long-term investigations between 1.4% and 3.7% (87,88). However, problems that are related to software and isotope changes were reported to elevate the CVs up to 6% (66,89,90). Especially the gradual decay of the isotope source, which must be changed every 18 months, may result in long-term drifts of the BMD measurements. Lumbar spine measurements by DPA are regularly influenced by osteophytes, hypertrophy of posterior elements, compression fractures with impacted bone or callus, and vascular calcifications, which superimpose the scanned field (91). These error sources, however, can be recognized by plain radiographs or computed tomography (92–94).

III. PRESENT METHODS

A. Dual X-ray Absorptiometry

In the past 6 years DPA has been replaced by dual x-ray absorptiometry (DXA). This technique is based on the same principle as DPA, but uses an x-ray tube instead of a radionuclide source. The concept has existed since the 1960s and 1970s, but it was not until 1987 that DXA was made commercially available (95–97). For this method various acronyms such as DER (dual-energy radiography), DRA (digital radiographic absorptiometry), QDR (quantitative digital radiography), and DEXA (dual-energy x-ray absorptiometry) have been used. The use of the acronym DXA has been proposed for this technique and is now generally accepted (98–100).

The main advantage of an x-ray system over a radionuclide source is the increased photon flux, facilitating a finer collimation of the beam of about 1.5 mm compared to 5–8 mm for DPA. The use of an x-ray system results in shorter scan time, greater accuracy and precision, higher resolution, and the lack of radionuclide decay. Additional technical improvements such as internal calibration have helped to improve the accuracy and precision further. The correlation between DPA and DXA was found to be excellent in spine and in hip (101). Correlation for the spine was r=0.98, with a standard error of the estimate (SEE) of 0.037 g/cm^2; for the femoral neck a correlation of r=0.95, with a standard error of the estimate (SEE) of 0.031 g/cm^2 was described (102). Because of the strong correlations between the two techniques, normative data generated with DPA can be extrapolated to DXA with appropriate calibration.

The usual locations for DXA measurements are the lumbar spine, proximal femur, and whole body. The forearm and the calcaneus can also be scanned. The digital image resulting from the measurement allows a gross survey of the examined region. The sophisticated software of all DXA devices facilitates identification of regions of interest with distinct compositions such as the femoral neck, Ward's triangle, and the ultradistal radius. At the lumbar spine every vertebral body can be measured separately, and fractured vertebrae can be excluded from the analysis.

The examination time for the earlier pencil beam devices ranges from 5 to 8 min for a PA spine measurement; a total body measurement with pencil beam technique requires about 10–20 min. The advanced generation of scanners such as the Hologic QDR 2000 or the newly introduced Lunar Expert use a fan beam and multidetector arrays instead of a pencil beam and single detector, decreasing the examination time by a factor of 4–5. An ultra-high-speed scanning mode on the Hologic QDR 2000 allows for 5-sec screening scans of the spine. A total body examination now requires less than 5 min. This advance reduces movement artifacts, improves the patient's comfort, and enhances patient throughput. Radiation dose for these investigations is very low. For a posterior-anterior (PA) lumbar spine measurement it is about 1 μSv for standard resolution examinations.

The in vivo precision of a PA DXA examination of the lumbar spine is generally about 1%. The accuracy error is on the order of 4–8%. Mazess et al. found that short-term in vivo precision was between 0.6% and 1.5% in the PA spine and between 1.2% and 2% in the hip, depending on the scanning speed (103). Similarly, Pacifici et al. obtained a short-term precision in vitro of 0.41% and in vivo of 1% (104). Glüer et al. found a long-term in vitro precision of 0.44% for DXA with a Hologic scanner (102). In less than 5 years DXA has taken the place of the DPA with a distribution of about 2,500 systems worldwide, thereby reaching great acceptance in clinical medicine and research (101–108).

B. Quantitative Computed Tomography

Quantitative computed tomography allows for a true three-dimensional bone density measurement without superimposition of other tissues, and therefore provides exact three-dimensional anatomic localization of the measured tissue. Bone density can be calculated separately in trabecular and cortical bone compartments. QCT makes possible, at least in theory, a direct measurement of density (g/cm^3) at any skeletal site. QCT is widely available now as a standard clinical examination of the bone density of the lumbar spine. Selective measurement of high-turnover trabecular bone such as the central portion of the vertebral body is of some advantage since it excludes cortical bone and extraosseous calcifications.

For vertebral measurements, first a lateral digital radiograph is obtained for slice selection at the midvertebral levels of three or four consecutive vertebral bodies (usually L1–L3, or L2–L4). Single midvertebral slices with a thickness of 8–10 mm are acquired parallel to the vertebral end plates. For calibration of a vertebral QCT scan, the technique developed at the University of California at San Francisco uses a mineral reference phantom (109–115). Two different calibration techniques exist: simultaneous and nonsimultaneous calibration. The method that is now routinely used in clinical applications is the simultaneous calibration (109). Simultaneous calibration corrects to a large extent for short-term and long-term scanner instabilities. Nonsimultaneous calibration, in which a quasianthropomorphic tissue equivalent phantom is scanned before or after the patient, has been used in several studies (116,117). This technique does not allow for correction of short-term instabilities. After performing the scans, the average attenuation in the region of interest is measured in the image, compared to the attenuation values of the reference standard, and finally expressed in mineral equivalents in mg/cm^3. Densities for the vertebrae are averaged and compared to those of a normal population.

A single-energy technique (single-energy quantitative CT, SEQCT) is usually applied for routine examinations. For SEQCT, a low-dose, low-energy setting should be selected resulting in an effective dose of typically 50 μSv (including the lateral digital radiograph) with essentially no gonadal exposure.

The absorption is not only influenced by bone, but also by other constituents. Bone marrow fat, which increases relatively with age, impacts the measured density, underestimating the actual bone mineral content by up to 15–20%. The clinical relevance of the fat error is small, however, due to the use of age matched databases (118). After performing the scans, the average attenuation in the region of interest is measured in the image, compared to the attenuation values of the reference standard, and finally expressed in mineral equivalents in mg/cm^3. Densities for the vertebrae are averaged and compared to those of a normal population.

For measurements of bone mineral content at the peripheral skeleton special purpose QCT scanners have been employed. The usual site for this technique is the ultradistal radius or distal tibia. Modern peripheral QCT (pQCT) scanners using a multislice technique offer short examination times, good precision error, and small radiation doses (119–121).

QCT provides information not only on bone mineral density but also on bone structure for the regions examined. High-resolution computed tomography can be the basis for future structural analysis with the potential of quantifying architectural changes in trabecular bone and improving fracture discrimination. Limitations of the method are its availability, greater complexity, higher costs, and radiation exposure compared to that of DXA measurements.

IV. FUTURE METHODS

A. Quantitative Ultrasound

Ultrasound techniques used to assess material properties are well known in industrial material testing. The first experiments to determine material properties of bone using ultrasound transmission velocity were performed in the 1960s (122,123). Though these experiments showed promising results, ultrasound techniques for the detection of osteoporosis were not employed widely until recently due to their limited practicability. The latest developments in hardware and software resulting in enhanced precision and ease of use have made these techniques a promising option for the assessment of material properties of the bone.

The ultrasound transmission velocity, or speed of sound (UTV; SOS), is calculated as the quotient of the transit time of an ultrasound wave through bone and the diameter of this bone and given in m/sec (124). SOS may be influenced by bone mass, distribution of trabecular and cortical bone, trabecular orientation, composition of organic and anorganic components, fatigue damage, etc. Accordingly, bone mass and qualitative characteristics of bone contribute to SOS. Abendschein and Hyatt found a significant correlation between SOS and elastic modulus ($r = 0.855$) or SOS and physical density ($r = 0.866$) (123). Tavakoli and Evans reported a correlation of 0.97 for SOS and bone mineral content of cancellous bone (125). The velocities measured in vitro have a wide range from 1,400–2,300 m/sec for cancellous bone to 3,000–3,600 m/sec for cortical bone (123,126,127).

Only a few in vivo studies have been performed to prove the diagnostic value of SOS for the detection of osteoporosis. Jergas et al. found a significant difference in the SOS as measured at the proximal phalanxes of the second and third fingers between osteoporotic and nonosteoporotic women (128). Heaney et al. stated that patellar SOS measurements have the ability to discriminate between normal and osteoporotic women as well as bone densitometry does in the axial skeleton (129). Brandenburger et al. reported that subjects with an SOS 1 SD or more below normal had a three to five times increased risk for vertebral crush fractures in the following two years than those with normal results (130).

Statements concerning correlations between SOS and BMD measurements at various skeletal sites have been controversial. Depending on the positioning of ultrasound transducers Zagzebski et al. reported a correlation of $r = 0.51$ to 0.72 between SOS and BMD, both measured at the os calcis (131). Herd et al. calculated a correlation coefficient of $r = 0.55$ between SOS at the os calcis and BMD of the lumbar spine, while Mazess et al. found a correlation coefficient of $r = 0.84$ for the same comparison (132,133). Other authors have reported only poor correlation for SOS measurements at the patella or fingers versus spinal or forearm BMD (128,134,135).

Attenuation measurements of ultrasound in humans were performed in the 1970s. The purpose of these early experiments was to establish a method for diagnostic ultrasound of the brain comparable to the CT scan (136). Reflection and absorption are the main components that contribute to the attenuation of the ultrasound penetrating a material (124). In addition, the attenuation of ultrasound strongly depends on the frequency of the ultrasound used. Using a low-frequency range (approx. 200–600 kHz), the attenuation is an almost linear function of frequency. With higher frequencies the attenuation is greater and nonlinear. In quantitative ultrasound techniques the attenuation of ultrasound is measured using the low-frequency range—e.g., 200–600 kHz. This technique is called broadband ultrasound attenuation (BUA). The slope of the regression line resulting is the BUA value and is given in units of dB/MHz.

In vitro studies showed significant correlations between physical density and BUA (137). Agren and co-workers were able to demonstrate a high correlation between BUA and trabecular bone volume (138). Zerwekh et al. stated that BUA appeared to provide a sensitive means of assessing changes in the material property of bone (139). Glüer et al. demonstrated a significant impact of trabecular orientation on BUA measurements, thus revealing the ability of BUA measurements to detect structural changes of the bone (140).

Clinical studies using BUA measurements have mainly concentrated on the os calcis as measurement site (Fig. 8). Resch et al. reported a good differentiation between osteoporotic and nonosteoporotic females using BUA (141). One prospective study demonstrated a significant association of BUA and fracture inci-

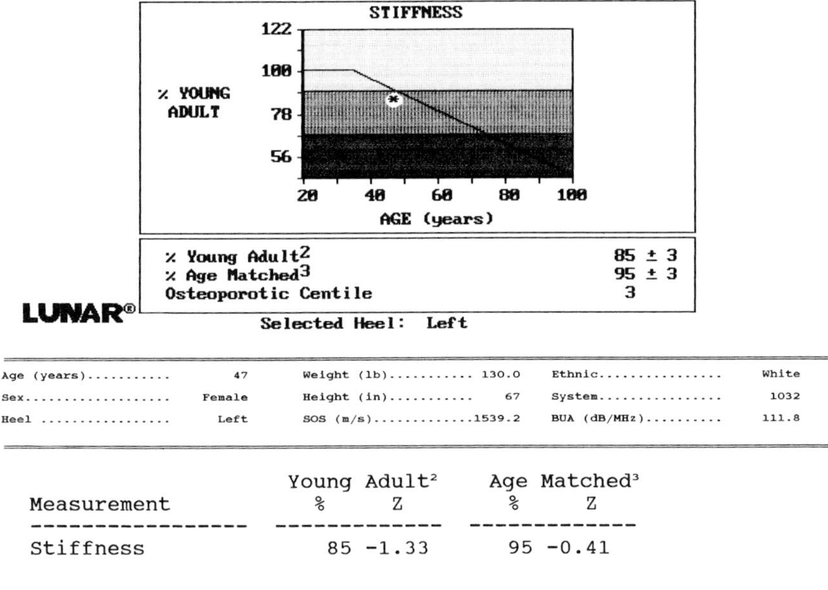

Age (years)...........	47	Weight (lb)...........	130.0	Ethnic................	White
Sex..................	Female	Height (in)...........	67	System................	1032
Heel	Left	SOS (m/s)..............	1539.2	BUA (dB/MHz)..........	111.8

Measurement	Young Adult[2] %	Young Adult[2] Z	Age Matched[3] %	Age Matched[3] Z
Stiffness	85	-1.33	95	-0.41

1 - See appendix E on precision and accuracy. Statistically 68% of repeat scans will fall within 1 SD.
2 - USA Reference Population, Ages 20-45.
3 - Matched for Age, Weight, Ethnic. See Appendices.

Figure 8 Printout of an ultrasound measurement of the calcaneus with a Lunar Achilles ultrasound scanner (Lunar Corp., Madison, Wisc). SOS and BUA results are given, and the calculated stiffness of the patient's calcaneus is automatically compared to that of a reference population.

dence (142). Baran et al. compared BUA with DPA measurements of vertebral bodies and femoral neck and found a significant decrease of BUA values in women with low bone mass. Although the spinal deformity index in osteoporosis was found to be unrelated to ultrasound measurements (143), Massie et al. as well as Young et al. found significant correlations between BMD results at the spine and hip measured by DXA and BUA of the os calcis (144,145). The diagnostic sensitivity and specificity of BUA measurements was found to be 80%. For patients with a femoral neck fracture sensitivity and specificity were still higher (146). Glüer et al. compared SXA (single x-ray absorptiometry) measurements with BUA measurements of the os calcis and found an overall correlation of $r = 0.58$ for a mixed population, and for a subgroup of women the correlation was $r = 0.72$, leaving about 50% of unexplained variability. The authors drew the conclusion that the unexplained 50% may relate to properties of the bone other than density, which may be assessed by ultrasound (147).

Comparing SOS and BUA, Ramalingham and co-workers found a correlation of $r = 0.81$. The correlation between BUA values using two devices of different manufacturers revealed a correlation of $r = 0.83$ (148).

Statements concerning the reproducibility of SOS and BUA measurements strongly depended on the devices used. The precision error (CV) for in vivo os calcis measurements using the most common devices was reported to be between 1.35% and 3.8% for BUA measurements and from 0.15% to 2.7% for measurements of the SOS (133,147,149–151). The in vitro precision error for measuring a phantom estimated by Schott et al. was 0.84% for BUA and 0.15% for SOS (149).

A main advantage of an ultrasound examination is the complete absence of radiation and the low cost of the equipment, but the uncertain relationship between bone mass, elastic properties of the bone and ultrasound, the influence of surrounding soft tissue, the path of the ultrasound wave when penetrating the bone and the effect of physical activity are issues that are still unsolved in the application of ultrasound as a diagnostic tool (126,137,143–145,152–156). Though a significant number of devices have already been distributed, some questions still need to be answered before ultrasound techniques are established as routine diagnostic tools for the clinical application.

B. Magnetic Resonance Imaging

Today, magnetic resonance (MR) is widely employed for medical imaging. MR has only recently been proposed as a method for providing information related to structure as well as density in the assessment of bone (157–168). Direct MR measurement of mineralized elements of bones has been relatively unsuccessful because bone tissue as a solid material has low mobile proton density and short T2 relaxation times, making detection by conventional MR imaging impracticable. Therefore information on cortical bone that can be acquired by MR is very limited. Trabecular bone can only be assessed by measurement of the surrounding bone marrow components. This method takes advantage of the fact that in trabecular bone the protons in the marrow are in a unique physical environment by being situated in the boundary zone of two physical phases of different magnetic susceptibility. Differences in magnetic susceptibility between bone marrow and trabecular bone result in a distortion in the lines of force, causing strong local inhomogeneities. Such field inhomogeneities result in dephasing of the transverse magnetization in marrow tissue with a decrease in marrow transverse relaxation time T2*, and consequently a reduction of signal intensity in gradient-echo images (Figs. 9, 10).

The relationships between bone formations in the marrow and MR T2* relaxation time measurements have been described for in vivo and in vitro situations in several studies. Davis et al. found in an in vitro study with bone powder (ground-up trabecular bone) that T2* decreased significantly for water-and-oil solutions as the bone density and surface-to-volume ratio of the bone solution increased (157). In another study, Rosenthal et al. measured a decrease in T2* relaxation time of

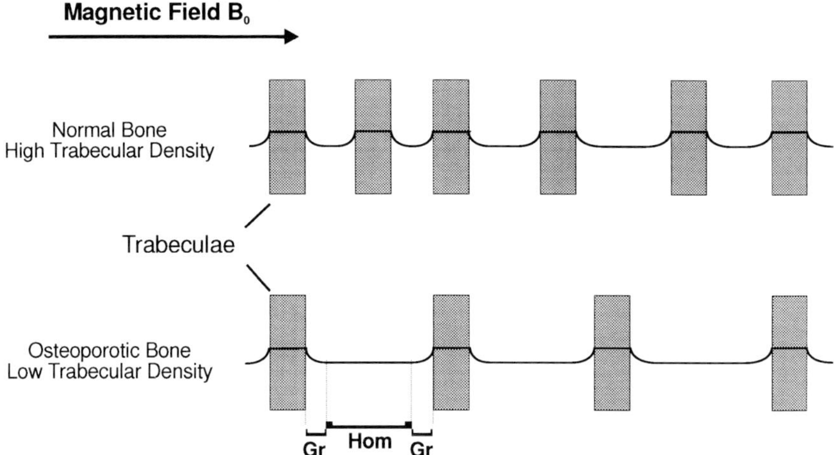

Figure 9 Principle of trabecular bone measurement by MR. Field inhomogeneities in the bone marrow are created by the presence of trabeculae, resulting in gradients (Gra) (upper line). Larger intertrabecular spaces allow for regions of magnetic homogeneity (Hom), thus lowering the transverse relaxation time T2* (lower line).

water in the trabecular spaces of vertebral specimen compared to T2* of extra-trabecular water (169). The results of these studies demonstrated that trabecular bone structure in the marrow space causes shortening of T2* relaxation time and accordingly signal loss in the given sequences. Consequently, these authors have stated that the presence of trabecular bone may affect the relaxation times of bone marrow in vivo. The in vitro studies of Majumdar et al., in which the effects of trabecular bone on the relaxation behavior of bone marrow in gradient-echo images were quantified, confirmed these results (159,160). Here the relaxation rate 1/T2* of saline in the presence of trabecular bone increased at a rate of 0.2 $s^{-1}/mg/cm^3$ due to the dephasing of the transverse magnetization in the magnetic field inhomogeneities. The in vivo influence of trabecular density in gradient-echo images was demonstrated by Sebag et al. Imaging the knee joint they found high signal intensity of the fat marrow in the diaphysis, where the trabecular density is relatively low. In the epiphysis, where more trabecular structure is present, low signal intensity was observed on gradient-echo images resulting from more pronounced T2* shortening at the trabecular-marrow interface (165). The same rate of change was found in a more recent study by Majumdar and Genant in which the distal radius and proximal tibia were investigated in vivo (170). The observation that T2* decreases as the degree of trabeculation increases was made in several studies using direct image-based T2* measurements as well as interferometry and localized spectroscopy (162,171–173). It has also been shown that T2* times

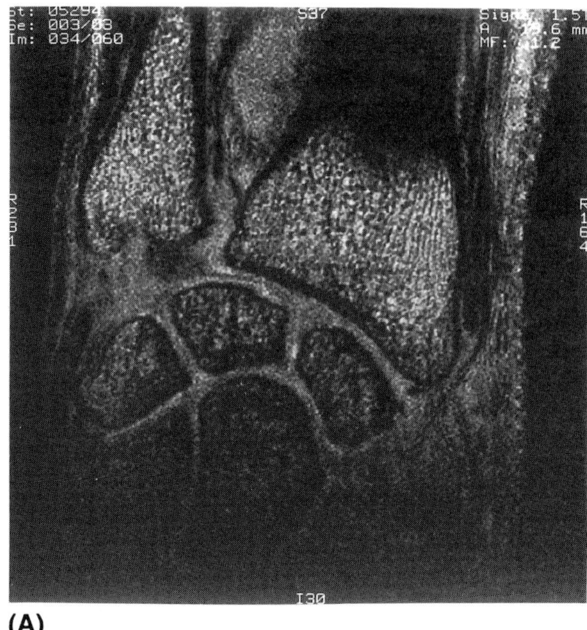

(A)

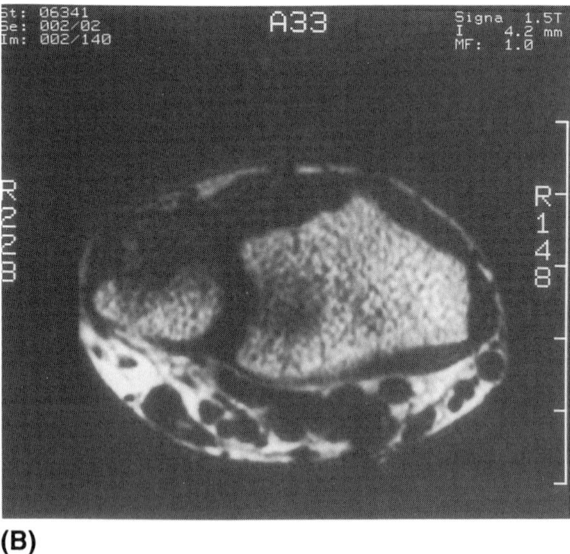

(B)

Figure 10 MR imaging at the distal radius with a 1.5 Tesla GE Signa scanner (General Electric, Milwaukee, Wisc). (A) Coronal slice though the distal radius—T2* weighted water-presaturated sequence. (B) Axial slice though the distal radius—T2* weighted water-presaturated sequence.

increased only slightly with age in healthy persons, whereas in patients with osteoporosis the T2* relaxation times were substantially increased, most likely caused by decrease of trabecular structure (174). In a study comparing BMD measurements using peripheral quantitative computed tomography with 1/T2* measurements using MR at the distal radius, Grampp et al. found a correlation coefficient of $r = 0.81$ between the two techniques (175). The potential of MR is further increased because, apart from trabecular bone density, trabecular architecture further affects the estimated T2* values (160,163,176).

The precision and reproducibility of bone marrow T2* measurements were previously investigated in an in vitro study. For this purpose, Majumdar and Genant used dried excised human vertebral bodies, immersed in physiologic saline. The specimens were measured three times (170). The coefficients of variation for the short-term precision of 1/T2* ranged from 2% to 11%, and the long-term precision was found to be between 20% and 50%. In an in vivo study Grampp et al. estimated precision errors between 3.3% and 12%, depending on the ROI placement, for the measurement at the distal radii of healthy volunteers (177).

In the near future MR imaging may be used to study changes in bone density and structure since MR imaging offers the potential of providing information about trabecular bone status (166,168,175,178). Especially for research applications it may be an important alternative method besides the x-ray-based techniques, yielding the potential of providing additional information.

C. Finite Element Analysis

The progress achieved in the computer sciences over the last few decades has also opened new horizons for the assessment of osteoporosis. Finite element analysis (FEA) of the human skeleton based on three-dimensional QCT or potentially MR of the trabecular network is a complex mathematical procedure that has been made possible with sophisticated software and modern microprocessor design. To describe the mechanical behavior of a structure with FEA, knowledge of its geometry, material properties, loading conditions, and applied forces is necessary (179–182). The method divides structures with unknown mechanical properties into a number of geometrically simplified elements. The qualities and behavior of each of these elements are calculated and combined. FEA was successfully employed in recent studies using three-dimensional volumetric computed tomography of the spine (Fig. 11) (183–186), the proximal femur (187–190), and prosthetic bone implants (191,192). In a study by Faulkner et al., CT examinations of lumbar vertebral bodies were used to calculate the strength of the vertebrae and to discriminate between osteoporotic and nonosteoporotic patients (186). They found large variations in estimated strength between vertebral bodies, which had very similar BMC and BMD results. Since these vertebrae contained similar amounts of calcified tissue, differences in estimated FEA strength were most likely caused by different distribution patterns of this tissue. In this study FEA

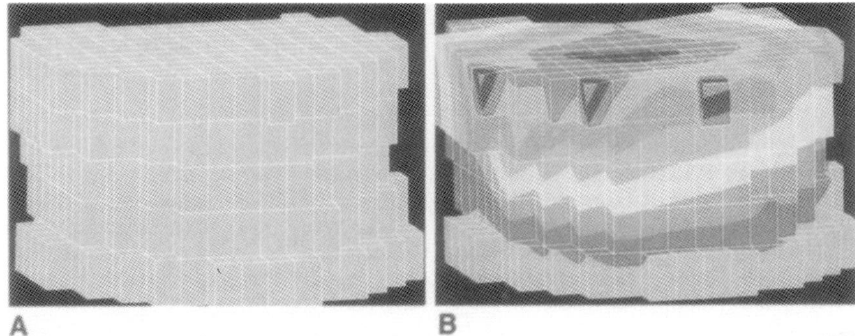

Figure 11 (A) Finite element mesh of a vertebral body calculated form a volumetric QCT dataset, consisting of 575 rectangular elements. (B) Deformed mesh plot of Figure 11A. Banded displacement contours demonstrate regions of minimal displacement at the lower model surface, where the object is contained not to move. Large amounts of displacements are visible at the higher surface of the object. These results can be used to estimate the compressive strength of the analyzed and remodeled vertebral body (with permission of [186]).

compared to QCT demonstrated a significantly improved ability to differentiate between osteoporotic and healthy patients.

FEA requires, however, a sophisticated computer environment and considerable computing time. Improvements in computer performance and software may help to establish this method, which seems to have potential for its improved discrimination of osteoporotic patients.

REFERENCES

1. Duboeuf F, Braillon P, Chapuy MC, et al. Bone mineral density of the hip measured with dual-energy x-ray absorptiometry in normal elderly women and in patients with hip fracture. Osteoporosis Int 1991; 1:242–249.
2. Black D, Cummings SR, Melton LJ. Appendicular bone mineral and a woman's lifetime risk of hip fracture. J Bone Miner Res 1992; 7:639–646.
3. Black D, Cummings SR, Genant HK, et al. Axial and appendicular bone density predict fractures in older women. J Bone Miner Res 1992; 7:633–638.
4. Hansson T, Roos B. The relation between bone mineral content, experimental compression fractures, and disc degeneration in lumbar vertebrae. Spine 1981; 6: 147–153.
5. Mosekilde L, Bentzen SM, Ørtoft G, and Jørgensen J. The predictive value of quantitative computed tomography for vertebral body compressive strength and ash density. Bone 1989; 10:465–470.
6. Dambacher MA, Ittner J, Rueegsegger P. Osteoporose—Pathogenese, Prophylaxe, Therapie. Internist 1989; 27:206–213.

7. Cummings SR, Kelsey JL, Nevitt MC, O'Dowd KJ. Epidemiology of osteoporosis and osteoporotic fractures. Epidemiol Rev 1985; 7:178–208.
8. Cummings SR, and Nevitt MC. Epidemiology of hip fractures and falls. In: Clinical Disorders of Bone and Mineral Metabolism: Proceedings of the Laurence and Dorothy Fallis International Symposium: 1989: 231–236.
9. Kelsey JL. The changing risk of disease in women: an epidemiologic approach. In: Gold EB, ed. Epidemiology of Osteoporosis. Baltimore: Johns Hopkins University. 1981:287–298.
10. Grampp S, Jergas M, Glüer CC, et al. Radiological diagnosis of osteoporosis: current methods and perspectives. Radiol Clin North Am 1993; 31:1133–1145.
11. Lang P, Steiger P, Faulkner KG, Glüer CC, Genant HK. Osteoporosis: current techniques and recent developments in quantitative bone densitometry. Radiol Clin North Am 1991; 29:49–76.
12. Ostlere SJ, Gold RH. Osteoporosis and bone density measurement methods. Clin Orthop Rel Res 1991; 271:149–163.
13. Fogelman I, Ryan P. Measurement of bone mass. Bone 1992; 13:S23–S28.
14. Johnston CC Jr, Slemenda CW, Melton LJ III. Clinical use of bone densitometry. N Engl J Med 1991; 324:1105–1109.
15. Johnston CC Jr. Noninvasive methods for quantitating appendicular bone mass. In: Miller P, ed. The Osteoporotic Syndrome: Detection, Prevention and Treatment. Boston: Little Brown; 1983:73–84.
16. Hangartner TN. The radiologic measurement of bone. J Can Assoc Radiol 1986; 37: 143–152.
17. Faulkner KG, Glüer CC, Majumdar S, et al. Noninvasive measurements of bone mass, structure, and strength: current methods and experimental techniques. Am J Radiol 1991; 157:1229–1237.
18. Genant HK, Block TE, Steiger P, Glüer CC, Ettinger B, Harris ST. Appropriate use of bone densitometry. Radiology 1989; 170:817–822.
19. Finsen V, Anda S. Accuracy of visually estimated bone mineralization in routine radiographs of the lower extremity. Skeletal Radiol 1988; 17:270–275.
20. Barnett E, Nordin BEC. The radiological diagnosis of osteoporosis: a new approach. Clin Radiol 1960; 11:166–174.
21. Singh YM, Nagrath AR, Maini PS. Changes in trabecular pattern of the upper end of the femur as an index of osteoporosis. J Bone Joint Surg 1970; 52A:457–467.
22. Herrs Nielsen VA, Pødenphant J, Martens S, Gotfredsen A, and Juel Riis B. Precision in assessment of osteoporosis from spine radiographs. Eur J Radiol 1991; 13: 11–14.
23. Cooper C, Barker DJP, Hall AJ. Evaluation of the Singh index and femoral calcar width as epidemiological methods for measuring bone mass in the femoral neck. Clin Radiol 1986; 37:123–125.
24. Meema HE, Meema S. Radiogrammetry. In: Cohn SH, ed. Non-invasive Measurements of Bone Mass. Boca Raton: CRC Press; 1981:5–50.
25. Dequeker J. Quantitative radiology: radiogrammetry of cortical bone. Br J Radiol 1976; 49:912–920.
26. Mazess RB. The noninvasive measurement of skeletal mass. Bone Miner Res Annu 1983; 1:223–273.

27. Meema HE, Meema S. Postmenopausal osteoporosis: simple screening method for diagnosis before structural failure. Radiology 1987; 164:405–410.
28. Garn SM. The earlier gain and later loss of cortical bone. In: Nutritional Perspective. Springfield: CC Thomas; 1970;146.
29. Van Hemert AM, Vandenbroucke JP, Birkenhäger JC. Prediction of osteoporotic fractures in the general population by a fracture risk score: a 9-year follow-up among middle-aged women. Am J Epidemiol 1990; 132:123–135.
30. Heuck F, Schmidt E. Die quantitative Bestimmung des Mineralgehaltes des Knochens aus dem Röntgenbild. Fortschr Röntgenstr 1960; 93:523–554.
31. Cosman F, Herrington B, Himmelstein S, Lindsay R. Radiographic absorptiometry: a simple method for determination of bone mass. Osteoporosis Int 1991; 2:34–38.
32. Hagiwara S, Yang S-O, Dhillon MS, et al. Precision and accuracy of radiographic absorptiometry: preliminary results. In: Proceedings of 4th International Symposium on Osteoporosis & Consensus Development Conference, Hong Kong; 1993:49.
33. Louis O, Van den Winckel P, Covens P, Schontens A, Osteaux M. Dual-energy x-ray absorptiometry of lumbar vertebrae; relative contribution of body and posterior elements and accuracy in relation with neutron activation analysis. Bone 1992; 13: 317–320.
34. Chow R, Harrison JE, Notarius C. Effect of two randomised exercise programmes on bone mass of healthy postmenopausal women. Br Med J 1987; 295:1441–1444.
35. Cohn SH. In-vivo neutron activation analysis: state of the art and future prospects. Med Phys 1981; 8:145–154.
36. Garnett ES, Kennett TJ, Kenyon DB, Webber CE. A photon scattering technique for the measurement of absolute bone density in man. Radiology 1973; 106:209–212.
37. Webber CE. Compton scattering methods. In: Cohn SH, ed. Non-invasive Measurements of Bone Mass and Their Clinical Application. Boca Raton: CRC Press; 1981: 101–120.
38. Maziere B, Kuntz D, Comar D, Ryckewaert A. In vivo analysis of bone calcium by local neutron activation of the hand: results in normal and osteoporotic subjects. J Nucl Med 1979; 20:85–91.
39. Smith MA, Tothill P, Kennedy NSJ, Eastell R. Total body calcium by neutron activation analysis. In: Dixon AJR, Russel G, Stamp TCB, eds. Osteoporosis: A Multidisciplinary Problem. Royal Society of Medicine International Congress and Symposium 1983; 55:121.
40. Williams ED, Boddy K, Harvey I, Haywood JK. Calibration and evaluation of a system for total body in vivo activation analysis using 14 MeV neutrons. Phys Med Biol 1978; 23:405.
41. Cohn SH, Ellis KJ, Wallach S, et al. Absolute and relative deficit in total-skeletal calcium and radial bone mineral in osteoporosis. J Nucl Med 1974; 15:428.
42. Cohn SH, Yasamura AS, Zanzi AI, Ellis KJ. Comparative skeletal mass and radial bone mineral content in black and white women. Metabolism 1977; 26:171–178.
43. Manzke E, Chestnut CH III, Wergedal JE, Baylink DJ, Nelp WB. Relationship between local and total bone mass in osteoporosis. Metabolism 1975; 24:605–615.
44. Aloia JF, Vaswani A, Atkins H, et al. Radiographic morphometry and osteopenia in spinal osteoporosis. J Nucl Med 1977; 18:425–431.

45. McNeill KG, Thomas BJ, Sturtridge WC, Harrison JE. In vivo neutron activation analysis for calcium in man. J Nucl Med 1973; 14:502.
46. Roberts JG, DiTomasso E, Webber CE. Photon scattering measurements of calcaneal bone density: results of in vivo cross-sectional studies. Immunol Rev 1982; 17: 20–28.
47. Margulies JY, Leichter I, Robin GC, Gazit D, Bab I. A correlative assessment of photon interaction and histomorphometric measurements of bone density. Arch Orthop Trauma Surg 1986; 105:239–242.
48. Webber CE, Kennett TJ. Bone density measured by photon scattering. I. A system for clinical use. Phys Med Biol 1976; 21:760–769.
49. Shukla S, Leichter I, Karellas A, Craven JD, Greenfield MA. Trabecular bone mineral density measurement in vivo: use of the ratio of coherent to Compton-scattered photons in the calcaneus. Radiology 1986; 158:695.
50. Kennett TJ, Webber CE. Bone density measured by photon scattering. II. Inherent sources of error. Phys Med Biol 1976; 21:770.
51. Battista JJ, Bronskill MR. Compton-scatter imaging of transverse sections: corrections for multiple scatter and attenuations. Phys Med Biol 1977; 22:229.
52. Battista JJ, Bronskill MR. Compton-scatter tissue densitometry: calculation of single and multiple scatter photon fluences. Phys Med Biol 1978; 23:1.
53. Hazan G, Leichter I, Loewinger E, Weinreb A, Robin GC. The early detection of osteoporosis by Compton gamma ray spectroscopy. Phys Med Biol 1977; 22:1073–1084.
54. Puumalainen P, Uimarihuhta A, Alhava EM, Olkkonen H. A new photon scattering method for bone mineral density measurements. Radiology 1976; 120:723.
55. Cohn SH, Vaswani AN, Zanzi I, Ellis KJ. Effect of aging on bone mass in adult women. Am J Physiol 1976; 230:143–148.
56. Ott SM, Murano R, Lewellen TK, Nelp WP, Chesnut CH III. Total body calcium by neutron activation analysis in normals and osteoporotic populations: a discriminator of significant bone loss. J Lab Clin Med 1983; 102:637.
57. Cohn SH, Aloia JF, Vaswani AN, et al. Women at risk for developing osteoporosis: determination by total body neutron activation analysis and photon absorptiometry. Calcif Tissue Int 1986; 38:9–15.
58. Cameron JR, Sorenson JA. Measurement of bone mineral in vivo: an improved method. Science 1963; 142:230–232.
59. Cameron JR, Mazess RB, Sorenson MS. Precision and accuracy of bone mineral determination by direct photon absorptiometry. Invest Radiol 1968; 3:141–150.
60. Strandjord NM, Lanzl LH. Iodine-125 bone densitometry. In: Progress in Development of Methods in Bone Densitometry. Washington, DC: National Aeronautics and Space Administration; 1965:111–124.
61. Schlenker RA, Von Seggen WW. The distribution of cortical and trabecular bone mass along the lengths of the radius and ulna and the implications for in vivo bone mass measurements. Calcif Tissue Res 1970; 20:41–52.
62. Vogel JM. Application principles and technical considerations in SPA. In: Genant HK, ed. Osteoporosis Update 1987. San Francisco: Radiology Research and Education Foundation; 1987:219–231.

63. Wahner HW, Eastell R, Riggs BL. Bone mineral density of the radius: where do we stand? J Nucl Med 1985; 26:1339–1341.
64. Awbrey BJ, Jacobson PC, Grubb SA, et al. Bone density in women: a modified procedure for measurement of distal radial density. J Orthop Res 1984; 2:314–321.
65. Nilas L, Borg J, Gotfredsen A, Christiansen C. Comparison of single- and dual-photon absorptiometry in postmenopausal bone mineral loss. J Nucl Med 1985; 26: 1257–1262.
66. Nilas L, Pødenphant J, Riis BJ, Gotfredsen A. Usefulness of regional bone measurements in patients with osteoporotic fractures of the spine and distal forearm. J Nucl Med 1987; 28:960–965.
67. Williams JA, Wagner J, Wasnich R, Heilbrun L. The effect of long-distance running upon appendicular bone mineral content. Med Sci Sports Exercise 1984; 16:223–227.
68. Suominen H, Heikkinen E, Vaino P, Lahtinen T. Mineral density of calcaneus in men at different ages: a population study with special reference to life-style factors. Age Ageing 1984; 13:273–281.
69. Yano K, Wasnich RD, Bogel JM, Heilbrun LK. Bone mineral measurements among middle-aged and elderly Japanese residents in Hawaii. Am J Epidemiol 1984; 119: 751–764.
70. Davis MR. Screening for postmenopausal osteoporosis. Am J Obstet Gynecol 1987; 156:1–5.
71. Ross PD, Wasnich RD, Heilbrun LK, Vogel JM. Definition of a spine fracture threshold based upon prospective fracture risk. Bone 1987; 8:271–278.
72. Vogel JM, Wasnich RD, Ross PD. The clinical relevance of calcaneus bone mineral measurements: a review. Bone Miner 1988; 5:35–58.
73. Wasnich RD, Ross PD, Heilbrun LK, Vogel JM. Prediction of postmenopausal fracture risk with use of bone mineral measurements. Am J Obstet Gynecol 1985; 153:745–751.
74. Wasnich RD, Ross PD, Heilbrun LK, Vogel JM. Selection of the optimal site for fracture risk prediction. Clin Orthop 1987; 216:262–268.
75. Cummings SR, Black DM, Nevitt MC, et al. Appendicular bone density and age predict hip fracture in women. JAMA 1990; 263:665–668.
76. Szücs J, Jonson R, Granhed H, Hansson T. Accuracy, precision, and homogeneity effects in the determination of the bone mineral content with dual photon absorptiometry in the heel bone. Bone 1992; 13:179–183.
77. Yamada M, Ito M, Hayashi K, Nakamura T. Calcaneus as a site for assessment of bone mineral density: evaluation in cadavers and healthy volunteers. Am J Roentgenol 1993; 161:621–627.
78. Mazess RB, Barden HS. Single- and dual-photon absorptiometry for bone measurement in osteoporosis. In: Genant HK, ed. Osteoporosis Update. San Francisco: Radiology Research and Education Foundation; 1987:73–80.
79. Gingold E, Hasegawa B. Systematic bias in basis meterial decomposition applied to quantitative dual-energy x-ray imaging. Med Phys 1992; 19:25–33.
80. Hassager C, Jensen SB, Gotfredsen A, Christiansen C. The impact of measurement errors on the diagnostic value of bone mass measurements: theoretical considerations. Osteoporosis Int 1991; 1:250–256.

81. Wilson CR. Bone mineral content of the femoral neck and spine versus the radius or ulna. J Bone Joint Surg (Am) 1977; 59A:665–669.
82. Feyerabend AJ, Lear JL. Regional variations in bone mineral density as assessed with dual-energy photon absorptiometry and dual x-ray absorptiometry. Radiology 1993; 186:467–469.
83. Slosman DO, Rizzoli R, Buchs B, et al. Comparative study of the performances of x-ray and gadolinium 153 bone densitometers at the level of the spine, femoral neck and femoral shaft. Eur J Nucl Med 1990; 17:3–9.
84. Stevenson JC, Lees B, Devenport M, Cust MP, Ganger KF. Determinants of bone density in normal women: risk factors for future osteoporosis? BMJ 1989; 298: 924–928.
85. Wahner H, Dunn WL. Non-invasive bone mineral measurements. Semin Nucl Med 1983; 13:282–289.
86. LeBlanc AD, Evans HJ, Marsh C, et al. Precision of dual photon absorptiometry measurements. J Nucl Med 1986; 27:1362–1365.
87. Slemenda CW, Johnston CC. Bone mass measurement: which site to measure? Am J Med 1988; 84:643–645.
88. Nilas L, Hassager C, Christiansen C. Long-term precision of dual-photon absorptiometry in the lumbar spine in clinical settings. Bone Miner 1988; 3:305–315.
89. Ross PD, Wasnich RD, Vogel JM. Precision errors in dual-photon absorptiometry related to source age. Radiology 1988; 166:523–527.
90. Dawson-Hughes B, Deehr MS, Berger PS, Dallal GE, Sadowski LJ. Correction of the effects of source, source strength, and soft-tissue thickness on spine dual-photon absorptiometry measurements. Calcif Tissue Int 1989; 44:251–257.
91. Cann CE, Rutt BK, Genant HK. Effect of extra-osseous calcifications on vertebral mineral measurements. Calcif Tissue Int 1983; 35:647.
92. Peel NFA, Johnson A, Barrington NA, Smith TWD, Eastell R. Impact of anomalous vertebral segmentation on measurements of bone mineral density. J Bone Miner Res 1993; 8:719–723.
93. Hurxthal LM, Vose GP, Dotter WE. Densitometric and visual observations of spinal radiographs. Geriatrics 1969; 24:93–106.
94. Ito M, Hayashi K, Yamada M, Uetani M, Nakamura T. Relationship of osteophytes to bone mineral density and spinal fracture in men. Radiology 1993; 189:497–502.
95. Gustavson L, Jacobson B, Kusoffsky L. X-ray spectrophotometry for bone mineral determinations. Med Biol Eng Comput 1974; 12:113–118.
96. Jacobson B. X-ray spectrophotometry in vivo. Am J Roentgenol 1964; 91:202–210.
97. Stein JA, Lazewatsky JL, Hochberg AM. Dual energy x-ray bone densitometer incorporating an internal reference system. Radiology 1987; 165(P):313.
98. Genant HK, Glüer CC, Faulkner KG, et al. Acronyms in bone densitometry. Radiology 1992; 184:878.
99. Glüer CC. Klinische Anwendung Absorptiometrischer Verfahren. In Schild HH, Heller M, eds. Osteoporose. Stuttgart: Thieme Verlag.
100. Wilson CR, Collier BD, Carrera GF, Jacobson DR. Acronym for dual-energy x-ray absorptiometry. Radiology 1990; 176:875–876.
101. Borders J, Kerr E, Sartoris DJ, et al. Quantitative dual energy radiographic absorp-

tiometry of the lumbar spine: in vivo comparison with dual-photon absorptiometry. Radiology 1989; 170:129–131.

102. Glüer CC, Steiger P, Selvidge R, et al. Comparative assessment of dual-photon-absorptiometry and dual-energy-radiography. Radiology 1990; 174:223–228.
103. Mazess RB, Collick B, Trempe J, Barden H, Hanson J. Performance evaluation of a dual energy x-ray bone densitometer. Calcif Tissue Int 1989; 44:228–232.
104. Pacifici R, Rupich R, Vered I, et al. Dual energy radiography (DER): a preliminary comparative study. Calcif Tissue Int 1988; 43:189–191.
105. Kelly TL, Slovik DM, Neer RM. Calibration and standardization of bone mineral densitometers. J Bone Miner Res 1989; 4(5):663–669.
106. Sartoris DJ, Resnick D. Dual energy radiographic absorptiometry for bone densitometry: current status and perspective. AJR 1989; 152:241–246.
107. Uebelhart D, Braillon P, Meunier PJ, Delmas PD. Lateral dual photon absorptiometry of the spine in vertebral osteoporosis and osteoarthritis. Comparison with quantitative computed tomography. J Bone Miner Res 1989; 4(suppl):S328 (abstract).
108. Wahner HW, Dunn WL, Brown ML, Morin RL, Riggs BL. Comparison of dual-energy x-ray absorptiometry and dual photon absorptiometry for bone mineral measurements of the lumbar spine. Mayo Clin Proc 1988; 63:1075–1084.
109. Cann CE, Genant HK. Precise measurement of vertebral mineral content using computed tomography. J Comp Assist Tomogr 1980; 4:493–500.
110. Cann CE, Genant HK. Single versus dual-energy CT for vertebral mineral quantification. J Comp Assist Tomogr 1983; 7:551–552.
111. Genant HK, Boyd DP. Quantitative bone mineral analysis using dual energy computed tomography. Invest Radiol 1977; 12:545–551.
112. Genant HK, Cann C. Vertebral mineral determination using quantitative computed tomography. In: Proceedings of Tenth Steenbock Symposium, Madison, Wisc. Baltimore: University Park Press; 1981:37–47.
113. Genant HK, Block JE, Steiger P, Glüer CC. Quantitative computed tomography in the assessment of osteoporosis. In: Genant HK, ed. Osteoporosis Update 1987. San Francisco: Radiology Research and Education Foundation; 1987:49–71.
114. Genant HK, Glüer CC, Steiger P, Faulkner KG. Quantitative computed tomography for the assessment of osteoporosis. In: Moss AA, Gamsu G, Genant HK, eds. Computed Tomography of the Body. Philadelphia: W.B. Saunders; 1992:2:523–549.
115. Laval-Jeantet AM, Cann CE, Roger BM, et al. A postprocessing dual-energy technique for vertebral CT densitometry. J Comp Assist Tomogr 1984; 9:1164–1167.
116. Abols Y, Genant HK, Rosenfled D, et al. Spinal bone mineral determination using computerized tomography in patients, controls, and phantoms. In: Mazess RB, ed. Washington, DC: US Government Printing Office; 1979:NIH:80-1928.
117. Cann CE. Quantitative computed tomography for bone mineral analysis: technical considerations. In: Genant HK, ed. Osteoporosis Update 1987. San Francisco: University of California Printing Services; 1987:131–145.
118. Glüer CC, Genant HK. Impact of marrow fat on accuracy of quantitative CT. J Comput Assist Tomogr 1989; 13:1023–1035.
119. Kaisel W, Rüegsegger P. 3D-QCT at peripheral measuring sites. Osteoporosis Int 1991; 1:193.

120. McClean BA, Overton TR, Hangartner TN, Rathee S. A special purpose x-ray fan beam CT scanner for trabecular bone density measurement in the appendicular skeleton. Phys Med Biol 1990; 35:11–19.
121. Rüegsegger P, Durand E, Dambacher MA. Localization of regional forearm bone loss from high resolution computed tomographic images. Osteoporosis Int 1991; 1: 76–80.
122. Floriani L, Debevoise N, Hyatt G. Mechanical properties of healing by the use of ultrasound. Surg Forum 1967; 18:468–470.
123. Abendschein W, Hyatt GW. Ultrasonics and selected physical properties of bone. Clin Orthop Rel Res 1970; 69:294–301.
124. Antich PP, Anderson JA, Ashman RB, et al. Measurement of mechanical properties of bone material in vitro by ultrasound reflection: methodology and comparison with ultrasound transmission. J Bone Miner Res 1991; 6:417–426.
125. Tavakoli MB, Evans JA. Dependence of the velocity and attenuation of ultrasound in bone on the mineral content. Phys Med Biol 1991; 36:1529–1537.
126. McCartney R, Jeffcott L. Combined 2.25 MHz ultrasound velocity and bone mineral density measurements in the equine metacarpus and their in vivo applications. Med Biol Eng Comput 1987; 25:620–626.
127. Turner CH, Eich M. Ultrasonic velocity as a predictor of strength in bovine cancellous bone. Calcif Tissue Int 1991; 49:116–119.
128. Jergas M, Uffmann M, Müller P, Köster O. Ultraschallgeschwindigkeitsmessungen zur Diagnose der postmenopausalen Osteoporose. Fortschr Röntgenstr 1993; 158: 207–213.
129. Heaney RP, Avioli LV, Chestnut CH, et al. Osteoporotic bone fragility: detection by ultrasound transmission velocity. JAMA 1989; 261:2986–2990.
130. Brandenburger GH, Kwon S, McDougall SW. Preliminary results from a longitudinal clinical study of ultrasound velocity. In: Proceedings of Third International Symposium on Osteoporosis, Copenhagen, Denmark; 1991:199.
131. Zagzebski JA, Rossmann PJ, Mesina C, Mazess RB, Madsen EL. Ultrasound transmission measurements through the os calcis. Calcif Tissue Int 1991; 49:107–111.
132. Herd RJM, Blake GM, Miller CG, Fogelman I. Can ultrasonic measurements in the calcaneus predict osteopenia in the axial skeleton? In: Ring EFG, ed. Proceedings of Current Research in Osteoporosis and Bone Mineral Measurement II: Bath, 1992. London: British Institute of Radiology; 1992:45.
133. Trempe J, Genske T, Wiener S, Mazess R. Ultrasound measurement of the os calcis. In: Ring EFG, ed. Proceedings of Current Research in Osteoporosis and Bone Mineral Measurement II: 1992, 1992. London: British Institute of Radiology; 1992: 43–44.
134. Klein K, Allolio B. A health promotion project "osteoporosis"—in cooperation with the insurance company "Deutsche Bank AG." In: Ring EFG, ed. Proceedings of Current Research in Osteoporosis and Bone Mineral Measurement II: Bath, 1992. London: British Institute of Radiology; 1992:97.
135. Agnusdei D, Camporeale A, Gennari C. La velocita di transmissione degli ultrasuoni nella patella in soggetti normali ed in pazienti con osteoporosi postmenopausale. Minerva Endocrinol 1991; 16:73–77.

136. Fry FJ, Barger JE. Acoustical properties of the human skull. J Acoust Soc Am 1978; 63:1576–1590.
137. McCloskey EV, Murray SA, Charlesworth D, et al. Assessment of broadband ultrasound attenuation in the os calcis in vitro. Clin Sci 1990; 78:221–225.
138. Agren M, Karellas A, Leahey D, Marks S, Baran D. Ultrasound attenuation of the calcaneus: a sensitive and specific discriminator of osteopenia in postmenopausal women. Calcif Tissue Int 1991; 48:240–244.
139. Zerwekh JE, Antich PP, Sakhaee K, et al. Assessment by reflection ultrasound method of the effect of intermittent slow-release sodium fluoride–calcium citrate therapy on material strength of bone. J Bone Miner Res 1991; 6:239–244.
140. Glüer CC, Wu CY, Genant HK. Broadband ultrasound attenuation signals depend on trabecular orientation: an in-vitro study. Osteoporosis Int 1993; 3:185–191.
141. Resch H, Pietschmann P, Bernecker P, Krexner E, Willvonseder R. Broadband ultrasound attenuation: a new diagnostic method in osteoporosis. Am J Radiol 1990; 155:825–828.
142. Porter R, Miller C, Grainger D, Palmer S. Prediction of hip fracture in elderly women: a prospective study. BMJ 1990; 301:638–641.
143. Bernecker P, Pietschmann P, Winkelbauer F, et al. The spine deformity index in osteoporosis is not related to bone mineral and ultrasound measurements. Br J Radiol 1992; 65:393–396.
144. Massie A, Reid DM, Porter RW. Screening for osteoporosis: comparison between dual energy x-ray absorptiometry and broadband ultrasound attenuation in 1000 perimenopausal women. Osteoporosis Int 1993; 3:107–110.
145. Young H, Howey S, Purdie DW. Broadband ultrasound attenuation compared with dual-energy x-ray absorptiometry in screening for postmenopausal low bone density. Osteoporosis Int 1993; 3:160–164.
146. Baran DT, Kelly AM, Karellas A, et al. Ultrasound attenuation of the os calcis in women with osteoporosis and hip fractures. Calcif Tissue Int 1988; 43:138–142.
147. Glüer CC, Vahlensieck M, Faulkner KG, et al. Site-matched calcaneal measurements of broadband ultrasound attenuation and single s-ray absorptiometry: do they measure different skeletal properties? J Bone Miner Res 1992; 7:1071–1079.
148. Ramalingham T, Herd RJM, Blake GM, Miller CG, Fogelman I. Ultrasonic measurements in the calcaneus: a comparison of two commercial scanners. In Ring EFG, ed. Proceedings of Current Research in Osteoporosis and Bone Mineral Measurement II: Bath, 1992. London: British Institute of Radiology; 1992:44.
149. Schott AM, Hans D, Sornay-Rendu E, Delmas PD, Meunier PJ. Ultrasound measurements on os calcis: precision and age-related changes in a normal female population. Osteoporosis Int 1993; 3:249–254.
150. Miller CG, Herd RJM, Ramalingam T, Fogelman I, Blake GM. Ultrasonic velocity measurements through the calcaneus: which velocity should be measured? Osteoporosis Int 1993; 3:31–35.
151. McKelvie ML, Fordham J, Clifford C, Palmer SB. In vitro comparison of quantitative computed tomography and broadband ultrasonic attenuation of trabecular bone. Bone 1989; 10:101–104.
152. Rubin C, Pratt G, Porter A, Lanyon L, Poss R. The use of ultrasound in vivo to

determine acute change in the mechanical properties of bone following intense physical activity. J Biomechanics 1987; 20:723–727.

153. Jergas M, Uffmann M, Wittenberg R, Müller P, Köster O. Ultraschallgeschwindigkeitsmessungen an belastungstragenden und nichtbelastungstragenden Stellen des peripheren Skeletts. Der Einfluß körperlicher Aktivität bei Fußballspielern. Fortschr Röntgenstr 1992; 157:420–424.
154. Jones PRM, Hardmann AE, Hudson A, Norgan NG. Influence of brisk walking on the ultrasonic attenuation of the calcaneus in previously sedentary women aged 30–61 years. Calcif Tissue Int 1991; 49:112–115.
155. Langton CM, Riggs CM, Evans GP. Pathway of ultrasound waves in the equine third metacarpal bone. J Biomed Eng 1991; 13:113–118.
156. McCloskey EV, Murray SA, Miller C, et al. Broadband ultrasound attenuation in the os calcis: relationship to bone mineral at other sites. Clin Sci 1990; 78:227–233.
157. Davis CA, Genant HK, Dunham JS. The effects of bone on proton NMR relaxation times of surrounding liquids. Invest Radiol 1986; 21:472–477.
158. Majumdar S, Thomasson D, Shimakawa A, Genant HK. Appearance of bone marrow in the presence of trabecular bone: quantitation of the susceptibility effects and correlation with bone density. Radiology 1990; 177(P):128–129.
159. Majumdar S, Thomasson D, Shimakawa A, Genant HK. Quantitation of the susceptibility difference between trabecular bone and bone marrow: experimental studies. Magn Reson Med 1991; 22:111–127.
160. Majumdar S. Quantitative study of the susceptibility differences between trabecular bone and bone marrow: computer simulations. Magn Reson Med 1991; 22:101–110.
161. Ford JC, Wehrli FW, Gusnard DA. Quantification of the intrinsic magnetic field inhomogeneity of trabecular bone. Magn Reson Imag 1990; 8S1:37.
162. Ford JC, Wehrli FW. In vivo quantitative characterization of trabecular bone by NMR interferometry and localized proton spectroscopy. Magn Reson Med 1991; 17: 543–551.
163. Ford JC, Wehrli FW, Chung H. Magnetic field distribution in models of trabecular bone. In: Proceedings of SMRM 92, Berlin, Germany; 1992:1302.
164. Ford JC, Wehrli FW, Chung H. Magnetic field distribution in models of trabecular bone. Mag Reson Med 1993; 30:373–379.
165. Sebag GH, Moore SG. Effect of trabecular bone on the appearance of marrow in gradient-echo imaging of the appendicular skeleton. Radiology 1990; 174:855–859.
166. Ito M, Hayashi K, Uetani M, et al. Bone mineral and other bone components in vertebrae evaluated by QCT and MRI. Skeletal Radiol 1993; 22:109–113.
167. Wehrli FW, Ford JC, Kaut-Watson C. Quantitative MR: a new method for in vivo characterization of trabecular bone structure. Radiology 1990; 177(P):245.
168. Wehrli FW, Ford JC, Chung HW, et al. Potential role of nuclear magnetic resonance for the evaluation of trabecular bone quality. Calcif Tissue Int 1993; 53(suppl 1): S162–S169.
169. Rosenthal H, Thulborn KR, Rosenthal DI, Rosen BR. Magnetic susceptibility effects of trabecular bone on magnetic resonance bone marrow imaging. Invest Radiol 1990; 25:173–178.
170. Majumdar S, Genant HK. In vivo relationship between marrow T2* and trabecular

bone density determined with a chemical shift-selective asymmetric spin-echo sequence. J Magn Reson Imaging 1992; 2:209–219.

171. Glazel JA, Lee KH. On the interpretation of water nuclear magnetic resonance relaxation times in heterogeneous systems. J Am Chem Soc 1974; 96:970–978.
172. Korczyk P, Hoszowski K, Jaworski M, Talajko A, Lorenc RS. Clinical precision and accuracy of ultrasound measurements of the calcaneus in diagnosis of osteopenia. In: Proceedings of 4th International Symposium on Osteoporosis & Consensus Development Conference, Hong Kong; 1993:59.
173. Dooms GC, Fisher MR, Hricak H, et al. Bone marrow imaging: magnetic resonance studies related to age and sex. Radiology 1985; 155:429–432.
174. Wehrli FW, Ford JC, Attie M, Kressel HY, Kaplan FS. Trabecular structure: preliminary application of MR interferometry. Radiology 1991; 179:615–621.
175. Grampp S, Majumdar S, Jergas M, Lang P, Genant HK. In vivo estimation of bone mineral density in the radius using magnetic resonance and peripheral quantitative computed tomography. Radiology 1993; 189(P):283.
176. Engelke K, Majumdar S, Genant H. Impact of trabecular structure on marrow relaxation time, T2*. In: Proceedings of 9th Int Workshop on Bone Densitometry, Traverse City, 1992.
177. Grampp S, Majumdar S, Jergas M, Huang Y, Genant HK. In vivo precision of bone marrow MR relaxation time. ECR 93, Book of Abstracts 1993; 108.
178. Jara H, Wehrli FW, Chung H, Ford JC. High-resolution variable flip angle 3D MR imaging of trabecular microstructure in vivo. Magn Reson Med 1993; 29:528–539.
179. Reddy JN. An Introduction to the Finite Element Method. New York: McGraw-Hill, 1984.
180. Brekelmans WAM, Poort HW, Sloof TJJH. A new method to analyse the mechanical behavior of skeletal parts. Acta Orthop Scand 1972; 43:301–317.
181. Rybicki EF. On the mathematical analysis of stress in the human femur. J Biomechanics 1972; 5:203–215.
182. Huiskes R, Chao EYS. A survey of finite element analysis in orthopedic biomechanics: the first decade. J Biomechanics 1983; 16:385–409.
183. Mizrahi J, Silva MJ, Eng M, et al. Finite-element stress analysis of the normal and osteoporotic lumbar vertebral body. Spine 1993; 18:2088–2096.
184. Faulkner KG, Cann CE. Patient-specific finite element models for analysis of vertebral strength. Radiology 1989; 173(P):415.
185. Faulkner KG, Cann CE. ROC analysis of vertebral finite element models for fracture prediction: comparison with QCT. In: Proceedings of Third International Symposium on Osteoporosis, Copenhagen, Denmark, 1990. Copenhagen: Osteopress; 1990:1029–1031.
186. Faulkner KG, Cann CE, Hasegawa BH. The effect of bone distribution on vertebral strength: assessment with patient-specific nonlinear finite element analysis. Radiology 1991; 179:669–674.
187. Faulkner KG, Grampp S, Glüer C-C, Genant HK. Patient specific finite element analysis of the proximal femur: comparison with compression tests in-vitro. J Bone Miner Res 1991; 6:344.
188. Rohlmann A, Mossner U, Bergmann G, Kobel R. Finite-element analysis and experimental investigation of stresses in a femur. J Biomed Eng 1982; 4:241–246.

189. Keyak JH, Meagher JM, Skinner HB, Mote CD. Automated three-dimensional finite element modelling of bone: a new method. J Biomed Eng 1990; 12:389–397.
190. Brown TD, DiGiola AM. A contact-coupled finite element analysis of the natural adult hip. J Biomechanics 1984; 17:437–448.
191. Scholten R, Roehrle H, Sollbach W. Analysis of stress distribution in natural and artificial hip joints using the finite element method. S Afr Mech Eng 1978; 28: 220–225.
192. Rybicki EF, Simonen FA. Mechanics of oblique fracture fixation using a finite element model. J Biomechanics 1983; 16:385–409.

9

Clinical Applications of Bone Mineral Measurements

JILL E. SPADIA and DAVID J. SARTORIS

University of California, San Diego, School of Medicine, and University of California, San Diego, Medical Center San Diego, California

HEINZ W. WAHNER

Mayo Clinic Rochester, Minnesota

I. WHY MEASURE BONE MINERAL DENSITY?

Osteoporosis, the most severe form of low bone mass, is a major medical problem with rising medical, social, and economic consequences. Osteoporosis is a multifactorial disease; the definition of osteoporosis has changed over the years to reflect changing insights into its complex mechanism (1). The definition used by a consensus development conference in 1991 (2) and accepted by a recent World Health Organization (WHO) study report (3) emphasizes a heterogeneity of skeletal and extraskeletal factors leading to bone fragility. Osteoporosis is defined as "a disease characterized by low bone mass and microarchitectural deterioration of bone tissue, leading to enhanced bone fragility and a consequent increase in fracture risk." This definition replaces fracture, which was an important diagnostic criterion in older definitions, by low bone mass. Thus it is now possible to diagnose osteoporosis prior to the occurrence of fracture.

The clinical syndrome of osteoporosis can be divided into primary and secondary forms. Primary osteoporosis is the most common. Primary osteoporosis can be further subclassified into type I (postmenopausal) and type II (senile) osteoporosis (4,5).

Type I, or postmenopausal osteoporosis, primarily involves the axial skeleton and trabecular bone. It is characterized by occurrence in the menopausal age and by spinal compression fractures. In general there is a high bone turnover state.

Type II, or senile osteoporosis, involves both trabecular and cortical bone and is characterized by axial and peripheral bone fractures. This form is present in older age groups. Generally there is low bone turnover.

Advanced type II osteoporosis, labeled type III, is similar to type II but with an etiology of decreased absorption of calcium. Calcium absorption can be improved by oral 1,25-hydroxycholecalciferol.

Secondary forms of osteoporosis are extremely rare. They include those associated with drugs; endocrine, gastrointestinal, renal, hepatic, and congenital diseases; organ transplantation; and immobility. In these cases, treatment is mainly directed at the underlying disease process. Lab tests such as serum calcium, phosphorus, alkaline phosphatase, PTH, urine calcium, urine phosphorus, hydroxyapatite, osteocalcin, and pyridinium derivatives are occasionally indicated to rule out secondary forms of osteoporosis. In a population of 286 older stationary patients with the clinical diagnosis of primary osteoporosis, Ringe et al. (6) found about 13% with abnormal laboratory values suggestive of secondary causes for the bone loss.

With the newer definitions of osteoporosis, which include those who have not yet experienced fractures but who have sufficiently low bone mass to place them at risk for fractures, the number of affected individuals is conservatively estimated at 14 million (49). Other estimates for this population have been as high as 25 million (7). Over 8 million Americans suffer from osteoporotic fractures. Osteoporosis, and in more general terms, low bone mass, is responsible for about 1.3 million skeletal fractures in the U.S. each year (8). An estimated 1.7 million hip fractures occurred in the world in 1990 (9). The lifetime cumulative fracture risk for a 50-year-old Caucasian woman without intervention approaches 60% (10). Worldwide, the number of hip fractures is increasing in both women and men (11,12). As many as 21% of nursing home patients are admitted with a diagnosis of hip fracture. Hip fracture is associated with an excess mortality of up to 20% and vertebral fracture, with an excess mortality of 4% (13). Survivors of both hip and vertebral fractures have severely compromised quality of life (14,15).

The National Osteoporosis Foundation (NOF) has estimated that the cost of treating osteoporosis in 1990 was US$10 billion (16). With the aging of the population, the increasing prevalence of osteoporosis, and the current patterns of inflation, the total direct medical cost alone is predicted to reach US$30–45 billion before the year 2020 (17). Prevention of osteoporotic fractures, with the attendant reductions in healthcare costs and excess morbidity and mortality, depends on identification of individuals at risk for fractures so that proper intervention (e.g., lifestyle decision, exercise, hormone or drug therapy) can be initiated before fractures occur. Historical risk factors alone have been shown to be inadequate for the prediction of low bone mass or fracture risk (18,19). However, several prospective studies have now shown that the relative risk of most appendicular and axial skeletal fracture increases exponentially with incremental reductions in bone mass, clearly establishing the utility of bone mass measurement in predicting a patient's future risk of fracture (18–28). In one study fracture risk for all fractures increased by 40–80% for each standard deviation of reduction in appendicular bone mass (29). This is particularly true in the elderly.

The identification of younger asymptomatic individuals who are at risk for osteoporotic fractures is imperative if the morbidity, mortality, and economic consequences of osteoporosis are to be reduced. Prevention of the first fracture is a concept that is important for several clinical reasons. First, asymptomatic nonfractured individuals with low bone mass (either due to low peak bone mass or bone loss of whatever etiology) have an increased fracture risk relative to individuals with normal bone mass. Second, identification of high-risk nonfractured individuals leads to discovery of possible secondary etiologies of low bone mass and initiation of appropriate intervention strategies. Results from bone mass measurements do not allow differentiation among the various forms of osteoporosis. But low bone mass values are generally the starting point in the differential diagnosis of low bone mass, which is most frequently, but not always, due to primary osteoporosis. Third, once the first fracture occurs, the relative risk of a second fracture increases fivefold, independent of bone mass, and the combination of low bone mass and just one vertebral fracture increases the relative risk of a second fracture 25-fold (30). Lastly, once these high-risk patients are identified and intervention strategies are initiated, bone mass can be maintained and prevention of the first fracture can be achieved in many patients. If these individuals are not identified, bone loss many continue unrecognized.

A. Estimate Risk

Thus to prevent fracture, individuals at risk for future fracture must be identified. Bone mass measurements have been shown to predict fracture risk as well as or better than cholesterol measurements predict the risk of heart diseases (21) or blood pressure measurements predict the risk of stroke (30). Fracture risk increases approximately 2–2.5 times for every 1.0 standard deviation (SD) an individual's bone mass is below the mean normal peak bone mass of healthy 25-to-35-year-old individuals (20–24). Furthermore, the relationship between decreasing bone mass and increasing fracture risk is exponential (Fig. 1) (31). This unique ability of bone mass measurement to predict fracture risk should be an important tool for disease prevention.

B. Quantitation

Bone densitometry is the only currently available technology for the accurate quantitative measurement of bone mass for the prediction of fracture risk. Standard radiographs of the thoracic and lumbar spine cannot be used for this purpose

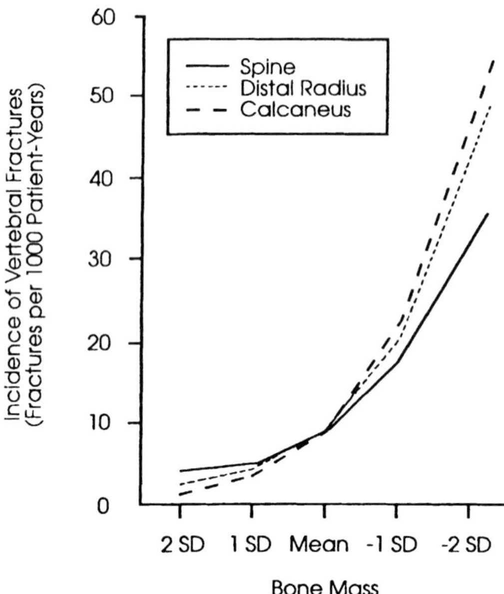

Figure 1 Exponential relationship between decreasing bone mass (mean ± SD; mean age, 63.7 years) and increasing incidence of vertebral fractures. Adapted from Wasnich et al. (31) with permission.

in the absence of preexisting fractures. More than 30% of spinal bone mass must be lost before decreased bone mass can be detected on plain radiographs. For this reason, bone mineral can be low when X-rays are still normal-appearing. Further, the determination of demineralization from plain radiographs is too subjective to be of value in determining bone mass, and no accurate quantitation of bone mass can be made under any circumstances. Radiographs are useful, however, to the extent that the existence of previous fractures does predict a higher risk of future fractures, independent of bone mass (20,24,30,32).

Using bone densitometry, bone mass can be quantitated and accurately compared to age-matched means and young adult reference means. Using the WHO study group recommendations, a normal value for bone mineral density (BMD) is within 1 SD of the young adult reference mean. Low bone mass (osteopenia) is present when BMD is between 1 and 2.5 SD below the young adult reference value. Osteoporosis can be defined by a value of equal to or greater than 2.5 SD below this reference value. Therefore, there should be a consensus to broaden the utilization of bone mass measurements to identify individuals with low bone mass and an increased risk of fracture.

Because of the lack of fully effective therapeutic intervention to replace lost bone and restore normal bone histomorphometry, emphasis is placed on early recognition and prevention of bone loss. Therefore bone mineral measurements are used to screen asymptomatic women in order to classify them as likely or unlikely to get fractures in the future (33–35). Rather than screen the entire population, a high-risk approach is generally practiced where women with clearly defined risk factors are screened. Screening the general population is not considered justified since the available risk-free interventions which would be prescribed for recognized individuals with low bone mass (i.e., stop smoking; exercise; get adequate nutrition) show only small benefit and have poor compliance.

In 1989, however, a subcommittee of the Scientific Advisory Board of the NOF described four clinical situations in which knowledge of the patient's bone mass or fracture risk could affect clinical management decisions (36,37): estrogen deficiency; vertebral abnormalities or suspected osteopoenia on plain radiography; asymptomatic primary hyperparathydroidism (to help identify possible surgical candidates); and long-term (greater than 1 month) corticosteroid therapy of a dose equal to or greater than 7.5 mg prednisone per day if dosage adjustments could be made or other treatment could be initiated to prevent bone loss. Additionally, knowledge of a pateint's bone mass may affect clnical management after organ transplantation (38). Lastly, as clinical experience in establishing the precision of newer bone mass measurement techniques has grown, serial measurement to determine the efficacy of treatments for osteoporosis is now feasible (7).

Estrogen-deficient women constitute one of the largest patient populations potentially affected by these recommendations. Women are more likely to initiate preventive measures for osteoporosis if they are aware of the presence of low bone mass (39). Thus, a bone mass measurement can help clarify the benefit-to-risk ratio of either estrogen or hormone replacement therapy (ERT or HRT) for women who are uncertain about whether to utilize it. To screen all women at the time of menopause in order to consider estrogen or hormone replacement therapy is controversial. Side effects of hormone therapy after menopause and the absence of a well-defined threshold of BMD below which treatment should be instituted, are major points of debate. However, screening women at the time of menopause who are undecided about starting HRT specifically to prevent bone mass loss has been recommended by the WHO panel. The decision to institute HRT may be based in part on or independent of a woman's perceived risk of osteoporosis. Yet such a decision made without knowledge of bone mass is an uninformed decision. HRT should not be prescribed for the sole purpose of preventing osteoporosis in the absence of bone mass measurements. An appropriate cutoff level for BMD is the lowest quintile of the normal range. Women at intermediate risk for later reevaluation can be defined as those with BMD in the next to the lowest quintile (40,41). Measurements of bone mass can be made at any time in estrogen-deficient women. However, the ideal time would be during the perimenopausal period when most decisions about initiation of hormone replacement therapy are made, because intervention to protect against bone loss is more effective the earlier applied.

II. DIAGNOSIS OF OSTEOPOROSIS

Before the advent of bone densitometry, the diagnosis of osteoporosis depended on the presence of a fragility fracture. With the ability to measure bone mass and the recognition of the relationship between reductions in bone mass and increases in fracture risk, the diagnosis of osteoporosis can and should be made based on the level of bone mass as determined by bone densitometry before fractures occur. Appropriate etiologies can then be investigated, appropriate interventions done, and appropriate longitudinal monitoring initiated.

In patients with nontraumatic spinal compression fractures, the diagnosis of osteoporosis is made on the basis of the X-ray findings, provided the clinical examination and laboratory procedures are in agreement. When BMD or BMC values are 2.5 SD or more below the mean value of young adults (age 20–30 years) of the same sex and race, the term established or severe osteoporosis is used (3,40). In this case bone mineral measurements help in the assessment of the severity of bone loss and selection of the appropriate therapy and can be used to monitor treatment. In the absence of compression fractures of other evidence of low bone mass on X-ray, bone mineral measurements are used to make the diagnosis of osteopenia (low bone mass) or osteoporosis.

The diagnostic bone mass threshold to define osteoporosis in nonfractured individuals is being clarified with increasing unanimity between various organizations concerned with this issue. Individuals whose bone mass is more than 2.5 SD below the mean normal peak bone mass (bone density) are termed osteoporotic, because over 95% of those who ultimately fracture have bone mass values below this level (22,40). However, it is important to recognize those individuals with lesser reductions in bone mass who are at risk for fracture and apply other diagnostic labels. The term osteopenia might be most appropriate to describe bone mass between 1.0 and 2.5 SD below mean normal peak bone mass, as suggested by the WHO (40). The diagnoses of osteoporosis and osteopenia that are based on levels of bone density have several appealing features. These diagnoses define the population at greatest risk for fracture (those with osteoporosis) but also emphasize the importance of identifying individuals with lesser reductions in bone density who nevertheless are at risk for fracture (those with oeteopenia) without attaching labels that might jeopardize insurability (particularly in the United States). The diagnostic threshold for osteopenia based on bone mass might also be useful as an intervention threshold. However, decisions about intervention are inherently more variable because of the wide range of individual clinical circumstances. Bone mass measurements again are analogous to measurements of blood pressure and cholesterol in asymptomatic individuals in whom the diagnostic threshold is also clearer than the intervention threshold.

The definitions of osteoporosis and osteopenia are based on comparisons of the measured bone density (as bone mineral content or bone mineral density) to the mean peak bone density of young normal individuals, usually expressed as T scores or young-adult Z scores (1,40). This is appropriate because the strength of the bone (and hence the individual's risk of fracture) is largely determined by its absolute mineral content (42). However, age is recognized as an independent risk factor for fracture (8,21). All of the current longitudinal studies relating bone mass to current fracture risk have been performed in patients with a mean age of approximately 65 years. These studies have shown that fracture prediction in this population is nearly as good as age-adjusted Z scores as with non-age-adjusted Z scores (23). Yet, osteoporosis and osteopenia cannot be defined in older patients based on age-matched Z scores. Many individuals who have already suffered fragility fractures will have low young-adult Z scores or T scores and normal age-matched Z scores. These individuals will be misdiagnosed as normal if only the age-matched Z scores are used.

To define osteoporosis on the basis of age-matched Z scores is illogical because that would imply that the prevalence of osteoporosis does not increase with age (40). However, the prevalence of osteoporosis does increase with age, and age is recognized as an independent risk factor for fracture. At the same time, younger individuals may be at greater risk for fracture during their lifetime than older individuals with equally low bone mass because they have a longer anticipated remaining life expectancy and therefore a longer duration of exposure to the effects of low bone mass (43,44). Consequently, a complete assessment of fracture risk and an estimation of benefit from interventions designed to reduce fracture risk should be based on an individual's current relative fracture risk, as determined by measured bone density, and remaining lifetime fracture probability (RLFP), which is influenced not only by bone mass but also by age and expected lifespan (45). A gradient-risk chart (Fig. 2) showing current and lifetime fracture risk based on age, bone mass, and duration of exposure to low bone mass will allow the clinician to estimate the expected benefit of recommended interventions in terms of fracture reduction.

A. How to Measure

Clinicians requesting or interpreting bone mass measurements should recognize that there are two categories into which these measurements generally fall: the quantitation of bone mass, and the assessment of fracture risk. Assessment of fracture risk may be global (general or skeletal) or site-specific. The choice of which site to measure and whether multiple sites are needed should be based on the intent of the assessment.

B. Quantitation of Bone Mass

Quantitation of bone mass permits the identification and/or confirmation of low bone mass. Bone mass measurements may also be performed to confirm the

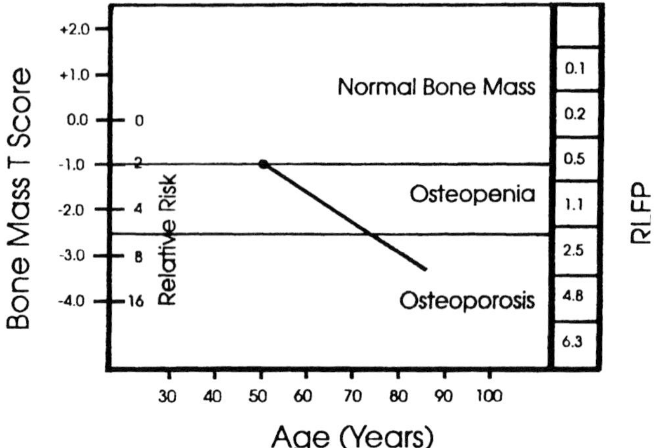

Figure 2 Gradient-risk chart showing current relative fracture risk and remaining lifetime fracture probability (RLFP) on the basis of bone mass (T-score) and age. T-score normalizes bone mass relative to the mean bone mass of young (age 25–35) normal adults (mean normal peak bone mass). Individuals whose bone mass is more than 1.0 SD but less than or equal to 2.5 SD *below* the mean (i.e., T-scores >1.0 but ≤2.5) are considered osteopenic; those whose bone mass is more than 2.5 SD *below* the mean (i.e., T-scores > 2.5) are considered osteoporotic (40). Current relative fracture risk approximately doubles for each SD reduction in bone mass. RLFP is the estimated mean number of fractures, both spine and nonspine, in remaining lifetime for individuals with a given age, initial bone mass, measured or expected rate of bone loss, and life expectancy (duration of exposure to low bone mass); nomograms for the estimation of RLFP have been published (45).

The line shown represents a hypothetical 50-year-old female patient with an initial bone mass measurement approximately 1 SD below mean normal peak bone mass. Based on her expected rate of bone loss and estimated life expectancy, this patient would be predicted to experience approximately 2.5 fractures in her remaining lifetime *if untreated.* However, if bone loss is completely prevented by intervention, the patient will be predicted to experience approximately 0.5 fractures, suggesting the potential to prevent two fractures.

radiologist's visual impression of osteopenia in patients with roentgenographic evidence of demineralization. Additionally, one can evaluate the effects of a certain disease process on the skeleton or the effects of a prescribed intervention, either good or ill, on bone mass. In such cases, the measurement site should ideally be the region of the skeleton in which the clinician is interested.

The choice of skeletal site may be based on the known effects of diseases on specific skeletal regions or types of bone and the relative composition of the various skeletal sites that can be measured. For example, in primary hyperparathyroidism, the greatest effect of excess parathyroid hormone may be on cortical bone in the appendicular skeleton (46,47). Therefore, the appropriate site at which to determine the deleterious skeletal effects of hyperparathyroidism may be the radius or femoral neck, which are primarily cortical bone. In Cushing's disease or with chronic corticosteroid therapy, the greatest effect will likely be seen in the spine (37,38,48), making this the preferred site of measurement. In the community, the diagnosis of osteopenia in asymptomatic nonfractured individuals younger than 65 years of age may be made more often by axial (spine) measurements or both axial and appendicular (wrist) measurements than by appendicular measurements alone (49). However, prediction of current fracture risk is similar by axial and appendicular measurements in the older population (65 years and over) (20).

Serial measurements may play a role in monitoring the skeletal effects of a disease process or therapeutic intervention over time (50). BMD measurements can be used repeatedly in cross-sectional studies or in individual patients to estimate the rate of bone loss when long periods are considered. Successively obtained data are linearly regressed on time for rate calculation. This has been reviewed (51).

The choice of which skeletal site to monitor longitudinally is again initially determined by the anticipated effects of the disease process. In disease states in which the effects on the skeleton are generalized, the choice of site for longitudinal testing is usually based on considerations of rates of change in bone mass within the skeleton itself (i.e., in general, sites of trabecular bone change more rapidly than those of cortical bone) and the precision of bone density testing at a particular site. In most circumstances, serial measurements are not obtained more often than once a year. The anticipated changes in bone mass are not great enough to be detected with confidence in a shorter period of time because of the effects of the magnitude of change and the precision error of bone mass measurements. An exception may be during the early stages of corticosteroid therapy, when the rates of bone loss may be rapid (38,52).

Clinicians must be aware of the precision of the currently available techniques for measuring bone mass to properly interpret an apparent change. The precision of a measurement (precision error) is generally expressed as a percent coefficient of variation, which by definition indicates the amount of random variation not caused by a biologic change in the patient. In other words, if a measurement is repeated under identical circumstances and no real change has occurred in the patient to cause a change in the actual bone mass being measured, the same result should be obtained every time. However, this is generally not the case in any clinical measurement because of random variation ("noise") in the measurement itself. Although clinicians have inherently appreciated precision in other quantitative measurements routinely employed in clinical practice, precision issues in bone mass measurements have been less well understood. Newer bone densitometry techniques have some of the lowest precision errors in quantitative medical testing today, but the precision error is not zero. Because the degree of changes in bone mass is generally small, precision becomes an important consideration in identifying skeletal sites for serial measurement, determining the timing of these measurements, choosing the technique to use, and interpreting the measured changes.

Rate of bone loss in expressed in terms of BMD or BMC as percent change of the first measurement (baseline) per year. In general, a practical clinical guideline is that the smallest measured change in bone density should be equal to or greater than 2.8 times the precision error (coefficient of variation) of the measurement technique for it to be considered "real" (with a 95% confidence). With currently available dual-energy X-ray absorptiometry (DXA) equipment, the precision error of a measurement of the anterior/posterior (AP) axial skeleton in clinical settings is usually 2–3% (53), so a change in bone mass of at least 5.6–8.4% is required for the measurement to be interpreted as meaningful. The precision error of DXA measurement of the femoral neck is 4–5% (53), indicating that a change of at least 11.2–14.0% is needed to be clinically meaningful. Better precision errors for DXA are possible with currently available equipment in expert hands. Measurement precision error can be improved to about 1% by performing duplicate measurements at each interval and using the mean value of the duplicate measurements for the rate of loss calculation. If precision values of 1% can thus be achieved, bone loss of 3% per year can be recognized with 95% confidence if two duplicate measurements are made 2 years apart.

If the precision error of a bone mass measurement of a given skeletal site is 2%, a change of 4% at that site over an interval of 1 year may not be clinically significant. Thus, changes in patient management should not necessarily be made based on one repeat measurement that falls within the statistical confidence of the precision error—i.e., less than 2.8 times the percent coefficient of variation. With a precision error of 2% for the measuring technique, the clinician should require a change of at least 5.6% before accepting that this change is real. However, a change in bone mass (especially a decline), even within the statistical confidence limits of the precision error of a particular technique at a particular skeletal site, should not necessarily be discounted as potentially meaningless. It may alert the clinician to the need to discuss issues of compliance (particularly with regard to hormone replacement therapy) and to justify continued longitudinal monitoring to detect a trend. In this model, if a patient on estrogen treatment for osteoporosis loses BMD at a rate of 3% per year of more, compliance with the drug regimen or the diagnosis may be in doubt.

Bone mass measurements of the wrist (cortical bone) (54) or calcaneus (trabecular bone) (103) by single-energy X-ray absorptiometry (SXA) have precision errors similar to those of measurements of the AP axial skeleton by DXA. Quantitative computerized tomography (QCT) of the spine can achieve a precision error of 3–4% (53) if the equipment is calibrated daily and calibration is repeated before each test for each patient. With this technique, a change in bone mass of at least 8.4–11.2% must be observed to be interpreted as clinically meaningful.

Interequipment variability may reduce precision sufficiently to make it difficult to reliably compare bone mass measurements obtained on different machines, even those from the same manufacturer, and caution must be emphasized in this context. Ideally, patients should be followed longitudinally on the same machine.

The manufacturers of equipment for measuring bone mass provide in vivo and in vitro precision values under ideal testing circumstances for the various skeletal sites. However, precision for the various skeletal sites and bone density equipment must be established by each clinical center, and strict compliance to calibration and quality control procedures is paramount to competent testing.

III. SITE-SPECIFIC VS. GLOBAL MEASUREMENTS

Global assessment of fracture risk by bone mass measurements estimates an individual's risk for any and all types of osteoporotic fracture. A clinician can thus assess a patient's risk of osteoporotic fracture in general but may not be able to precisely assess the risk of a specific type of osteoporotic fracture. Many studies of selected populations have shown that lower than normal bone mass measured at any of the currently measured sites (distal radius, midradius, calcaneus, spine, and proximal femur) is indicative of an increased fracture risk at all skeletal sites (20,22,55–57). This is the basis for using peripheral bone measurements to estimate fracture risk in the axial skeleton. Therefore, for a clinician who wishes a global fracture risk assessment, the choice of a site or sites may be based on those that available equipment can measure with acceptable precision and a knowledge of any artifactual changes such as osteophytes, sclerosis, or existing fractures, which may falsely elevate certain bone mass measurements.

The potential limitations of global fracture risk assessments based on bone mass measurements of one skeletal site are in the possible misclassification of fracture risk and misdiagnosis of low bone mass. Bone mass measurements at multiple skeletal sites are concordant in 85% of cases in the older population (104). However, two studies in perimenopausal women have shown discordant bone mass (measured as bone mineral density) of the spine and hip (58,105). Although the majority of women in these studies were correctly classified as "at risk" or "not at risk" on the basis of either a spine or femoral neck bone mass measurement, between 8% and 18% would have been classified incorrectly if only the femoral neck measurement was considered and between 10% and 30% would have been misclassified if only the spine measurement was considered.

A rationale for bone mass measurements of multiple skeletal sites exists even if bone mass of the initially measured site is found to be low. If bone mass is normal at one site and low at a second site, the actual fracture risk is intermediate, and bone mass measurements should be given equal weight (56). Some patients may be rapid losers at the hip and slow losers at the spine or vice versa (57,58). Some women receiving estrogen replacement therapy may maintain bone mass at the spine but exhibit bone loss at the hip (59). Therefore, because bone loss can be selective rather than generalized in individual patients, longitudinal monitoring of multiple skeletal sites may be justified.

A site-specific assessment of fracture risk by bone mass measurements refers to an assessment of risk for a specific type of fracture—e.g., vertebral compression fracture or femoral neck fracture. Site-specific approaches are more logical in the clinical setting in which patients may present with site-specific clinical problems (e.g., height loss or prediction of future fracture risk at a site of clinical concern).

The diagnostic sensitivity of bone mass measurements for fracture prediction is further improved when bone mineral is measured at the site of frequent non-traumatic fractures (29). Thus L-spine (thoracic and lumbar spine compression fractures) and hip (hip fractures) are clinically the most interesting sampling sites when osteoporosis is considered. A large prospective longitudinal study demonstrated that measurements of the proximal femur are superior to measurements of other sites for prediction of hip fracture risk (23). Spinal bone mineral is less accurate for predicting fractures in the trochanter or the femur, and even less so for femoral neck fractures when compared with direct measurements of the hip.

If measurement of bone mass at either the spine or hip indicates an increase in fracture risk, the other site may not need to be measured. However, if the first site measured does not indicate an increased fracture risk, measurement of a second site should be considered because of the possible discordance between sites, as previously discussed (57,58).

In general, if a site-specific assessment of fracture risk is desired, that specific site should be measured unless artifactual changes at that site prevent an accurate measurement. Occasionally, because of deformity, severe degenerative disease, aortic calcification, or surgical interventions in the L-spine, bone mineral in the L-spine is difficult to interpret in terms of fracture risk or presence of osteopenia (53). In this case, bone mineral in the hip, the radius, or calcaneus must be used as an alternative sampling site to predict spinal fracture risk. Possible contraindications to the use of bone mineral measurements are listed in Table 1. Such information is obtained from the clinical history, radiographs, or the scan image itself.

Important extraskeletal factors are also involved in fractures. The factors most studied are frequency and type of falls in the elderly (60). Conditions associated with an increased risk of falling such as neuromuscular disorders, poor coordination, or poor eyesight therefore have to be considered in addition to bone mineral when fracture risk is evaluated. Such factors may be responsible, when fractures occur with normal or almost normal bone mineral.

Table 1 Possible Contraindications for Using Bone Mineral[a] Measurements

Local spine or hip disease
• Compression fractures in L-spine, previous fracture in hip
• Other focal diseases such as Paget's disease, metastasis, tumors
• Severe deformities or congenital abnormalities
Conditions after surgery or trauma
• Laminectomy (if more than L4)
• Harrington rod
• Hip arthroplasty
Interference with measurements may occur with
• Severe aortic calcification (L-spine)
• Contrast medium in GI tract (L-spine)
• Prior isotope study (spine and hip)
• Undissolved calcium tablets (L-spine)
• Soft-tissue artifacts (metal) (spine and hip)

[a]For a detailed discussion see reference 53.

IV. TECHNIQUES

Efforts to measure the mineral content of bone noninvasively to diagnose and monitor bone disease have a long history. Since the beginning of such attempts, dating back about half a century, X-ray-based procedures have played a major role. Specifically, X-ray absorptiometry procedures have been used in technically increasing sophistication. To date, procedures of clinical interest for the measurement of bone mineral include dual- and single-energy X-ray absorptiometry (DXA and SXA, respectively), dual-photon absorptiometry (DPA), and quantitative computed tomography (QCT). In addition, several techniques based on ultrasound (velocity, attenuation, or reflection) are attractive. However, clinical usefulness is not yet well defined.

Bone density measurements are of clinical importance in the diagnosis and management of osteoporosis and to a lesser degree in a host of other clinical conditions where bone fractures and skeletal deformities contribute to morbidity. It is the only approach to estimate present fracture risk at specific skeletal sites and the estimation of lifetime fracture risk (44). In addition, bone mineral measurements are widely used as research tools for the testing of new drugs and in studies of the epidemiology and mechanism of bone loss and bone formation. For research applications, noninvasive measurements in small animals and assessment of bone mineral changes around metal implants are possible. Total body and regional bone mass, body fat, and lean tissue mass can also be estimated with DXA or DPA. The DXA technique has been extended to measurements of bone strength in vivo, based on bone mass and bone geometry. Morphometry of spinal vertebrae can be performed for the early recognition and documentation of vertebral compression fractures on newer instruments.

The techniques for measuring bone mineral currently in use and readily available for clinical applications are listed in Table 2. In 1984, the American College of Physicians (ACP) reviewed the available photon absorptiometry techniques, the skeletal sites at which they were appropriately used, and their precision, accuracy, and safety (61). The ACP concluded that dual-photon absorptiometry appeared more advantageous than the other techniques. However, dual-energy X-ray absorptiometry was not available at the time of that report.

Currently, DXA is the most widely used technique for measurement of axial bone mass in most countries and, because of its greater precision, has begun to replace DPA in most centers (62). DXA has low radiation exposure and excellent precision for longitudinal monitoring and can be used to measure bone mass in both the spine (anterior/posterior and lateral) and hip. The majority of the cross-sectional and longitudinal bone mass data used to establish the diagnosis of osteoporosis in nonfractured individuals and for the prediction of fracture risk have been obtained with appendicular bone mass measurements by SPA or SXA and axial measurements by DPA or DXA (20–23). Vertebral QCT is also valuable in the prediction of risk (24). SXA of the wrist or calcaneus and peripheral quantitative computerized tomography (pQCT) of the wrist are beginning to challenge SPA in the measurement of appendicular bone mass and are accepted techniques to predict fracture risk. Prospective longitudinal data for the appendicular skeleton (wrist and calcaneus) by SPA or SXA and the axial skeleton (spine) by DPA, DXA, or QCT appear to have equivalent value in the prediction of fracture risk at any skeletal site in the older population (20–22,24). For monitoring longitudinal changes in bone mass, the technique should be chosen based on the precision of measurement at the site that was initially measured and/or initially low and the technique originally used. Ideally, the best technique would be that which can measure the desired skeletal site with the highest precision (i.e., lowest precision error).

In some instances, a particular technique may be selected based on the anticipated validity and quality of the scan. For example, in elderly individuals, osteophytes or sclerosis of posterior facets frequently falsely elevate and invalidate the AP measurement of axial (spine) bone mass by DXA or DPA. These artifacts may also be seen in younger individuals with rheumatologic diseases that cause axial arthropathies. In those cases, a diagnosis of osteopenia or osteoporosis could be missed with a measurement of only AP axial bone mass by DXA or DPA. However, measurement of axial (spine) bone mass by QCT and lateral spine bone mass by DXA have advantages because these abnormalities do not influence those

Table 2 Comparison of Techniques for Bone Mineral Measurements

Name of technique	Information	Instrument cost	Remarks
Single-energy photon absorptiometry (SPA)	Restricted to appendicular bone. Predominantly trabecular (diaphysis) or cortical bone sites (metaphysis) as integral bone.	\$20,000	Replaced by DXA technology. Commercial instruments using ^{125}I sources available for radius and calcaneus.
Single energy X-ray absorptiometry (SXA)			
Dual-energy X-ray absorptiometry DXA) (X-ray source)	Standard sites are spine (L2–L4), hip (neck, trochanter, Ward's triangle), and total skeleton. Integral bone is measured.	\$60,000–180,000	Technique with widest application and best performance characteristics.
Quantitative computed tomography (single- and dual-energy)	Spine (T12–L3), trabecular bone. Future applications in the hip. Dedicated instruments for radius are available.	For spine measurements, software and reference phantom for most commercial CT scanners are available \$20,000	

techniques at those sites (63,64). Alternatively, SPA or SXA could be used to measure the wrist or calcaneus, or DPA or DXA could be used to measure the proximal femur, provided the clinician recognizes the limitations of extrapolation of data between sites.

Whatever technique is selected to measure bone mass, quality control must be strictly maintained. Daily phantom quantitation and scheduled calibration and maintenance must be performed according to manufacturers' guidelines to ensure accurate and precise results. Technician training in patient positioning, equipment operation, and scan analysis is also critical. The bone densitometry facility should be able to provide information on its quality control program.

A. Single-Photon Absorptiometry

SPA is used for measurement of bone mineral content (BMC) in cortical and trabecular bone at various sites of the appendicular skeleton, usually the radius or calcaneus. Results are expressed in terms of gram bone ash in a cross section of the tubal bone, 1 cm in axial length (g/cm). The measurements are obtained by scanning with a small, well-collimated beam of photons, usually from a 200-mCi source of ^{125}I (35 keV, half-life 60 days) once or repeatedly across the bone. BMC is derived from measurements of the attenuation of the photon beam as it traverses bone and soft tissue versus attenuation of soft tissue alone. The thickness of the soft tissue is standardized by immersion of the extremity in a water bath or cuffing with a fluid-filled bag. BMD, normalized for bone size, in units of g/cm^2, can be obtained by dividing BMC by bone diameter at the scanning site. By choosing the scanning site to be along the axis of a long bone, such as the radius (distal end or midshaft), or selecting certain bones for their structural composition (e.g., trabecular bone in the calcaneus), predominantly trabecular or cortical bone sites of the appendicular skeleton can be assessed (65,66).

Commercial instruments for radius or heel measurements are simple to operate and maintain. Radius type instruments are versatile for measurements at different sites in the appendicular skeleton and are used in the neonate. Instruments for measurements at the calcaneus are dedicated machines. For measurements on the upper arm or thigh, gamma rays with higher energy, such as available from Isotope Americium, are used.

Measurement reproducibility is very dependent on accurate repositioning. Automatic site selection using anatomical markers of ulna and radius is used in the latest instruments. Comparison of data is only possible if exactly identical sites are compared. Varying fat content of the tissue surrounding bone leads to errors in measurement accuracy also. Corrections are applied in some instruments. Calibration and quality control are based on commercially available phantoms supplied with each instrument. These phantoms are generally specific for the brand and are not interchangeable among different brands of SPA instruments. The phantoms are measured daily when the instrument is in use. They are also used to measure precision and accuracy of a given instrument and to document measurement stability over time (53). A reference standard (European forearm phantom) has been developed by an international panel to facilitate cross calibration of different brand instruments.

Appendicular bone mineral measurements are also possible with dual-energy X-ray absorptiometry (DXA) (67). DXA instruments and instruments based on single-energy X-ray absorptiometry have replaced most SPA instruments in recent years. Dedicated instruments based on the principle of quantitative computed tomography (QCT) are also commercially available to measure trabecular, cortical, or integral bone separately at the distal radius (68). Advanced instruments of this type have a high measurement precision and are used in research, where small rates of bone loss or gain have to be detected. QCT-based instruments for forearm measurement have never been popular in the U.S. but are more frequently used in some European countries.

B. Dual-Energy X-Ray Absorptiometry

DXA can be used for accurate and precise determination of bone mineral in the axial and peripheral skeleton. Total skeletal bone mass or density can also be assessed using DXA. Because of the differences in composition and thickness of soft tissue surrounding the axial skeleton, calculation of bone mineral requires simultaneous attenuation measurements of two photon or gamma rays. In DXA this is achieved by scanning with two X-rays of different energies. This is done either by using an energy switching X-ray source (Hologic, Inc. instruments) or by using a constant-potential X-ray source combined with rare earth filters to produce two energy levels (Lunar, Norland, Sopha instruments).

The unit of measurement is grams of ashed bone or equivalent hydroxyapatite in the projected bone area (g/cm^2). This is defined as the bone mineral density (BMD). The area is defined by the selected region of interest (ROI) on the computer screen. The term "areal density" is used to emphasize that the bone mineral contained in a given projected area of bone is measured bidimensionally, but the true bone volume is not available. This makes the measurement somewhat dependent on bone thickness (69,70). This inherent error is minimized if bones at similar sites are compared.

The ROI, such as spine or hip (or the entire body), is scanned in a rectilinear fashion, and transmitted low- and high-energy photons are recorded on a pixel-by-pixel basis for BMD calculation (53,71,72). For clinical use, measurements on the L-spine (L2–L4) and the hip (femur neck, trochanter, Ward's triangle) are preferred since these are common sites of nontraumatic fractures when bone loss occurs in osteoporosis (73).

Newer developments in DXA instruments include a lateral scanning approach to the spine. This allows the exclusion of the posterior portion of the vertebra where the facet joints are frequent sites of degenerative changes resulting in focal mineral increase, particularly in the elderly (63,74). Earlier attempts to use lateral scans with systems based on isotope sources (DPA) were frustrated by the relatively low source intensity. Lateral spine scans can be performed on standard DXA instruments with the patient in the lateral decubitus position (75). However, because of the relative proximity of iliac crest and costal margin in the older person with osteoporosis, only two lumbar vertebral bodies, or at best three, can be scanned with this approach. Due to the greater abdominal thickness in the lateral decubitus position when compared to the standard supine position, there is greater difficulty in positioning and a larger effect of fat on the measurements. The small sampling site (ROI) generally leads to a decrease in measurement precision (3–4%) and accuracy (10–12%) when compared with the standard approach (75,76).

Newer DXA instruments have a movable C-arm which allows lateral scans with the patient supine. The higher proportion of trabecular bone in the vertebral body when compared with the entire vertebra explains the higher bone loss with age in cross-sectional studies noted with these measurements. Anteroposterior lumbar spine measurements show mean BMD values in patients with spinal fractures (osteoporosis) of −3.1 SD when compared with young-adult reference values, and −1.2 SD when compared with age-matched controls. For lateral spine measurements, these values are −2.8 SD and −1.2 SD, respectively. Since AP spine scans are a better discriminator of low bone mass, it is doubtful that lateral scans will replace or compete with the standard AP scan of L2–L4 in clinical practice. The high measurement reproducibility of spinal BMD measurements of about 1% (CV) and better accuracy make the AP approach with DXA the best method available for clinical measurements.

Concern that area density varies with bone size and that low BMD in patients with osteoporosis may be due in part to smaller vertebrae in these patients stimulated efforts to develop volumetric density measurements (g/cm^3) with DXA. Efforts to calculate vertebral depth from AP scans with a vertebral model approach and then calculate vertebral volume did not result in improved discrimination of osteoporotic populations. More sophisticated approaches including estimates of vertebral compressive strength have been tried with promising results.

More recently, however, lateral measurements of vertebral bodies which allow better estimates of vertebral depth together with the information from the AP scan have been used to estimate vertebral volume. The resultant measurement is referred to as volumetric density and expressed in g/cm^3. In one study volumetric density based on lateral and AP scans with DXA (like volumetric density from QCT) increased the discrimination between normal and osteoporotic populations (77,78). Further studies are necessary.

As described with SPA, DXA instruments are calibrated with phantoms which differ among manufacturers. A typical quality control protocol requires daily measurements of a spine phantom. The data are entered into a quality control database for analysis. A typical protocol for a multicenter study and results have been described in detail (79,80). A cross calibration phantom is available for comparison of different types and brands of instruments. The different phantoms available have been reviewed (53,81).

A typical DXA instrument is illustrated in Figure 3. Data output for a bone mineral measurement at the L-spine contain an image of the area scanned, region of interest (L2 to L4 as selected by the algorithm), biographical data, calibration data for the instrument, and measurement results (Figs. 4–6). The results are plotted onto a normal range (sex, age, and race adjusted) and expressed in terms of Z-scores, T-scores, and cumulative percentiles. Z-scores are numbers of standard deviations below (−) or above (+) the population mean adjusted for age, sex, and race. T-scores are numbers of standard deviations below or above the mean value of the maximal bone mass in young adults (age 20–35). The relationship between commonly used percentile values and standard deviations commonly used in Z-scores and T-scores are given in Figure 7.

The BMD results from L-spine measurements are only useful for fracture risk estimation or bone mass assessment when bone mineral is distributed uniformly throughout the spine and the measured vertebrae are representative of the remaining spinal column with respect to BMD. In the presence of degenerative changes, deformity, or postoperative spinal changes, the hip should be selected as the measuring site. The thoracic spine, the site of most of the fractures, cannot be measured directly with comparable accuracy and precision since the overlying sternum and ribs interfere with measurements. Failure load of thoracic vertebrae, however, does correlate with lumbar spine BMD (82).

In the hip, ROIs are the femoral neck, trochanter, Ward's triangle, intertrochanter region, and total proximal femur. When using hip scans, clinical decisions are usually based on results from the femur neck ROI (Fig. 8).

C. Quantitative Computed Tomography

Most commercial computed tomography instruments can be adapted for QCT by the purchase of a software package and calibration phantom (83). Quality controls for these measurements exceed those usually necessary for imaging procedures, and meticulous observation of details regarding patient positioning and instrument performance is required (84). The results are of comparable value or marginally better when compared with DXA for fracture prediction and most other clinical indications. QCT may be preferable in older subjects with marked degenerative changes in the spine where lateral scans with DXA are now being evaluated. Results are expressed in terms of physical density—that is, mg/cm^3 of trabecular bone in the center of the vertebral body. A normal range that is generally reproducible in different laboratories is supplied with the software. With this method, the

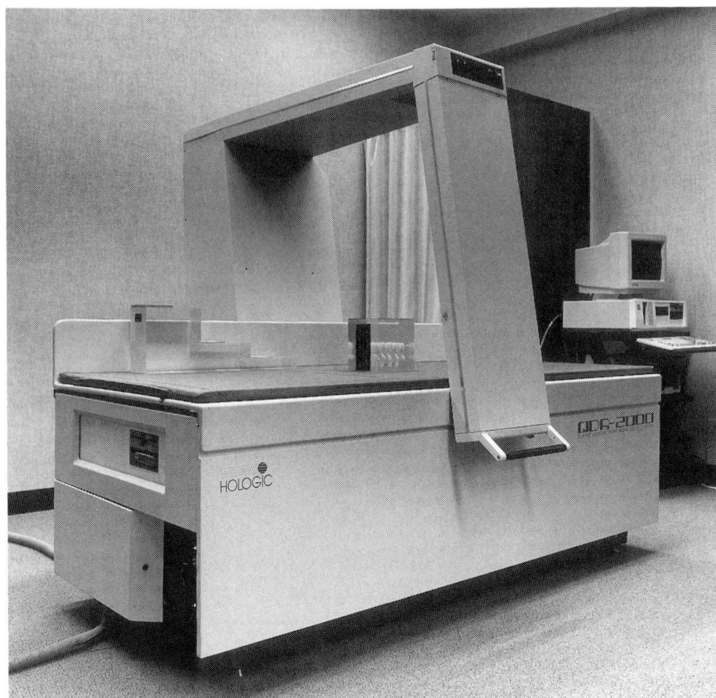

Figure 3 Commercial instrument for bone mineral measurements in the L-spine (Hologic, Inc., Waltham, MA, model QDR-2000). The C-arm with a bank of detectors (above table) and collimated X-ray source (below tabletop) move across the area to be scanned.

annual loss of density in trabecular bone of the L-spine in women is 1.2%/year by percent cubic regression (menopausal loss). By age 75, the density is reduced to 50% of maximum at young adult age and about 90 mg/cm^3. When compared with DXA, QCT has a relatively high radiation dose (Table 3). This, together with a greater accuracy error with QCT, makes DXA the method of choice for longitudinal studies and for measurements on normal populations and children. For clinical use, the local expertise and instrumentation available often decides which instrument is used. The techniques are compared in Table 3.

D. Other Methods

Computer-enhanced X-rays of the hand (radiogramography or radiographic absorptiometry) (85) and ultrasound bone densitometry of the calcaneus (86) are being used as investigational tools. However, they have limited clinical applicability because of a lack of sufficient longitudinal data to establish their precision

Table 3 Comparison of Densitometry Techniques

Technique[a]	Bone site	Bone type measured	Precision[b] (%)	Accuracy (%)	Time of exam (min)	Radiation		Cost per test ($)
						Source	Absorbed dose (mrem/scan)	
SPA	Distal radius, mid-radius, calcaneus	Integral	1–3	5–8	15	^{125}I (35 keV)	5–10 (to scan site)	50–75
DXA	Spine, hip (femur neck, Ward's triangle, trochanter), total body	Integral	0.8–1.5 2–3	4–6	3–6 3–6	X-ray (70, 140 keV)	2–20 2–20	150–200
QCT	Spine	Trabecular, cortical	2–6	5–15	10	X-ray (85 keV)	200–1,000	300–400

[a]SPA, single-photon absorptiometry; DXA, dual-energy X-ray absorptiometry; QCT, quantitative computed tomography (single energy).
[b]Shown as coefficient of variation (CV).

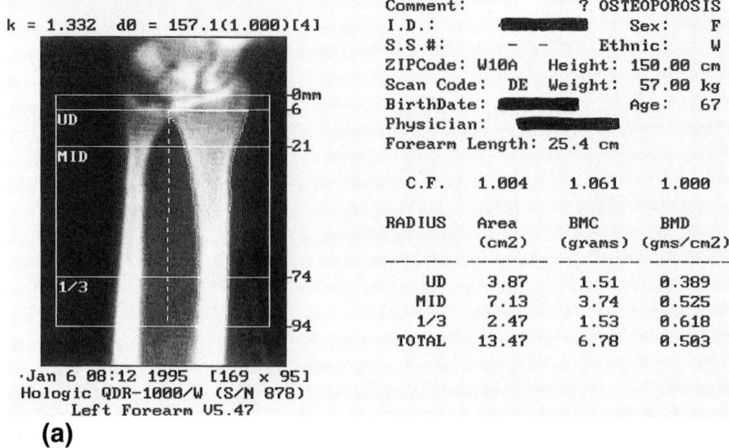

Figure 4 (a) DXA scan of the radius. The most commonly used ROI is the ultradistal (UD) site, representing predominantly trabecular bone. Other ROIs are midradius (MID) and one-third of the radius length (⅓). Note that MID does not correspond to the middle of the radius. The "⅓ ROI" represents predominantly cortical bone. Patient information and results are given to the right of the scan image (Hologic, Inc., Waltham, MA, model QDR 1000/W). (b) Data from a radius scan continued. The normal range for the "⅓ ROI" is given in the upper left corner, data below. Mean values ± 2 SD is listed. The stippled line represents the "fracture threshold" at a point −2 SD below the mean value of young adult BMD. (c) Normal values for white women age 20–80 years for four ROIs at the radius (from Hologic, Inc.)

and, therefore, their ability to monitor treatment or predict future fracture risk in prospective studies (87,88). Eventually, these techniques may provide data comparable to those generated by the established techniques available.

V. INTERPRETATION

Physicians performing densitometry testing come from a variety of medical specialties. There is no one specialty whose members are uniquely qualified to perform densitometry testing and interpretation. The densitometrist should be generally versed in radiographic anatomy, skeletal development and composition, metabolic bone disease, the concept of fracture gradients, and statistical issues pertaining to quantitative measures such as accuracy and precision.

The present level of familiarity with bone mass data in the general medical community is such that computer-generated data alone are insufficient as a reporting tool for the densitometrist or primary care clinician. Computer-generated data should be accompanied by a written clinical report in which the data are inter-

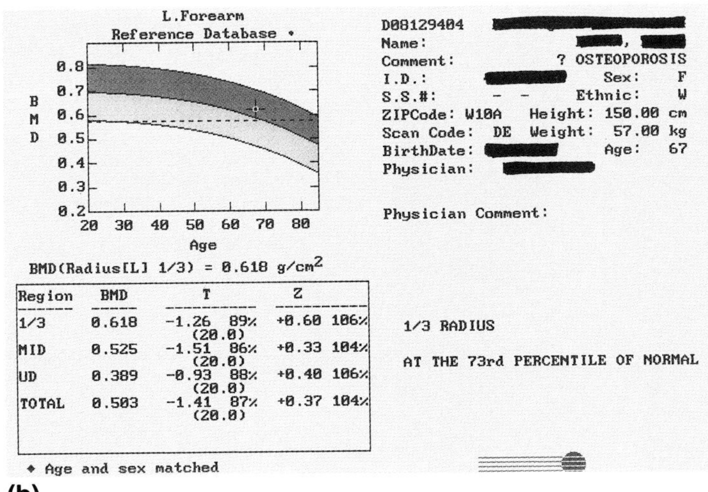

L.Forearm
Reference Database ◆

D08129404
Name:
Comment: ? OSTEOPOROSIS
I.D.: Sex: F
S.S.#: - - Ethnic: W
ZIPCode: W10A Height: 150.00 cm
Scan Code: DE Weight: 57.00 kg
BirthDate: Age: 67
Physician:

Physician Comment:

BMD(Radius[L] 1/3) = 0.618 g/cm^2

Region	BMD	T		Z	
1/3	0.618	-1.26 (20.0)	89%	+0.60	106%
MID	0.525	-1.51 (20.0)	86%	+0.33	104%
UD	0.389	-0.93 (20.0)	88%	+0.40	106%
TOTAL	0.503	-1.41 (20.0)	87%	+0.37	104%

1/3 RADIUS

AT THE 73rd PERCENTILE OF NORMAL

◆ Age and sex matched

(b)

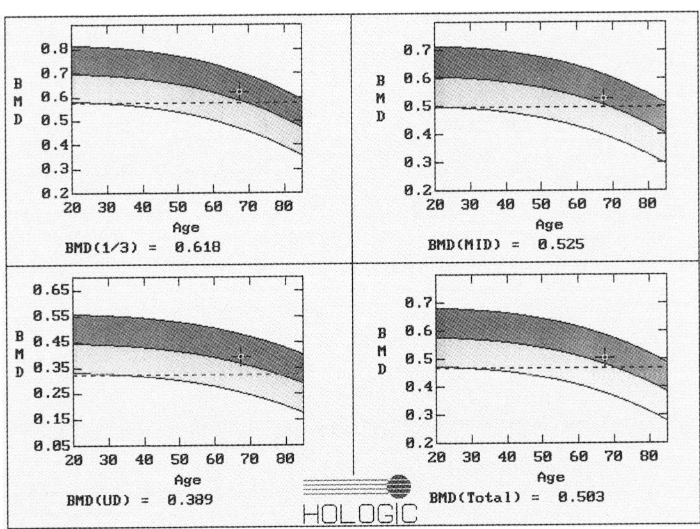

(c)

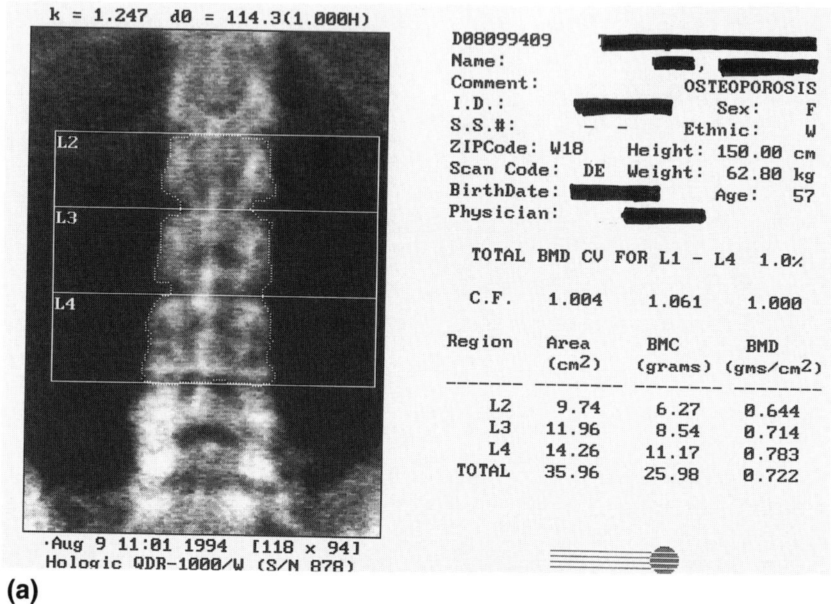

(a)

Figure 5 (a) Data printout from a lumbar spine measurement. Note the scan image on the left with ROIs indicated. Standard ROI is L2-4 or L1-4. The global ROI (outer box) should include sufficient soft tissue. The dimension of the global ROI is given in millimeters below the image. Bibliographic data are given in the right upper corner of the report, followed by the data referring to the calibration of the instrument (CF). Results are listed in the right lower corner (Hologic, Inc., Waltham, MA). (b) Continued from Figure 5a, showing the normal range and fracture threshold (stippled line) for white women.

preted by the densitometrist in light of relevant aspects of the patient's clinical circumstances and medical history.

Review of bone mass data and historical data, obtained by the densitometry technician or the primary care clinician and documented on an appropriately designed patient questionnaire (Table 4), can permit the densitometrist to make broad and often specific clinical recommendations on patient management to the referring clinician. In addition, this review may provide insight into potential etiologies of low bone mass and possible interventions. In the absence of such a clinical interpretation, bone mass measurements have diminished utility for the clinical management of a patient with bone loss or established osteoporosis.

Information obtained from plain radiographic films of the spine may enhance interpretation of densitometry data. Structural changes visible on plain films, such as fractures, osteophyte formation, aortic calcification, and facet sclerosis, may

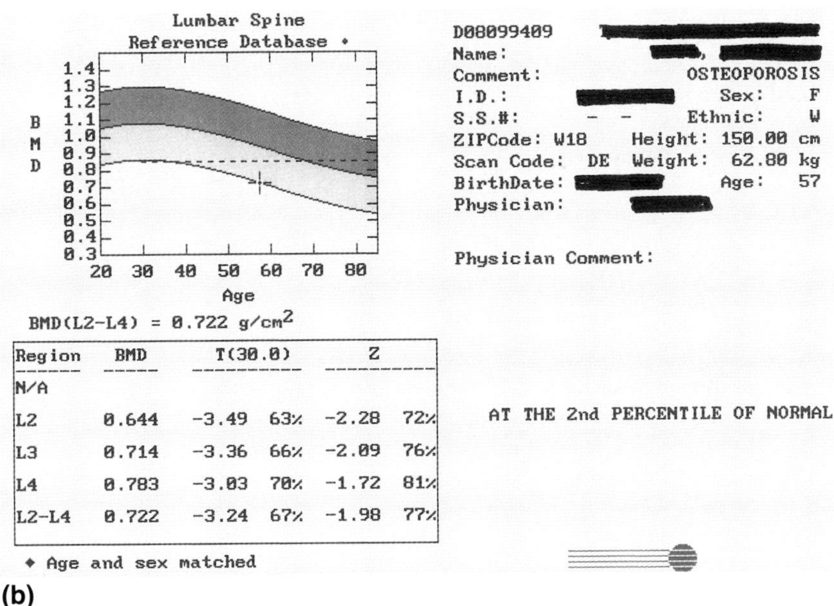

BMD(L2-L4) = 0.722 g/cm²

D08099409
Name:
Comment: OSTEOPOROSIS
I.D.: Sex: F
S.S.#: - - Ethnic: W
ZIPCode: W18 Height: 150.00 cm
Scan Code: DE Weight: 62.80 kg
BirthDate: Age: 57
Physician:

Physician Comment:

Region	BMD	T(30.0)		Z	
N/A					
L2	0.644	-3.49	63%	-2.28	72%
L3	0.714	-3.36	66%	-2.09	76%
L4	0.783	-3.03	70%	-1.72	81%
L2-L4	0.722	-3.24	67%	-1.98	77%

AT THE 2nd PERCENTILE OF NORMAL

• Age and sex matched

(b)

affect the accuracy and interpretation of densitometry results. The presence of a fragility fracture increases the relative risk of fracture over and above the risk assigned based on densitometry data alone (20,24). For example, the presence of wrist fractures increases the risk of spine fractures (32), and the presence of spine fractures increases the risk of hip fractures (89). Consequently, information from plain films of the skeleton should be provided to the densitometrist by the referring clinician, whenever possible. Alternatively, the densitometrist may, in some circumstances, appropriately request plain films of the spine or other skeletal regions to permit a more complete interpretation of the densitometry data.

A. Bone Mass Changes Throughout Life

Throughout life, the skeleton shows several distinct developmental phases which have to be recognized in the clinical interpretation of bone mineral measurements (90). Each phase has different clinical disease entities, technical demands for bone mineral measurements, and specific clinical interpretations. The neonatal, prepubertal, and pubertal skeletons each show distinct physiological changes (91,92). In these age groups, clinical relevance of BMD measurements is more limited than in the skeleton of the older adult, and absorptiometry measurements are used only in specialty clinics for rare clinical disorders. Of importance is the varying size of the bone, particularly the vertebra, and its effect on area density measurements.

Table 4 Important Patient Information for Clinician and Densitometrist Evaluation of Bone-Mass Measurements

General patient information
- Name and address
- Patient identification number
- Sex
- Age
- Height
- Weight

Hospital/site information
- Site number
- Referring clinician

Previous scan information
- Previous scan(s) (date[s], skeletal region[s])
- Instrument(s) used for and hospital/site(s) of previous scan(s)
- Findings of previous scan(s)

Present scan information
- Reason for present scan
- Scheduled date and time for present scan
- Densitometry technician for present scan
- Densitometrist (interpreting physician) for present scan
- Instrument used for present scan

Changes in clinical circumstances since previous scan
- Fractures: date, skeletal region, classification (traumatic/nontraumatic)
- Height loss: extent, time period
- Medications: changes in drug(s) and/or dosage(s) (list previous and new)
- Other

Lifestyle factors
- Smoking status: Current smoker (duration and quantity/day); nonsmoker (never smoked); nonsmoker/quitter (how long since cessation; duration and quantity/day before cessation)
- Exercise: type, duration, frequency, history (e.g., low-impact aerobics for 30 min/day, 2/week for 6 months)

Medical history
- General history: adult nontraumatic fractures (date, skeletal region); allergies; calcium/dairy intake; family history of osteoporosis; height loss (extent, time period); lactose intolerance; menopausal status (time of menopause or last menstrual period); sekeletal pain (chronic/acute, skeletal region, duration, etiology if known)
- Disease history: arthritis; diabetes; kidney disease; thyroid disease; other
- Surgical history: abdominal surgery; hysterectomy; oophorectomy; organ transplantation; orthopedic surgery; other
- Medication history: name(s) of drug(s), dosage, duration, and reason(s) for use; note especially use of calcium, estrogen or hormone replacement therapy, multivitamins, steroids, thyroid hormone replacement therapy, vitamin D, other (e.g., antihypertensive drugs, antiarthritic drugs, antidepressant drugs, cardiac drugs, diuretics)

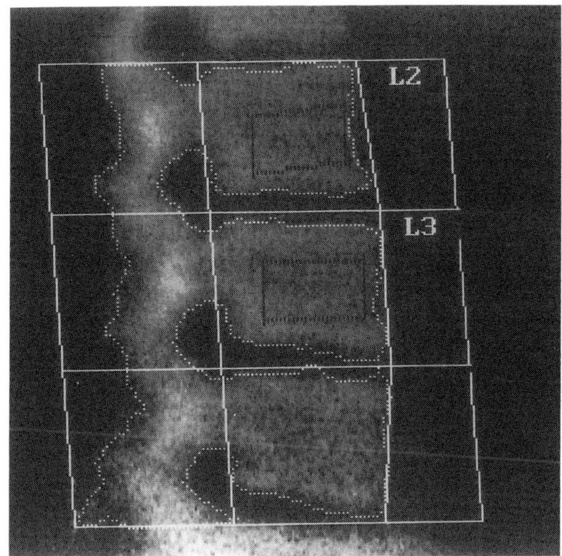

Figure 6 Lateral L-spine scan showing ROIs in the vertebral bodies excluding the end plates (mid-ROI). Scan obtained with patient in supine position. ROIs including the entire vertebral body are included for comparison.

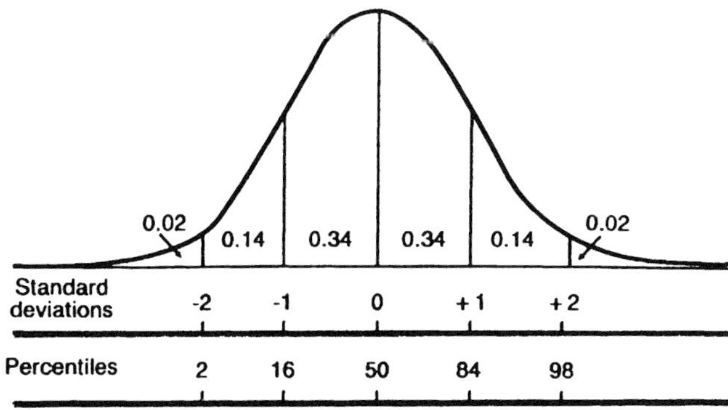

Figure 7 Relationship between standard deviations and cumulative percentiles in a showing a normal distribution. Occasionally data are reported in terms of percent of the mean values, where the mean value of bone mineral for age is given as 100% (from Moro et al. [82], by permission).

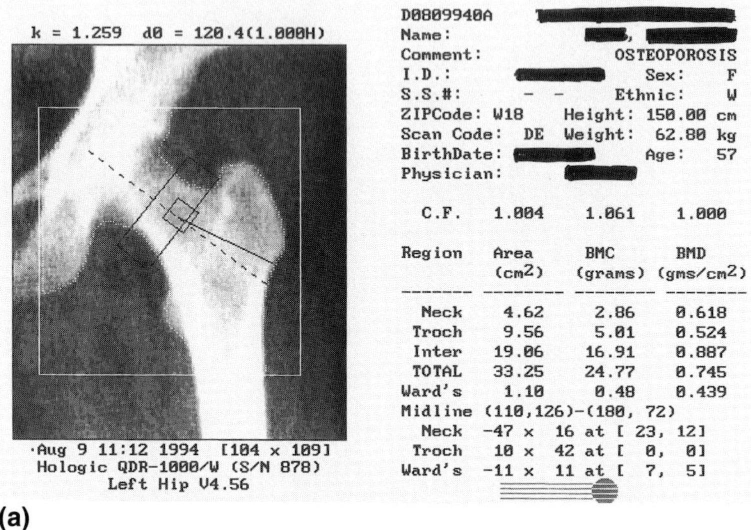

(a)

Figure 8 (a) Data from the scan of the left hip. ROIs are femur neck, trochanter, Ward's triange, intertrochanter, and total. (b) Normal data for BMD at the femur neck for white women, fracture threshold and data summary from a hip scan. (c) Normal BMD values for the remaining ROIs.

Most of the information on neonates and small children is from SPA measurements on the forearm.

The adult skeleton consists of compact, cortical (80%) and trabecular (20%) bone. The marrow cavity is filled with red (cellular elements) or yellow (fat) bone marrow. These three components of bone vary with the skeletal site and the age of the subject. Generally, there is predominantly trabecular bone in the axial skeleton and more cortical bone in the peripheral skeleton. Trabecular bone is metabolically more active and undergoes normal and abnormal changes more rapidly than cortical bone. Bone marrow, particularly its fat component, introduces a small measurement error by reducing the measured bone mineral. This error is small for DXA and generally neglected, but corrections are routinely made when QCT is used. Replacement of red marrow with fat occurs during aging at a different rate in different bones, making corrections impractical when multiple sites are evaluated as commonly done with DXA.

Bone loss in trabecular bone occurs by reduction in thickness of trabecules as well as by loss of trabecules. In cortical bone, bone loss is accompanied by decreasing cortical thickness (increase of the internal diameter and decrease of the external diameter) as well as by porosis—i.e., the formation of small holes in the

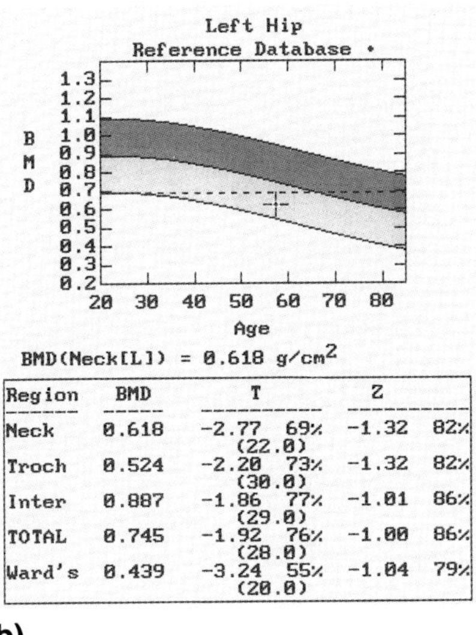

Region	BMD	T		Z	
Neck	0.618	-2.77 (22.0)	69%	-1.32	82%
Troch	0.524	-2.20 (30.0)	73%	-1.32	82%
Inter	0.887	-1.86 (29.0)	77%	-1.01	86%
TOTAL	0.745	-1.92 (28.0)	76%	-1.00	86%
Ward's	0.439	-3.24 (20.0)	55%	-1.04	79%

(b)

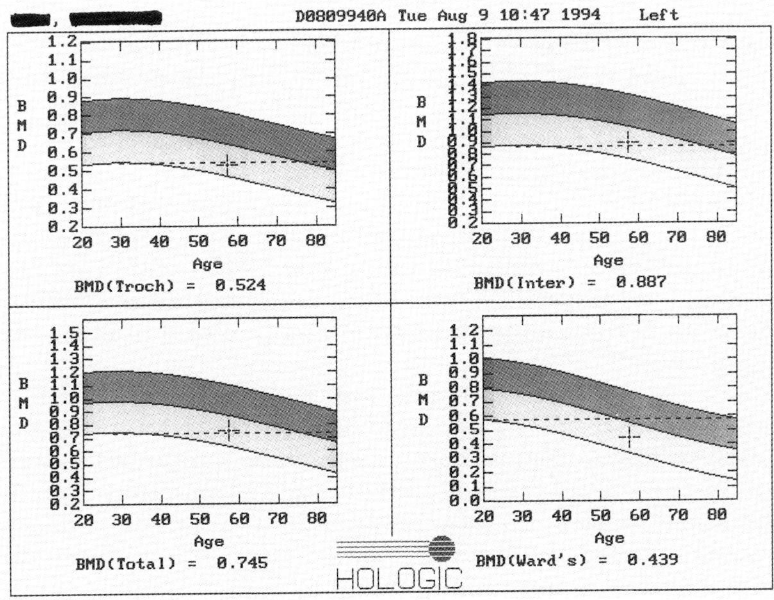

(c)

cortex. Thus, bone loss with age and disease shows a loss in bone mass (measured by DXA) as well as a change in bone structure (not measured by DXA). It is important to recognize that though bone strength is dependent on bone mass and bone structure, only bone mass is measured by absorptiometry techniques and used as the basis for fracture risk estimation.

In adults, maximal bone mass is reached in young adult age (20–30 years). Men have 10–50% greater bone mass than women depending on bone site measured. Cross-sectional studies of normal populations show a bone loss with age in men of about 0.3–0.5% per year. In women, bone mass decreases minimally prior to menopause. Then, there is a period of 5–10 years of accelerated bone loss in which the rate of loss may reach 2–6% per year (average 2%) at the spine (93–95). A similar bone loss is seen after oophorectomy. Postmenopausal bone loss varies, ranigng from 1% to 5% per year. Some studies have shown a group of "fast losers" (25–30%) and "slow losers." With available techniques, seasonal changes in the rate of bone loss are only recognizable in cross-sectional studies of some large populations.

B. Bone Strength and Architecture

An understanding of the relationship between bone mass and bone strength and of the factors leading to fracture is necessary for the interpretation of bone mineral results in clinical practice (90,96).

In excised bones, ash weight of bone, which is an equivalent of bone mineral measured by absorptiometry, is proportional to the compressive strength of bone (97,98). The correlation between bone density measured with densitometry techniques and bone strength is high. Comparatively small changes in bone density are associated with large changes in strength. In vitro 70–80% of the variability in bone strength is determined by bone mineral density or bone mineral content. Measurements of bone mineral thus serve to estimate bone strength and risk of fracture.

While bone mass appears to be the most important single factor in bone strength, other skeletal factors such as the shape or microarchitecture of a bone also contribute to bone strength. The shape of the proximal femur (bone geometry) is of particular theoretical interest as much potentially relevant information is now available from current bone mineral measurement techniques (99,100). Simple measurements such as femur neck length and femur neck angle are readily available from the scan images. Complex approaches which calculate actual bone strength from both bone mineral data and bone geometry are under investigation (101). An association of a longer femur neck axis or a greater femur neck angle with increased fracture risk has been suggested (102). These studies are of interest only to the epidemiologist at this time. It has been suggested that fracture risk prediction can perhaps be improved by incorporating these geometric data. In clinical applications, a bone mass measurement is the only current practical approach to estimate fracture risk.

REFERENCES

1. Nordin BEC. The definition and diagnosis of osteoporosis. Calcif Tissue Int 1987; 40:57–58.
2. Consensus Development Conference. Diagnosis, prophylaxis, and treatment of osteoporosis. Am J Med 1991; 90:107.
3. WHO Study Group. Assessment of fracture risk and its application to screening for postmenopausal osteoporosis. WHO Technical Report Series 843. Geneva: WHO, 1994.
4. Riggs BL, Melton LJ III. Evidence for two distinct syndromes of involutional osteoporosis. Am J Med 1983; 75:899.
5. Riggs BL, Melton LJ III. Involutional osteoporosis. N Engl J Med 1986; 314:1676.
6. Ringe JD, Mäckelburg U, Meyer-Baumgartner HP. Häufige Verkennung sekundärer Osteoporosen im geriatrischen patientengut. Z Geriat 1989; 2:23.
7. National Osteoporosis Foundation Advisory Board. Physician's Resource Manual of Osteoporosis. Washington, DC: National Osteoporosis Foundation; 1994:7.
8. Cummings SL, Black DM, Nevitt MC, et al. Appendicular bone density and age predict hip fracture in women. JAMA 1990; 263:665–668.
9. Cooper C, Campion G, Melton LJ III. Hip fractures in the elderly: a world-wide projection. Osteoporos Int 1992; 2:285.
10. Cummings SR, Black DM, Rubin SM. Lifetime risks of hip, Colles' or vertebral fracture and coronary heart disease among white postmenopausal women. Arch Intern Med 1989; 149:2445–2448.
11. Melton LJ III. Osteoporosis: a worldwide problem. In: Proceedings of the Third International Symposium on Osteoporosis, Washington, DC, March 2–5, 1994. Washington DC: National Osteoporosis Foundation/National Institutes of Health; 1994:23.
12. Seeman E. Epidemiology and diagnosis of osteoporosis in men. In: Christiansen C, Riis B, eds. Proceedings of the Fourth International Symposium on Osteoporosis and Consensus Development Conference, Hong Kong, March 27–April 2, 1993. Rødovre, Denmark: Fourth International Symposium on Osteoporosis; 1993:186–189.
13. Cooper C, Atkinson EJ, Jacobsen SJ, O'Fallon WM, Melton LJ III. Population-based study of survival after osteoporotic fracture. Am J Epidemiol. 1993; 137: 1001–1005.
14. Cook DJ, Guyatt GH, Adachi JD, et al. Quality of life issues in women with vertebral fractures due to osteoporosis. Arthritis Rheum 1993; 36:50–56.
15. Lyles KW, Gold DT, Shipp KM, Pieper CF, Martinez S. Association of osteoporotic vertebral compression fractures with impaired functional status. Am J Med 1993; 94:595–601.
16. Repa-Eschen L. Prevention and treatment of osteoporosis in our health care delivery system. In: Avioli LV, ed. The Osteoporotic Syndrome. New York: Wiley-Liss; 1993:197.

17. Chrischilles E, Shireman T, Wallace R. Costs of health effects of osteoporotic fractures. Bone 1994; 15:377–386.
18. Pouilles JM, Ribot C, Tremollieres F, Bonneu M, Brun S. Risk factors of vertebral osteoporosis. Results of a study of 2279 women referred to a menopause clinic. Rev Rheum Mal Osteoarticularies. 1991; 58:96–101.
19. Slemenda CW, Hui SL, Longcope C, Wellman H, Johnston CC Jr. Predictors of bone mass in peri-menopausal women. Ann Intern Med 1990; 112:96–101.
20. Ross PD, Davis JW, Epstein RS, Wasnich RD. Pre-existing fractures and bone mass predict vertebral fracture incidence in women. Ann Intern Med 1991; 114:919–923.
21. Hui SL, Slemenda CW, Johnston CC Jr. Age and bone mass as predictors of fracture in a prospective study. J Clin Invest 1988; 81:1804–1809.
22. Melton LJ III, Atkinson EJ, O'Fallon WM, Wahner HW, Riggs BL. Long-term fracture prediction by bone mineral assessed at different skeletal sites. J Bone Miner Res 1993; 8:1227–1233.
23. Cummings SR, Black DM, Nevitt MC, et al. Bone density at various sites for prediction of hip fractures. Lancet 1993; 341:72–75.
24. Ross PD, Genant HK, Davis JW, Miller PD, Wasnich RD. Predicting vertebral fracture incidence from prevalent fractures and bone density among non-black, osteoporotic women. Osteoporos Int 1993; 3:120–126.
25. Black D et al. Axial and appendicular bone density predict fractures in older women. J Bone Miner Res 1992; 7:633.
26. Hui SL, Slemenda CW, Johnston CC. Baseline measurement of bone mass predicts fracture in white women. Ann Intern Med 1989; 111:355.
27. Ross P et al. A critical review of bone mass and the risk of fractures in osteoporosis. Calcif Tissue Int 1990; 46:149.
28. Wasnich RD et al. Prediction of postmenopausal fracture risk with use of bone mineral measurements. Am J Obstet Gynecol 1985; 153:745.
29. Seely D, Browner WS, Nevitt MC, Genant HK, Scott JC, Cummings SR. Which fractures are associated with low appendicular bone mass in elderly women? Ann Intern Med 1991; 115(11):837–842.
30. Wasnich RD. Fracture prediction with bone mass measurements. In: Genant HK, ed. Osteoporosis Update. Berkeley, CA: University Press; 1987:95–101.
31. Wasnich RD, Ross PD, Davis JW, Vogel JM. A comparison of single and multi-site BMC measurements for assessment of spine fracture probability. J Nucl Med 1989; 30:1166–1171.
32. Wasnich RD, Davis JW, Ross PD. Spine fracture risk is predicted by non-spine fractures. Osteoporos Int 1994; 4:1–5.
33. Law MR, Wold NJ, Meade TW. Strategies for prevention of osteoporosis and hip fracture. Br Med J 1991; 303:453.
34. Melton LJ III, Eddy DM, Johnston CC. Screening for osteoporosis. Ann Intern Med 1990; 112:516.
35. Raffles AE. Report on bone mass screening for osteoporosis: a review of reviews. Bristol, UK: University of Bristol, 1992.
36. Johnston CC, Melton LJ III, Lindsay R, Eddy DM. Clinical indications for bone mass measurements. A report from the Scientific Advisory Board of the National Osteoporosis Foundation. J Bone Miner Res 1989; 4(suppl 2):1–28.

37. Johnston CC Jr, Slemenda CW, Melton LJ III. Clinical use of bone densitometry. N Engl J Med 1991; 324:1105–1109.
38. Julian BA, Laskow DA, Dubovsky J, Dubovsky EV, Curtis JJ, Quarles LD. Rapid loss of vertebral mineral density after renal transplantation. N Engl J Med 1991; 325:544–550.
39. Rubin SM, Cummings SR. Results of bone densimetry affect women's decisions about taking measures to prevent fractures. Ann Intern Med 1992; 116:990–995.
40. Kanis JA, Melton LJ III, Christiansen C, Johnston CC, Khaltaev N. The diagnosis of osteoporosis. J Bone Miner Res 1994; 9:1137–1141.
41. Mazess RB. Bone density in diagnosis of osteoporosis: thresholds and breakpoints. Calcif Tissue Int 1987; 41:117.
42. Ott SM. When bone mass fails to predict bone failure. Calcif Tissue Int 1993; 53(suppl 1):S139–S142.
43. Black DM, Cummings SR, Melton LJ III. Appendicular bone mineral and a woman's lifetime risk of hip fracture. J Bone Miner Res 1992; 7:639–646.
44. Melton LJ III et al. Lifetime fracture risk: an approach to hip fracture risk assessment based on bone mineral density and age. J Clin Epidemiol 1988; 41:985–994.
45. Wasnich RD, Ross PD, Vogel JM, Davis JW. Osteoporosis. Critique and Practicum. Honolulu: Banyon Press; 1989:133–136, 154–159.
46. Silverberg SJ, Shane E, de la Cruz L, et al. Skeletal disease in primary hyperparathyroidism. J Bone Miner Res 1989; 4:283–291.
47. Wilson RJ, Rao S, Ellis B, Kleerekoper M, Parfitt AM. Mild asymptomatic primary hyperparathyroidism is not a risk factor for vertebral fractures. Ann Intern Med 1988; 109:959–962.
48. Reid IR, Evans MC, Wattie DJ, Ames R, Cundy TF. Bone mineral density of the proximal femur and lumbar spine in glucocorticoid-treated asthmatic patients. Osteoporos Int 1992; 2:103–105.
49. Melton LJ III, Chrischilles EA, Cooper C, Lane AW, Riggs BL. Perspective: how many women have osteoporosis? J Bone Miner Res 1992; 7:1005–1010.
50. He Y-F, Ross PD, Davis JW, Epstein RS, Vogel JM, Wasnich RD. When should bone mass measurements be repeated? Calcif Tissue Int 1994; 55:243–248.
51. Wahner HW. Assessment of bone loss with repeated bone mineral measurements: application to measurements on the individual patient. Nucl Compact 1987; 18:7.
52. LoCascia V, Bonnucci E, Imbimbo B, et al. Bone loss in resonse to long-term glucocorticoid therapy. Bone Miner 1990; 8:39–51.
53. Wahner HW, Fogelman I, eds. The Evaluation of Osteoporosis: Dual Energy X-Ray Absorptiometry in Clinical Practice. London: Martin Dunitz, Ltd., 1994:22, 23, 178–195.
54. Kelly TL, Crane G, Baran DT. Single X-ray absorptiometry of the forearm: precision, correlation, and reference data. Calcif Tissue Int 1994; 54:212–218.
55. Melton LJ, Wahner HW. Defining osteoporosis. (Editorial.) Calcif Tissue Int 1989; 45:263.
56. Ross PD, Wasnich RD, Vogel JM. Detection of prefracture spinal osteoporosis using bone mineral absorptiometry. J Bone Miner Res 1988; 3:1.
57. Vogel JM, Wasnich RD, Ross PD. The clinical relevance of calcaneus bone mineral measurements: a review. Bone Miner 1988; 5:35.

58. Lai D, Rencken M, Drinkwater B, Chesnut CH III. Site of bone density measurement may affect therapy decision. Calcif Tissue Int 1993; 53:225–228.
59. Stevenson JC, Cust MP, Gangar KF, Hillard TC, Lees B, Whitehead MI. Effects of transdermal versus oral hormone replacement therapy on bone density in spine and proximal femur in postmenopausal women. Lancet 1990; 335:265–269.
60. Cummings SR, Nevitt MC. A hypothesis: the cause of hip fracture. J Gerontol 1989; 44:107.
61. Health and Public Policy Committee, American College of Physicians (Kimmel PL). Radiologic methods to evaluate bone mineral content. Ann Intern Med 1984; 100:908–911.
62. Fogelman I, Ryan P. Measurement of bone mass. Bone 1992; 13(suppl 1):S23–S28.
63. Uebelhart D, Duboeuf F, Meunier PJ, Delmas PD. Lateral dual-photon absorptiometry: a new technique to measure the bone mineral density at the lumbar spine. J Bone Miner Res 1990; 5:525–531.
64. Finkelstein JS, Cleary RL, Butler JP, et al. A comparison of lateral versus anterior-posterior spine dual energy X-ray absorptiometry for the diagnosis of osteopenia. J Clin Endocrinol Metab 1994; 78:724–730.
65. Wahner HW. Single- and dual-photon absorptiometry in osteoporosis and osteomalacia. Semin Nucl Med 1987; 4:305.
66. Wahner HW, Dunn WL, Riggs BL. Assessment of bone mineral. Parts I and II. J Nucl Med 1984; 25:1134, 1241.
67. Larcos G, Wahner HW. An evaluation of forearm bone mineral measurement with dual energy X-ray absorptiometry. J Nucl Med 1991; 32:2101.
68. Schneider P et al. Getrennte Messung von Kompakta- und Spongiosadichte mit einem Transversal-rotations-scanner. Fortschr mit einem Röntgenstr 1985; 143:178.
69. Gilsanz V, Loro ML, Roe TF, et al. Vertebral size in elderly women with osteoporosis. J Clin Invest 1995; 95:2332.
70. Prentice A, Parsons TJ, Cole TJ. Uncritical use of bone mineral density in absorptiometry may lead to size related artifacts in the identification of bone mineral determinants. Am J Clin Nutr 1994; 60:837.
71. Stein JA, Lazewatsky JL, Hochberg AM. Dual-energy X-ray bone densitometer incorporating an internal reference system. (Abstract.) Radiology 1987; 165(suppl):313.
72. Wahner HW et al. Comparison of dual energy X-ray absorptiometry for bone mineraurements of the lumbar spine. Mayo Clin Proc 1988; 63:1075.
73. Eastell R et al. Unequal decrease in bone denf lumbar spine and ultradistal radius in Colles' and vertebral fracture syndromes. J Clin Invest 1989; 83:168.
74. Mazess RB et al. DEXA measurement of spine density in the lateral projection. I. Methodology. Calcif Tissue Int 1991; 49:235.
75. Slosman DO et al. Vertebral bone density measured laterally by dual energy X-ray absorptiometry. Osteoporos Int 1990; 1:23.
76. Bjarnason K, Nilas L, Hassager C, et al. Dual energy X-ray absorptiometry of the spine—decubitus lateral versus anteroposterior projection in osteoporotic women: comparison to single energy X-ray absorptiometry of the forearm. Bone 1995; 16:225.

77. Jergas M, Breitenseher M, Gluer CC, et al. Estimates of volumetric bone density from projectional measurements improve the discrimination capability of dual X-ray absorptiometry. J Bone Miner Res 1995; 10:1011.
78. Sabin MA, Blake GM, MacLaughlin-Black SM, et al. The accuracy of the volumetric bone density measurements in dual X-ray absorptiometry. Calcif Tissue Int 1995; 56:210.
79. Orwoll ES, Oviatt SA, Biddle JA. Precision of dual energy X-ray absorptiometry: development of quality control rules and their application in longitudinal studies. J Bone Miner Res 1993; 8:693.
80. Wahner HW, Looker A, Dunn WL, et al. Quality control of bone densitometry in a National Health Survey (NHANES III) using three mobile examination centers. J Bone Miner Res 1994; 9:951.
81. Kalendar WA. A phantom for standardization and quality control in spinal bone mineral measurements by QCT and DXA: design considerations and specifications. Med Physics 1992; 19:583.
82. Moro M, Hecker AT, Bouxsein ML, et al. Failure load of thoracic vertebrae correlates with lumbar bone mineral density measured by DXA. Calcif Tissue Int 1995; 56:206.
83. Cann CE. Quantitative computed tomography for bone mineral analysis: technical considerations. In: Genant HD, ed. Osteoporosis Update. San Francisco: Radiology Research and Education Foundation; 1987:131.
84. Zamenhof RGA. Optimization of spinal bone density measurement using computerized tomography. In: Genant HD, ed. Osteoporosis Update. San Francisco: Radiology Research and Education Foundation; 1987:131.
85. Cosman F, Herrington B, Himmelstein S, Lindsay R. Radiographic absorptiometry: a simple method of determination of bone mass. Osteoporos Int 1991; 2:34–38.
86. Kaufman JJ, Einhorn TA. Ultrasound assessment of bone. J Bone Miner Res 1993; 8:517–525.
87. Massie A, Reid DM, Porter RW. Screening for osteoporosis: comparison between dual energy X-ray absorptiometry and broadband ultrasound attenuation in 1000 perimenopausal women. Osteoporos Int 1993; 3:107–110.
88. Stewart A, Reid DM, Proter RW. Broadband ultrasound attenuation and dual energy X-ray absorptiometry in patients with hip fractures: which technique discriminates fracture risk. Calcif Tissue Int 1994; 54:466–469.
89. Kotowicz MA, Melton LJ III, Cooper C, Atkinson EJ, O'Fallon WM, Riggs BL. Risk of hip fracture in women with vertebral fracture. J Bone Miner Res 1994; 9:599–605.
90. Chestnut CH III. Theoretical overview: bone development, peak bone mass, bone loss, and fracture risk. Am J Med 1991; 91(suppl 5B):2S.
91. Greer FR, McCormick A. Bone mineral content and growth in the very low birth weight premature infants. Am J Dis Child 1987; 141:179.
92. Bonjour J et al. Critical years and stages of puberty for spinal and femoral bone mass accumulation during adolescence. J Clin Endocrinol Metab 1991; 73:555.
93. Buchs B et al. Bone mineral density of the lumbar spine, the femoral neck, and

femoral diaphysis in a Genevian population sample. Schweiz med Wchshr 1992; 122:1129.

94. Hui SL et al. A prospective study of change in bone mass with age in postmenopausal women. J Chron Dis 1982; 35:715.
95. Falch JA, Sandvik L. Perimenopausal appendicular bone loss: a ten year prospective study. Bone 1990; 11:425.
96. Adami S, Vajis JA. Assessment of involutional bone loss: methodological and conceptional problems. J Bone Miner Res 1995: 10:511.
97. Ericksson SAV, Isberg BO, Lindgren JU. Prediction of vertebral strength by dual photon absorptiometry and quantitative computed tomography. Calcif Tissue Int 1989; 44:243.
98. Hayes WC, Gerhart TN. Biomechanics of bone: applications for assessment of bone strength. J Bone Miner Res 1985; 3:259.
99. Faulkner KG, McClung M, Cummings SE. Automated evaluation of hip axis length of predicting hip fracture. J Bone Miner Res 1994; 9:1065.
100. Yoshikawa T, Turner CH, Peacock M, et al. Geometric structure of the femoral neck measured using dual-energy X-ray absorptiometry. J Bone Miner Res 1994; 9:1053.
101. Beck UJ, Ruff CB, Warden KE, et al. Predicting femoral neck strength from bone mineral data. A structural approach. Invest Radiol 1990: 25:6.
102. Nakamura T, Turner CH, Yoshikawa T, et al. Do variations in hip geometry explain differences in hip fracture risk between Japanese and white Americans? J Bone Miner Res 1994; 9:1071.
103. Gluer CC, Vahlensieck M, Faulkner KG, Engelke K, Black D, Genant HK. Site-matched calcaneal measurements of broad-band ultrasound attenuation and single X-ray absorptiometry: do they measure different skeletal properties? J Bone Miner Res 1992; 7:1071–1079.
104. Davis JW, Ross PD, Wasnich RD. Evidence for both generalized and regional low bone mass among elderly women. J Bone Miner Res 1994; 9:305–309.
105. Pouilles JM, Tremollieres R, Ribot C. Spine and femur densitometry at the menopause: are both sites necessary in the assessment of the risk of osteoporosis? Calcif Tissue Int 1993; 52:344–347.

10

Current and Future Concepts in Osteoporosis Therapy

REIMER ANDRESEN

Behring Municipal Hospital
Free University of Berlin
Berlin, Germany

BRUCE WOLLMAN

University of California, San Diego,
School of Medicine
San Diego, California

DAVID J. SARTORIS

University of California, San Diego,
School of Medicine, and University of
California, San Diego, Medical Center
San Diego, California

I. THERAPEUTIC STRATEGIES FOR OSTEOPOROSIS

Therapies for osteoporosis usually act by a mechanism of increased formation or decreased resorption. These effects are summarized in Table 1. Other proposed means of treating osteoporosis include calcium, exercise, and growth hormone.

II. THERAPIES THAT INCREASE BONE FORMATION

A. Fluoride

The effect of fluoride is to increase the number, lifespan, and activity of osteoblasts. Fluoride has been used for decades to provide significant increases in spinal BMD (5–10%/year) and trabecular bone (10–20%/year) (1,2,35) and subsequent decreased rates of vertebral fracture (3,8). Furthermore, fluoride is unpatented and hence a relatively inexpensive therapy (4,62).

Although high doses of immediate-release fluoride increase BMD (8), lower doses or delayed-release has been found to be more effective in decreasing the risk of vertebral fracture (45). Monofluorophosphate may thus be more effective since

Table 1 Common Osteoporosis Therapy Strategies

Strategy	Decrease resorption	Increase formation
Effect on bone mass	Stabilize	Increase
Effect on bone cells	Decrease osteoclast activity	Increase osteoblast activity
Examples	Estrogen, calcitonin, bisphosphonates	Fluoride, vitamin D, parathyroid hormone (PTH)

it is more bioavailable (60) and also exists in an enteric-coated (sustained-release) form (61). Also, since vitamin D potentiates the stimulation of osteoblasts by fluoride (63), the two could be given concurrently in order to lessen the dose of each and hence possibly decrease side effects.

There are concerns that fluoride therapy, especially after long-term use, may cause poor connectivity in new trabecular bone or an increase in compact bone porosity leading to a higher risk of nonspinal fractures. While the results of recent research vary on this issue, a dosing schedule such as a 14-month cycle with 2 months off after every year on therapy may be advised (68). In addition, the response to fluoride is often diverse, and nonresponders and patients with very low BMD initially may still have a significant risk of fracture even after therapy (60).

For the last two decades there has been concern that sodium fluoride, even though it increases the density of axial trabecular bone, may not contribute to bone strength. First, fluorotic bone is not as strong as normal bone, and secondly, the trabecular bone that is formed may not proliferate at structurally important locations. Finally, the preservation of compact bone, rather than purely trabecular bone, may be important to the structure of the spine, the femur, and peripheral sites. If fluoride therapy does not stabilize compact bone, or if it increases structural abnormalities in compact bone, it could be deleterious.

Numerous studies have shown that fluoride therapy increases bone density and decreases the fracture rate in the spine (1–8). Recent studies have been collected in a special supplement to the March 1990 J Bone Miner Res (9). Even the negative studies from Mayo Clinic (8) and Henry Ford Hospital showed some decreases of spinal deformation, though less than those demonstrated in previous studies. The peculiar finding from the latter studies seems to be that high-dose calcium (1,500 mg/day above the usual intake for a total of > 2,000 mg/day) had an unexpectedly large effect in diminishing spinal deformation. On the other hand, those studies and others have suggested increases of fractures elsewhere in the skeleton. Hedlund and Gallagher (10) showed that the risk of hip fracture increased threefold with fluoride therapy, but a survey by Riggs et al. (11) showed no increase. Nonspine fractures (excluding stress fractures) doubled in the Mayo Clinic study (9). The results with hip fractures and peripheral fractures may result from the known effects of fluoride on cortical remodeling (12).

At recent meetings this ambivalence has led some leaders to indicate that physicians who treat with fluoride put their patients at risk and are themselves at risk for litigation. The evidence is not clear and physicians must carefully review the literature in order to ascertain if and when such treatment is reasonable. Current consensus among leaders in the U.S. is that fluoride should not be used for treatment of osteoporosis outside of clinical trials, although it may be useful short-term if preferential spinal osteopenia is present. In Europe and elsewhere a less cautious, more optimistic view prevails.

Recent studies from the Mayo Clinic and Henry Ford hospitals have shown that sodium fluoride was very effective in increasing spinal BMD (in %/year) and maintaining femoral BMD. However, there was not a significant decrease in the rate of vertebral fractures in these studies (8). These studies contrast with numerous studies in the U.S. and elsewhere showing that fluoride increases spinal bone density and decreases fracture rates (2,3,7,13–17).

Now, several studies have indicated that this difference in efficacy may be associated with dose form. The Mayo Clinic/Henry Ford studies used 75 mg NaF in an immediate-release form. European and U.S. researchers with positive results tend to use sustained-release forms or monofluorophosphate. Two recent studies (18,19) have shown that the serum fluoride levels are twice as high with immediate-release forms as with slow-release forms. Given this, the 75-mg immediate-release form would probably have serum levels five times higher than the 30-mg sustained-release form.

Advocates of slow-release fluoride suggest that these high levels of fluoride produce osteoblastic overstimulation and weak bone. The evidence for efficacy of the slow-release forms is just as compelling as the evidence for ineffectiveness of high-dose immediate-release NaF. Still, additional large-scale studies will be needed to overcome the caution flags raised by the recent U.S. studies.

Controversy with regard to sodium fluoride is intense and ongoing. New studies continue to show that sodium fluoride increases spinal BMD but has little effect on the peripheral skeleton. A recent report by Pouilles et al. (20) demonstrated a 3% annual increase of spinal BMD in a fluoride-treated (50 mg/day with calcium and vitamin D) group over 2 years. Half the group were responders who increased at an annual rate of 5.8%, and half were "nonresponders" in terms of bone. Both responders and nonresponders showed a 50% increase of osteocalcin, but no change in alkaline phosphatase. Bone loss from the femoral neck and trochanter was identical in the treated group, whether responders or not, and in controls (who received 1 g/day of calcium supplement). About 12–18 months was needed to identify the fluoride responders. Diversity in response also was shown by others (5,16,21). Fluoride at moderate doses does not adversely affect the structure or mechanical properties of trabecular bone (22–24); however, cortical bone may become more porous (25). The degree of cortical porosity seems dependent on fluoride dose, and this may explain differing findings on vertebral fracture rates (8,21,26). A recent multicommunity study in the U.S. showed elevated fracture rates over a 5-year period with high-fluoride (2.2×) and high-calcium (1.6×) intakes (27). Radial and femoral BMD values were lower in the high-fluoride area but did not show a larger aging decrease.

Debate on the use of sodium fluoride in osteoporosis continues. Recent summaries by Gruber and Baylink (28) and Kleerekoper and Balena (29) outlined major results and concerns regarding fluoride, and both concluded that fluoride should not have routine clinical use. Just a few years ago, a consensus panel of experts stated that fluoride was a positive agent (1). Fluoride is questioned today because of the negative results obtained in some prospective trials in which it was used at high doses (75 mg/day) (8,30). Fluoride produces a preferential increase (5–10%/year) of trabecular bone, which is relatively normal in structure and perhaps even stronger than untreated bone (23). In contrast, fluoride has little effect on the mass of compact bone, but it does increase cortical porosity, particularly in subjects who show the largest trabecular increases (25). Since the compact shell of the vertebral body is responsible for 50% of vertebral strength (31), fluoride-induced increases of trabecular bone might only slightly decrease vertebral fracture if strength of compact bone is offset by an increased cortical porosity. Conceivably, fluoride could be given at lower doses, or combined with an agent like estrogen that affects compact bone positively. Raymakers et al (32) confirmed earlier reports that combined fluoride and antiresorptive therapy (estradiol or pamidronate) for 3–4 years was no more effective than NaF alone on bone density, but fracture data were not reported.

Fluoride could be useful in conditions with an accelerated loss of trabecular bone, for example, corticosteroids (33). A recent study by Rico et al. (34) found that 50 mg/day of NaF was effective in increasing the usually depressed osteocalcin levels. They also found that a low dose of 1, alpha-D_3 (0.5 μg/day) had an effect similar to sodium fluoride. Even with the short half-life of vitamin D (under 24 hours), and its negligible side effects at this physiological dose, it may be preferred to fluoride. Paradoxically, calcitonin has also been effective in corticosteroid osteoporosis. The effectiveness of fluoride or vitamin D on fracture rates in corticosteroid osteoporosis remains to be demonstrated.

Fluoride continues to be a controversial therapy even though it increases trabecular density by 5–15% annually (35). At low doses, fluoride stimulates osteoblast formation, but at high doses, it depresses osteoblast activity and mineralization (36). Fluoride also can increase mineral density distribution of compact bone (37). A recent NIH workshop provided a summary of therapeutic trials and outlined the effects of water fluoridation (38). The Mayo Clinic (51) study of fluoride led many U.S. clinicians to reject this therapy, though it is used in France and Germany, where sustained-release formulations are available. As noted previously, the U.S. studies have been criticized for using a high-dose (75 mg/day), immediate-release formulation that produces large increases (8%/year) of histologically abnormal bone. Presumably, the high dose was responsible for the finding of no difference in spinal deformation in the fluoride-treated and calcium-treated groups. Both treatments decreased "fracture" rate by 20%, but a larger decrease in fracture rate for fluoride was expected based on the 32% increase of spine BMD, and a lesser decrease in fracturing would be expected for calcium, which had little effect on the spine. Studies using sustained-release fluoride or monoflurophosphate usually increase spine BMD by only 3–5%/year (39). At the ICCRH, Riggs reported on an additional 2-year follow-up (40), including results at lower doses. Patients at a dose of < 38 mg/day had a fracture rate of 24/100 patient-years, while those with a dose of 38–59 mg/day had a fracture rate of 30/100 patient-years. This was well below the rate of 45/100 patient-years in women receiving 60 mg/day (and the 50–80/100 patient-years usually seen in untreated controls). This confirms many other studies showing that immediate-release fluoride given at doses of 30–50 mg/day halves fracture rates. These new findings may encourage those who look to fluoride as an answer for patients with excessive spinal osteopenia, but they do not address potential adverse effects, at least with immediate-release sodium fluoride, on nonspine fractures

Fluoride is one of the most effective compounds in increasing spinal bone density; it can produce increases of 5% to 10% to 20%/year of purely trabecular bone of the spine (1,35). Fluoride has almost no effect, however, on either compact or trabecular bone of the peripheral skeleton. Lower doses of sodium fluoride (30–50 mg/day), preferably in sustained-release form, produce smaller bone increases but have far fewer side effects (1,19,35). Fluoride gave the first demonstration of the spine-specific response now recognized with many therapeutic agents in osteoporosis. The smaller spine BMD increases that occur with low-dose or sustained-release fluoride decrease fracture rates, but high doses of immediate-release fluoride do not. This led to questions about the strength of fluoride-treated bone (41). Two of the concerns about strength have been that the newly formed trabecular bone had poor connectivity, and that compact bone might develop increased porosity. Histological studies have shown that fluoride therapy thickens trabeculae without adversely affecting bone structure (23,42). Similarly, compact bone does not have increased porosity when slow-release fluoride is used (43), so the bone is stronger (44).

Researchers from Loma Linda University (45) have presented a retrospective study of 389 osteoporotic patients treated with sodium fluoride. Spinal fracture rate decreased as a function of time on therapy and was inversely related to spinal BMD. Patients who had a fracture during the fluoride therapy in general were those who 1. were not responsive, 2. were older, 3. had more fractures prior to initiation of therapy, and 4. had lower initial spine densities. This study of an osteoporotic group showed that spinal bone density was an important determinant of fracture risk both initially and in response to therapy. Fluoride has also been shown to be effective in preventing bone loss in primary biliary cirrhosis (46).

Fluoride is one of the few agents to stimulate osteoblastic number, activity, and lifespan. This can cause increases of 5–10% annually in the amount of bone (35). Several studies have shown that fluoride does decrease vertebral fracture rates if used in a low-dose or delayed-release formulation (45). High-dose fluoride in immediate-release formulation has limited effect, however, on fractures, even though it does increase BMD (8). Factors other than dose and formulation may influence the effectiveness of fluoride. Exposure to sodium fluoride in vitro does not modify the activity or proliferation of human osteoblast cells in primary cultures, according to a recent study (47). This suggests that the mechanism of action is more complex and indirect than previously thought. Biological cofactors could be needed to produce positive skeletal effects. There also may be critical thresholds of bone concentration that need to be reached before therapeutic (or toxic) effects are seen. A recent model for fluoride uptake by the skeleton should aid investigation (48).

Sodium fluoride continues to be of interest for postmenopausal osteoporosis (49, 50). It is one of a few drugs that affect bone formation positively by affecting osteoblasts (51). Recent evidence suggests that fluoride affects osteoblast progenitors and/or operates through a cofactor, since osteoblast proliferation and activity are not increased by exposure in vitro (52), but are increased subsequent to exposure in vivo, at least in those who respond with increased bone formation (51).

It is clear that fluoride increases trabecular bone in the axial skeleton, and there is even some suggestion that the peripheral trabecular bone, at least that in the lower limbs, also may be increased (53,54). However, neither the proximal femur nor trabecular bone in the distal radius is affected by conventional doses (20,54). Still, spinal fracture rates are decreased by 30% or more in treated subjects given moderate doses; even the Mayo Clinic trial, which is widely quoted as showing no effect, demonstrated a 35% reduced fracture rate in fluoride-treated patients over the last 3 years of the trial compared to calcium-treated controls (8). If there are any adverse effects of fluoride on bone strength, they occur only with high doses after long-term administration.

Among the problems with fluoride at high doses have been a negative effect on bone quality and strength (76,77), and accumulation of stress fractures. This may be due to differences in bioavailability of fluoride, absorption, and bone avidity (55). It is difficult to ascertain susceptibility to side affects except by detailed individual monitoring. Advocates of fluoride, however, point out that use of low doses in a sustained-release formulation should minimize side effects (56,57). Monofluorophosphate also appears to have equal efficacy and low side effects (58). Use of cyclical treatment, with dose tailored to the patient response, is another alternative (57).

As yet, detailed studies have not been done using fluoride in combination with compounds other than estrogen (78). Investigations of fluoride and estrogens have suggested that there may be some synergistic effect (59). The use of fluoride and bisphosphonates, or fluoride and calcitonin, has not been systematically investigated. Perhaps more important, the effect of a short course of fluoride followed by antiresorptive or estrogen therapy needs to be determined. It is quite possible that fluoride could be used for a year to augment bone density; the increased bone could then be stabilized using antiresorptive therapy.

Until recently, fluoride was the only agent that could be used in osteoporosis to provide rapid, sustained increases in spinal BMD (5–10%/year) (35,45,50). Decreased vertebral fracture rates accompany the increased spine BMD. Sustained-release forms (enteric-coated) are preferred but may compromise bioavailability. Monofluorophosphate is an active alternative form that may be more bioavailable (60). There is now even a sustained-release monofluorophosphate (61). Kanis (62) recently reviewed fluoride therapy and pointed out that controversy may exist because many of the studies with fluoride were done a decade or two ago when clinical trials were less rigorous. He also notes that contemporary trials are not likely to be undertaken because the treatment is both inexpensive and unpatented.

Vitamin D potentiates the effects of fluoride on osteoblasts (63,78). This suggests that active forms of vitamin D could be used together with fluoride to minimize fluoride dose (78). This could potentially diminish side effects. In addition, the vitamin D would stimulate calcium absorption and minimize the extent of calcium supplementation needed. Fracture efficacy in U.S. studies of fluoride may have been compromised by failure to include vitamin D as well as use of high-dose fluoride.

Fluoride continues to be of interest to many researchers and clinicians because of clear evidence that it can increase spinal BMD (50). An NIH-sponsored study with high-dose fluoride at the Mayo Clinic showed a large increase of spine BMD, but the decrease of fractures that occurred over the total 4-year period was not significant or different from calcium-treated controls (8). There was a significant decrease in spinal fractures in treated patients during the final 3 years of the trial, but this finding was obscured because of the increased fracture rate during the first year. A reevaluation of the Mayo Clinic trial has appeared (64). That reevaluation showed that treated patients, excluding those with excessive fluoride accumulation, had a reduction in fracture rate. Excessive fluoride could produce poor-quality bone. However, normal fluoride accumulation with aging does not decrease bone strength (65). There is evidence that moderate supplements *do not* adversely affect bone quality short-term, but over 5 years of continuous accumulation bone strength and quality were decreased by 40% (66).

The Mayo Clinic study has been criticized for using a high dose of fluoride in an immediate-release formulation. In contrast, other studies have used lower doses and/or slow-release formulation. Such studies have shown decreased fracture rates (66,67). One new study by Pak et al. (68) with a slow-release formulation (25 mg twice daily), repeated 14-month cycles (12 months on treatment followed by 2 months off) showed an increase in spine BMD and a decrease in new vertebral fractures. This confirms an earlier study, that was not well controlled, demonstrating similar results (3). Heaney, in an accompanying editorial (69), pointed out the importance of this study and the deficiencies of the Mayo

Clinic trial. Reevaluation of the original Mayo Clinic trial, coupled with the new study by Pak et al., shows that fluoride has potent antifracture efficacy, at least for the spine. There is still controversy about the effects on femur or radius BMD after 2 years' treatment, even though spine BMD increased by 10%. Bisphosphonates, like vitamin D and PTH, do affect nonspine areas (70). Also, high-dose fluoride can produce porosity in compact bone which decreases its strength. There appears to be a narrow window of safety for fluoride that will ultimately inhibit its long-term use. It could be used short-term to correct spinal osteopenia.

Fluoride produces demonstrated increases in spine BMD by stimulation of bone formation (69). Low-dose fluoride therapy, particularly with a sustained-release formulation or monofluorophosphate, increases spine BMD by 2–5%/year but has no effect on peripheral bone (68,70); the response of femur BMD is variable, with some studies showing no effect and others showing a small effect. Unlike antiresorptives, spine BMD remains elevated after treatment is terminated rather than undergoing accelerated loss.

Many researchers are concerned about potential adverse effects of fluoride based on problems with immediate-release formulations at high doses (64). Fluoride therapy over a few years does not have negative effects on blood chemistries (71) or on bone histology (72). Use of fluoride for a few years may, in fact, prevent trabecular perforation and maintain connectivity (72,73) and thereby reduce the rate of vertebral fracture. However, fluoride produces large mineral crystals that are abnormally located (74). Long-term treatment (5 years) apparently leads to decreased bone strength and quality (66), which suggests that fluoride therapy be used for only a few years. Such adverse effects are not evident in normal bone from subjects using fluoridated water (65,75).

B. Antiestrogens

There is increasing interest in the use of "antiestrogens" in osteoporosis. One antiestrogen, tamoxifen, is being studied for the prevention of breast cancer in women who have a high risk of cancer, and even in normal women. A major study in the U.S. is being undertaken in 16,000 women over 10 years to examine the possibility of cancer prevention, as well as reduction of cardiovascular risk (79,80). There are objections because tamoxifen causes some endometrial proliferation and increases cancer risk (81,82); however, tamoxifen could be taken with a low-dose progestin, perhaps given every 6 months, in order to prevent dangerous sequelae. Preliminary studies with tamoxifen showed a reduction of cardiovascular disease (83), and a new study from Sweden, in 2,365 women followed over 6 years (84), conclusively demonstrates a 30–60% reduction in cardiac disease in women treated with adjuvant tamoxifen for breast cancer; there was no increase in thromboembolic disease. Tamoxifen stabilizes spine and femur BMD (85–87), but the increase at both sites appears lower than observed with estrogen. It therefore appears that tamoxifen could be as effective as estrogen for the heart, even though it is somewhat less effective on bone.

Tamoxifen, a widely used antiestrogen, can delay or prevent recurrence in women with breast cancer (88–91). Antiestrogens were initially thought to be damaging to bone because of a possible interference with estrogen action. Pure estrogen antagonists, in fact, can cause loss of bone (92). However, studies done with tamoxifen have demonstrated bone preservation, not loss (85,87,93,94). Tamoxifen's estrogenic properties are manifest not only by protection of bone, but by lowering lipids and protection against cardiovascular risk (95,96). Tamoxifen has a particular effect on lipoprotein (a), a particularly atherogenic low-density lipoprotein (97). At the same time, however, there is endometrial stimulation which leads to an increased risk of cancer (98–100). This has raised the level of concern about use of this drug (101,102). In response to recent studies showing that tamoxifen increases cancer risk, labeling has been changed in the U.S. and elsewhere. The new U.S. labeling adds that the FDA and the National Cancer Institute have indicated that women taking tamoxifen face a risk of uterine cancer, about 2–3× higher than the risk for untreated women. However, the overall benefits of tamoxifen seem to outweigh the potential risks for breast cancer patients (90,91). Moreover, it is relatively easy to overcome the endometrial stimulation by either continuous low-dose progestins or episodic progestational ablation. There is still substantial controversy about ongoing studies in the U.S. and Europe to provide tamoxifen to high-risk women in order to prevent the initial appearance of breast cancer. Several women's groups oppose this testing because of 1. the risk of endometrial cancer, and 2. deficient informed consent. There has been a temporary halt since March 1994 on the $70 million, 5-year study in the U.S. as a consequence of unrelated events (a scandal over research fraud and auditing of results in an earlier breast cancer study). However, it is likely the tamoxifen prevention trial will go forward. Raloxifene, a similar agent with mildly estrogenic properties, is undergoing increased evaluation because it has less endometrial effect yet preserves bone and lowers cholesterol (103,104).

C. Bisphosphonates

Bisphosphonates have become one of the most studied therapies for osteoporosis (173,174). These compounds have potent antiresorptive effects and are especially useful for the first 5 years after menopause or other high-turnover osteoporosis.

One of these compounds, cyclic etidronate, has been used for two decades for hypercalcemia of Paget's disease and neoplasm and also decreases immobilization-induced bone loss. For osteoporosis, this drug has demonstrated a slight increase in spine and femoral neck BMD, and the effect on fracture rate is positive (177). However, in November 1994 a medical advisory panel to the Food and Drug Administration decided against registering etidronate in the United States. Newer bisphosphonates such as pamidronate and alendronate may have more positive results. Over a 1- to 2-year course, they result in an increased BMD of the spine (by up to 5% per year), femoral neck, and other peripheral sites (70,179). After 2 years, it appears that continued therapy does not provide an additional increase in BMD but does stabilize the bone (112).

Possible side effects of bisphosphonates are gastrointestinal disturbances, mineralization defects, and immune function depression (141). For example, high doses of cyclic etidronate (10–20 mg/kg) given continuously for long periods of time can lead to increased fracture rates and osteomalacia (109,110). For treatment of osteoporosis, the drug should be given in lower doses (7 mg/kg) and on an intermittent basis.

In addition, there have been concerns that these drugs may not be as effective on compact bone osteoclasts (125). In fact, paradoxical accelerated peripheral bone loss has been observed (145). Although this may also depend on the dose received, it has been recommended that other drugs that stabilize compact bone be given concurrently. Furthermore, simulations of bone remodeling have suggested that the positive effects of antiresorptives are transient and that termination of treatment may result in rapid bone loss (208).

Bisphosphonates, chiefly etidronate and second-generation drugs like APD, are now widely used in the treatment of high-turnover Paget's disease (105) but are not yet used for osteoporosis. A recent study in Denmark (106) and a multicenter study in the U.S. (107) have indicated that the cyclical administration of etidronate in doses under 10 mg/kg is effective in retarding bone loss in osteoporotic patients and diminishing spinal fracture rates. Histomorphometry did not indicate the mineralization defect (108) that is seen with high-dose continuous administration.

Continuous doses of 10–20 mg/kg for periods of 6–18 months cause osteomalacia and are associated with increased fracture rates (109,110). For osteoporosis, the drug is given at low doses (400 mg, or about 7 mg/kg) for only 2 weeks every 13 weeks, or effectively 2 months during any 1 year. Calcium supplements are given during the intervening periods. The accumulated dose is 10–20 times lower than that for Paget's disease.

In the multicenter study (107), the net bone increase above that in the control group over 2 years was about 3% for the spine BMD; about 1% for femoral neck BMD; about two-thirds of the increase was seen in the first 6 months. A similar pattern of small spinal increase, stabilizing by the second year of therapy, has been seen in other studies with bisphosphonates (111–114) and is the expected temporal pattern seen with pure antiresorptive agents. A small bone increase with subsequent stabilization is similar to the pattern observed with either calcitonin or estrogen (115,116).

Devogelaer and Nagant (112) reported at the ASBMR on long-term use of pamidronate, an APD. There was about a 5% increase in spinal and peripheral BMD in the first 2 years of therapy, which was stable for the succeeding 3 years.

Apparently, this 5% increase represents the magnitude of bone change that can be produced by any antiresorptive agent (estrogen, calcitonin, or bisphosphonates).

Etidronate, which has been used over the past 20 years, will probably be an alternative to estrogen in preventing bone loss in osteoporotic patients. Riggs, in his accompanying editorial in NEJM (117), indicated that additional studies are needed to show that long-term skeletal retention of etidronate does not eventually produce adverse effects on bone cell activity or bone strength, since etidronate, once bound to bone, will remain in the skeleton. Riggs also suggested that second- and third-generation bisphosphonates might have advantages. Finally, he noted that bisphosphonates need to be compared directly to estrogens and vitamin D, both of which have been shown to reduce fracture rates.

Bisphosphonates have also been shown to be useful in reducing the high turnover associated with multiple myeloma (118) and cyclosporine (119). Bisphosphonates might optimally be combined with vitamin D, as well as calcium, because there is at least a suggestion that bisphosphonates decrease production and increase catabolism of 1,25-D_3 (120).

The recent publication of positive clinical trials with etidronate (106,107,111) has convinced even skeptics of the value of intermittent cyclical treatment at low doses. This avoids the problems of mineralization defects seen at high, continuous doses, and provides bone stabilization. At a recent meeting, additional results were presented on longer-term treatment. Questions remained, like those on calcitonin, about special effectiveness in high-turnover patients and possible lack of effectiveness, or even negative effects, in a small minority of low turnover patients. Alternative bisphosphonates are under development (113,114). Many leading researchers, however, are now using etidronate, which is widely marketed for treatment of Paget's disease, to treat a portion of their osteoporotic caseload.

Bisphosphonates have a profound effect on decreasing resorption and turnover in trabecular bone, but seem to have a much smaller effect on compact bone. As a consequence, treatment of osteoporosis often causes a transient increase of spinal density by several percent, with most of the increase occurring in the first year. Although bisphosphonates can induce mineralization defects at high doses, the low-dose, intermittent therapy used in osteoporosis has no such side effect. Newer agents, such as risedronate and alendronate, may have even less impact on mineralization (121,122). Alendronate, which is being developed by Merck, prevents bone loss in oophorectomized rats and baboons (123,124). Clinical trials of alendronate are now commencing in the U.S. and elsewhere.

Bisphosphonates have a preferential effect in decreasing osteoclastic resorption, but they also tend to depress osteoblastic activity and overall turnover. A report by Chappard et al. (125) now shows that osteoclasts from trabecular bone differ markedly from those in compact bone in sensitivity to etidronate. Trabecular osteoclasts were increased in untreated subjects after bed rest, but they were decreased in subjects treated with etidronate. There was no effect on osteoclasts from compact bone. This may explain why bisphosphonates affect spinal bone density but have little or no effect on compact bone (107–127). In fact, in high-turnover patients, etidronate can produce spinal increases that parallel fluoride (127).

Bisphosphonates do not adversely influence bone quality or strength (128–130); in fact, strength in animal studies (rats, monkeys) was increased. This may mitigate concerns about the fracture efficacy of these agents that have a long skeletal retention. The positive skeletal effects of bisphosphonates might be enhanced by concomitant agents, such as estrogen, which stabilize compact bone. Compact bone is apparently important for bone strength and fracture susceptibility.

Bisphosphonates are currently the most widely investigated class of drugs for osteoporosis therapy. Etidronate, which was pioneered by Norwich, has been available for 20 years for treating hypercalcemia of malignancy and Paget's disease; it also reduces bone loss associated with immobilization. Several clinical trials have reported that etidronate slows the loss of spinal BMD in postmenopausal women (106,107). However, etidronate failed to achieve U.S. FDA approval in 1995 because spine fracture results were equivocal. The FDA has expressed their uncertainties with regard to both long-term safety and efficacy in preventing fractures. A major part of the problem in demonstrating fracture prevention was that the initial fracture rate in the multicenter etidronate trial was very low (< 10/100 patient-years versus a typical figure of ~ 70/100 patient-years in established osteoporosis). Consequently a much larger sample would be required to unequivocally demonstrate a lowering of fracture rate. A Danish study (106) had a higher initial fracture rate, and a significant decrease was demonstrated—from 50 to 15/100 patient-years. This decrease has been seen in a crossover of the controls to etidronate, as well as in the fifth year of treatment (131). In effect the U.S. etidronate study was a prevention trial rather than a therapeutic intervention in patients with established osteoporosis. Etidronate, as a preventive agent, should be judged on prevention of bone loss rather than fractures. Other concerns of the FDA were the long-term retention of bisphosphonates and their effect on bone structure and strength. A recent report (132) indicates that the half-life of etidronate in bone is about 3 years when used at low dose. Reports on structure and strength have also begun to appear (133).

Many other bisphosphonate compounds are in clinical trials in the U.S. and abroad. Experts believe that alendronate (Merck) is the most likely candidate for approval in the U.S. in the near future. Positive results have been reported for other bisphosphonates: pamidronate, tiludronate, risedronate, and clodronate.

Bisphosphonates are used mostly for Paget's disease (134–136) and for hypercalcemia of malignancy (137). Efforts are being undertaken by at least a dozen pharmaceutical companies to use bisphosphonates in osteoporosis, but to date, bisphosphonates have been approved only recently in some countries for osteoporosis. Bisphosphonates depress bone resorption, but they also may have a direct effect on depressing bone formation through recruitment of osteoblasts. Bisphosphonates suppress the anabolic function of estrogens (138), but trabecular bone formed in rats by prostaglandin E_2 treatment is maintained by subsequent bisphosphonate treatment (139). Clinical trials indicate that bisphosphonates increase spinal BMD in older women and osteoporotic patients but have little effect on peripheral bone density (107,140,184). Fracture rates appear to be reduced by bisphosphonate treatment, but questions have been raised with regard to the consequences of long-term depression of bone turnover. This could potentially result in accumulation of fatigue fractures. Newer agents, which have a higher specific antiresorptive action, may provide advantages. One such agent, risedronate, which was developed as a follow-up to etidronate by Norwich/Procter & Gamble, will now be codeveloped by Pfizer.

Side effects could also possibly differentiate some of the bisphosphonates. Most show little influence on renal, hematologic, or hepatic toxicity, but gastrointestinal disturbances often occur and there may be differences among agents. One complicating side effect of bisphosphonates is depression of immune function (141). This may be particularly acute for amino-containing compounds. Alendronate, which is well ahead of other bisphosphonates in clinical studies, may require additional data to show that immune function is not compromised. One study in Paget's patients showed that 3 of 10 patients developed a transient fever associated with a decrease in the total and differential white cell count (134). The first bisphosphonate to demonstrate efficacy, and absence of side effects, should be widely accepted throughout the world following regulatory approval.

Bisphosphonates are likely to become accepted for prevention of osteoporosis over the next decade in the U.S. and Europe, although at present they have limited use (140). Bisphosphonates inhibit osteoclastic resorption and depress bone turnover; as a consequence, agents such as etidronate have been used for the hypercalcemia of malignancy and for Paget's disease (137). Bisphosphonates also inhibit axial, but not peripheral, bone loss associated with corticosteroids (126, 142,143). They might be considered especially appropriate for the high-turnover phase occurring in the 5 years after menopause.

One of the concerns with long-term use of bisphosphonates is that profound depression of turnover may lead to osteomalacia and histological abnormalities. This apparently does not occur with intermittent, low-dose etidronate. Storm et al. (144) have shown that bone in iliac crest biopsies of patients after long-term (3-year) treatment with intermittent etidronate was normal. There was no change in trabecular bone volume, but formation was depressed. While resorption was depressed at 1 year, it had returned to pretreatment levels at 3 years. Longer-term studies may be needed to see if this adverse circumstance leads to long-term loss. An additional concern with bisphosphonates is that positive effects seem limited to axial trabecular bone and do not occur in peripheral trabecular bone or in compact bone (106,107). This is probably because cortical osteoclasts are less sensitive to bisphosphonates (125). Several studies have even shown paradoxical accelerated loss of peripheral bone. A recent report will raise additional concerns about possible peripheral osteopenia. Price et al. (145) found that lumbar spine BMD was increased in pagetic patients treated over 6 months with pamidronate; even nonpagetic portions (80%) of the lumbar spine increased by 5%. In contrast, forearm BMD decreased by 8% in those with active disease. This may relate to the dose received and/or to the extent of secondary hyperparathyroidism. In any event, it heightens concerns regarding peripheral osteopenia in other patient groups receiving bisphosphonates.

Use of bisphosphonates for the prevention of postmenopausal bone loss and for the therapy of osteoporosis is enjoying a newfound respect following studies over the past decade (105,140,146–150). Bisphosphonates inhibit bone resorption, perhaps through the mediation of osteoblasts as well as by osteoclast inhibition (151). Bisphosphonates, especially etidronate, have been available for the past 20 years for treatment of hypercalcemia of malignancy and for Paget's disease. Newer bisphosphonates, like pamidronate, clodronate, tiludronate, risedronate, and alendronate, are more potent and have been effective in Paget's disease that is resistant to conventional treatment with etidronate or calcitonin (152). Pamidronate and alendronate are also effective in preventing bone loss associated with thyroid hormone excess (153–155). Such new bisphosphonates are a primary focus today in clinical research on osteoporosis treatment.

Etidronate is safe when used at low doses in an intermittent cyclic fashion. It prevents loss of bone from the spine in GnRH (156) and corticosteroid-induced bone loss (157,158). Both etidronate and clodronate prevent spinal BMD decreases in the immediate postmenopausal period (159,160) and in established osteoporosis (107,161–163). At the ASBMR, it was reported that when the control group in the multicenter clinical trial of etidronate was crossed over to treatment, it showed a spine BMD increase of 4% over 2 years (161). However, not all research centers have shown positive spine effects with intermittent etidronate (164); some have suggested that the spine BMD increases in the multicenter study may be particularly large (15%) in one or two centers and small (1–3%) in others. These differences could arise if certain patient groups, for example those with high turnover, show particularly large responses, or if different modes of administration (for example, night administration) have a better effect. Still, the increased spine BMD does decrease spine fracture rate by 30%, or about half the magnitude of the decrease seen in estrogen-treated patients with similar spine BMD changes (162,163). However, bisphosphonates have been less effective in preventing loss of compact bone (157) and in preventing hip fractures. This may be because bisphosphonates have a lesser effect on osteoclasts from compact bone (125). For example, there was little effect on femur BMD in the U.S. multicenter clinical trial (156); presumably there was no effect on radius BMD in most studies, although these data have usually not been reported.

Newer bisphosphonates, with greater potency yet less inhibition of bone mineralization, are considered better than etidronate; they do appear to have a small effect on femur neck BMD. Chief among these is alendronate, which appears to prevent or reverse spine loss at the menopause and in established osteoporosis (165–167). Alendronate has about twice the effect of etidronate on spine BMD and also has a positive effect on femoral BMD (about half the magnitude of the spine increase). Alendronate does not alter the mechanical properties of bone (168–170). A detailed prospective trial (171) involving 6,000 women has been initiated by Merck to test the effects of alendronate on fracture, as well as safety. The negative immune effects of amino-containing bisphosphonates may inhibit long-term use of these products even if safety is demonstrated in short-term studies. An even larger trial of risedronate, another alternative, is being undertaken by Procter & Gamble. Experts feel large-scale, long-term studies are needed to show safety for hip fracture since activation frequency is depressed by all bisphosphonates (150).

Bisphosphonates are replacing calcitonin for the treatment of both Paget's disease and hypercalcemia (172). Bisphosphonates also are the most-investigated agents today for osteoporosis (173,174). A recent review by Herbert Fleisch (175) covers the entire area in detail, including the registration status of agents throughout the world. A major trial is under way of alendronate (Merck) (176), and another is scheduled for risedronate (Procter & Gamble). Each of these trials involves thousands of patients. Up until a few years ago, the largest trial of an osteoporosis therapy was another bisphosphonate, etidronate (107), but this involved only 450 patients, or 20–40× less than current trials.

A report on the 4-year follow-up of the above with intermittent cyclic etidronate recently appeared (177). Spinal BMD was stabilized at year 3 at a value 4% above control; femoral neck BMD was about 2% above control values. Of special interest was the fact that vertebral fracture rate was reduced, as was the case in the Danish trial (106). Marcus (178) notes that the effects on BMD were not impressive, and that treated patients actually had an increased fracture rate in the third year of the trial. Alendronate has greater effects than etidronate, and they occur much more rapidly. At 1 year of treatment with doses from 5 to 20 mg/day, there is a 5% increase of spine BMD and a 3% increase of femoral neck BMD (165–167,179). Several reports on alendronate appeared in a special supplement to *Osteoporosis International* (179–183). Reports continue to appear on newer agents and new uses (147,148,187–189). In contrast to calcitonin, bisphosphonates may be effective in stopping bone loss in the 5-year period immediately following menopause (159,160). One new application of bisphosphonates may be their use as an analgesic. Bisphosphonates, particularly alendronate, can apparently reduce back pain (190).

The first several years have seen an upsurge in research on bisphosphonates for osteoporosis and other metabolic bone diseases (140,146,147,149,150). Bisphosphonates are effective antiresorptives and decrease bone turnover (191); hence, they can be effective in high-turnover osteoporosis. One new application may be suppression of thyroid-stimulated osteopenia (153–155, 192). A variety of new bisphosphonates are being investigated (clodronate, alendronate, pamidronate, tiludronate, risedronate) (148,184,185,193,194); these may be particularly important in Paget's disease as a more powerful alternative to etironate. Their potential in osteoporosis is good (186). Intravenous pamidronate recently was shown to increase spine BMD by 10% over 2 years, which was comparable to the increase seen with fluoride (70). Unlike fluoride, pamidronate also increased femoral neck and radius BMD. Similar or better skeletal effects have been reported with alendronate (179,186).

Evidence is accumulating that etidronate might be effective in preventing bone loss, but the FDA has rejected the etidronate registration for osteoporosis in the U.S. There were initially some small positive studies in Europe, but a large multicenter study in the U.S. (107) failed to demonstrate a significant reduction in fracture rate, even though loss of BMD was prevented. The 4-year follow-up showed that spine BMD and femoral neck BMD were 4% and 2%, respectively, above control values (177). Fracture rate actually increased during the third year of the trial. Kanis (195) recently questioned the fracture end point used in this trial and others. Many false-positives can occur in clinical trials, which can decrease the apparent efficacy of a truly effective treatment. In a study of clodronate in breast cancer patients, a liberal definition of fracture produced many false-positives which obscured the decrease of fracture rate observed with a stringent fracture criterion. This alternative seems more reasonable than the view that etidronate produced poor-quality bone that was susceptible to fracture. Histomorphometry done in that multicenter study has been reported (196). Biopsies done at three centers showed that etidronate depressed activation frequency but did not produce osteomalacia. There were surprising differences in trabecular bone volume (11% in Denver, 15% in Atlanta, and 19% in Seattle); i.e., the first sample was at the level of severely osteoporotic women, the second at the level of elderly women, while the third was close to normal young women. The diversity of patients in the etidronate multicenter trial may have obscured the efficacy of etidronate in osteoporosis. There were not any significant increases of bone volume in the group as a while, but reportedly osteoporotic patients do respond. Etidronate may have to be reconsidered in a better-controlled study that is limited to truly osteoporotic patients, a group that is the most likely to respond positively.

Interest in bisphosphonates for treatment of osteoporosis has been high for the past several years (197). Etidronate is the best-studied bisphosphonate (198–203); it has been approved for treatment of osteoporosis in several countries, but a medical advisory panel to the FDA rejected registration in the U.S. in November 1994. Researchers today are focusing on alendronate. Alendronate appears to have a fairly wide therapeutic window, is relatively safe, and is effective in preventing bone loss (177,184,185,193,204). Regulatory approvals have been submitted in at least 25 countries for alendronate, and experts expect U.S. approval in 1995.

A multicenter study of etidronate treatment for established osteoporosis in the U.S. demonstrated increases in both spine and femoral BMD over a 4-year period (177). The inclusion of relatively normal postmenopausal women rather than osteoporotic subjects at two or more of the research sites probably confounded the positive results from the other sites where truly osteoporotic patients were treated. Etidronate appears to have a narrower therapeutic window than alendronate, and has to be used in a cyclical fashion to avoid mineralization defects. Histomorphometry results from the multicenter study demonstrated that cyclical etidronate did not compromise bone histology (205).

Risedronate, like alendronate, appears to have a more rapid and dramatic effect on axial bone than etidronate (206,207). Etidronate increases spine BMD by a few percent; it has small effects on the femur and almost no effect on the long bones (177,199,202). The newer bisphosphonates depress remodeling faster and produce some rapid remodeling transients, but may also have minimal effects on total skeletal mineral and calcium balance (199). Bisphosphonates at best cause a 1% increase of total skeletal mass or 15–20 g of mineral. This is equivalent to 6–8 g of Ca, which is equal to a positive calcium balance of ~ 10 mg/day over 2 years of therapy (201,207). The typical 4% increase in trabecular bone seen with bisphosphonates probably affects no more than 10% (or 200 g of mineral) of the total skeleton (the 4% increase of 200 g equals about 8 g of mineral). Thus, nearly half of the net positive effect of bisphosphonates on the total skeleton is due to reduction of the remodeling space in trabecular bone of the axial skeleton. There is little if any positive effect on compact bone itself, probably because the turnover of compact bone and the remodeling space in it are much lower than that of trabecular bone.

Researchers have attempted to model bone changes over the past decade, and several groups have recently published on this (73,191,208). Antiresorptive drugs, like the bisphosphonates, are expected to produce a bone gain due to depression of remodeling. However, Heaney (208) suggested this is a temporary transient that can disappear rapidly, leaving the skeleton compromised. Long-term trials with bisphosphonates may be demanded by alarmed regulatory agencies because the models suggest a rapid bone loss when treatment is terminated and remodeling returns to normal (73,208). In fact, bone loss does accelerate after termination of estrogen therapy but not after bisphosphonate therapy. One model developed by researchers at Procter & Gamble (191) showed that bone density could be maintained over 10 years of treatment with a bisphosphonate.

Bisphosphonates have been used to treat the hypercalcemia of malignancy and Paget's disease, but they are also effective in a high-turnover condition such as thyroid hormone-induced bone loss. They also appear effective to prevent, or even reverse, bone loss due to steroids (209,210), gastrectomy (198), hyperparathyroidism (211), Gaucher's disease (212), immobilization, and cerebral palsy (213).

D. Calcium

Calcium supplements increase bone mass prior to puberty, but this may be due to accelerated growth rather than an increased maximum value (238). In adult life, the theory behind increasing calcium intake is that postmenopausal and osteoporotic women have been shown to be in negative calcium balance of 60–80 mg/day (216). However, measurement of this balance is very inaccurate (error of up to 70 mg/day), and even premenopausal women in positive bone balance have a negative calcium balance as well, about 30–60 mg/day (217).

Because of these facts, it is no surprise that calcium intake and skeletal status are not correlated, and supplementation has not been shown to be effective in preventing bone loss (245–248). Although small studies occasionally demonstrate a positive effect of calcium supplementation on BMD (251), in general this effect decreases as sample size increases. One problem may be that the elderly lack the ability to absorb most of the calcium; concurrent supplementation of vitamin D may be more useful. Calcium for older patients with a nutritional deficiency (less than 400 mg/day), especially when combined with vitamin D, would seem to be particularly valuable (220).

Although the benefits of calcium supplements are mostly insignificant, it is one of the most commonly prescribed agents for postmenopausal women. Yet this may bring additional risks. Some supplements of natural origin (such as oyster shells) have trace amounts of lead or other toxic substances that may cause concern for safety (266). Furthermore, recent research, including a 10-year prospective trial of 60,000 women, showed increased fracture rates in females with high intakes of calcium (253–255).

Over the past 30 years, calcium has been used as a placebo in clinical trials of osteoporosis drugs, and as a nostrum in clinical practice. Physicians are sometimes not ready to undertake the more aggressive therapies used by experts (estrogens, bisphosphonates, calcitonin, vitamin D, or fluoride). They recognize that a calcium supplement may be helpful and that an excess will do little harm. A vocal minority over the years have claimed that calcium deficiency is the cause of osteoporosis, and that calcium supplementation is effective therapy (214,215). This speculation was based on studies like the recent work of Hasling et al. (216), showing that postmenopausal and osteoporotic women are in negative calcium balance (60–80 mg/day). It is now recognized that calcium "balance" methods are grossly inaccurate (error 70 mg/day). Even premenopausal women who are in positive bone balance, are in negative calcium balance by −30 to 40 mg/day, which is half the deficit seen in older patients (217).

Studies using contemporary densitometry, with a few exceptions (227,228), have been unable to detect an effect of calcium supplementation. The evaluation of calcium effects has been complicated by the wide diversity of both calcium absorption and dietary intakes. Some elderly women with the lowest calcium intakes or low absorption may respond positively to calcium supplementation. The exact proportion of such women entering studies has varied, and hence the results of studies over the past two decades have been equivocal because small samples have been used, so the effects of prior dietary intake and/or absorption could not be isolated.

A definitive large-scale study at the Nutritional Research Center of Tufts University has demonstrated that calcium supplementation (500 mg/day) is modestly effective for those older women (> 6 years postmenopausal) with a daily intake under 400 mg/day (220). Radius and femoral neck BMD were stabilized by calcium supplementation, particularly CCM (the calcium citrate maleate developed by Procter & Gamble). There was no significant effect of calcium supplementation at any skeletal site for women with intakes of 400–650 mg/day, or for women within 5 years of the menopause. The interpretation of these results will be controversial. Undoubtedly, proponents will justify calcium supplements for all women since they are effective at some skeletal sites in a minority. In the Tufts study, even though all subjects were below the median calcium intake for postmenopausal women (650 mg/day), there was no value of calcium supplements until dietary intake was < 400 mg/day. Calcium is not expected to benefit women with adequate intakes. In an elderly population, calcium supplements could be helpful in the 15% or so of women with calcium intakes under 400 mg/day. Presumably supplements may depress the rate of bone loss from compact bone. Calcium supplements can cost as much as estrogen, so there may be a difficult choice for concerned physicians. Women with intakes below 400 mg/day could reasonably benefit from supplementation. It is also reasonable to provide adequate calcium during growth and development to ensure an adequate substrate for bone formation (229).

Recent studies suggest a lack of influence of calcium intake on aging bone loss. Anderson et al. (222) reported that bone density loss over 5 years was not associated with calcium intake in 400 elderly white women. The loss rate in the lowest decile was identical to that in the highest decile (1%/year). Kanis (223) has pointed out cogently that intake shows a spurious correlation with calcium balance. Also, as intake increases, balance has to increase as the fixed influence of imperceptible calcium loss becomes relatively smaller. A positive balance does not necessarily mean that calcium is going to bone; some calcium may be stored in muscle. Most excess calcium simply is not absorbed and appears in the feces. Now Heaney (224) has shown that calcium intake correlates highly ($r = .9$) with fecal density. This may allow researchers to check on long-term compliance with calcium supplementation.

Calcium continues to be a major preventive used by physicians, even though there is little direct evidence for its efficacy in the elderly except in those with a low intake (225). A recent study by Dawson-Hughes (220) showed some inhibition of bone loss in women with intakes of 400 mg/day. In a second large study,

Elders et al. (226) found that supplements of 1,000 or 2,000 mg elemental calcium inhibited spinal bone loss but had no effect on losses from compact bone. A supplement to the *American Journal of Clinical Nutrition* contained summaries on the effects of calcium on balance, bone, blood pressure, and growth (227,228).

Calcium is the most commonly used nutritional supplement given to postmenopausal women and patients with osteoporosis. Studies continue to show that calcium supplements are not effective in preventing postmenopausal bone loss or reversing osteoporosis. At the same time, postmenopausal women with a calcium deficiency (intake < 400 mg/day) have shown reduced bone loss with supplementation (220). Reid et al. (229) reported on a 2-year trial of a 1,000 mg/day supplement in 120 women (58 ± 5 years). The loss rate of total body BMD (LUNAR DPX) declined from 0.91%/year to 0.51%/year. Elders et al. (230) gave calcium (1,000–2,000 mg/day) to over 200 women in the perimenopausal and immediate postmenopausal years for 3 years. Supplementation in the years immediately before cessation of menses inhibited spine loss, but not in women who had ceased menstruating. However, loss of compact bone was reduced by 30% in both peri- and postmenopausal groups. These studies amplify earlier findings suggesting that calcium may be more important for compact than trabecular bone. For example, a recent report showed a 6% annual loss of vertebral trabecular bone using 1,000 mg/day calcium in a control group of osteoporotic women (231). Since compact bone is important for fracture, calcium should be considered, along with agents that affect trabecular bone.

A recent symposium containing review articles appeared in the *Journal of Internal Medicine* (232–236). Calcium intake may be most important during the period of growth and development to allow achievement of peak bone mass (237).

Calcium deficiency, particularly that due to malabsorption, can lead to altered bone growth and even osteomalacia. However, it is uncertain that variation of calcium intake, within normal limits, is important for development of peak bone mass, for the maintenance of the adult skeleton, and for the evolution of aging bone loss (232,233,237,238). Calcium deficiency may slow the attainment of peak bone mass, but it does not necessarily alter the peak level achieved (233,237). Supplements do increase bone mass, at least prior to puberty (238,239). However, this may merely accelerate growth, not increase peak values. There is *no* correlation between calcium intake and skeletal status in adults, even on a grouped basis where subjects are stratified by intake level.

Calcium supplements have often been recommended (232), although there has been little direct evidence of efficacy. Reid et al. (240) recently reported that supplementation with 1,000 mg/day inhibited bone loss. The study involved 122 postmenopausal women (58 ± 3 years) who received 5 g calcium gluconate and 800 mg calcium carbonate. At the end of 2 years, the calcium-treated women had higher BMD levels than the controls: 1% for spine and femoral neck BMD, and 0.5% for total body BMD. An earlier trial reported by Dawson-Hughes et al. (220)

found that supplements of 500 mg/day inhibited bone loss in women with customary intakes below 400 mg/day, but had no effect in those with higher intakes. It is difficult to reconcile these results with the many trials that have demonstrated high bone loss in postmenopausal and osteoporotic women supplemented with calcium. Villareal et al. (231), for example, gave 1,000 mg/day calcium and found a 6% annual loss of trabecular bone. Every study to date has shown that calcium is *not* effective in stopping bone loss in the first 5 years after menopause, when estrogens are recommended (230). However, the new studies do suggest that calcium could be useful later. One of the problems in older subjects, however, may be poor calcium absorption. This may explain why supplements have been ineffective in clinical trials, and why calcium has been shown to have no effect on hip fracture in a recent multicenter WHO study (241). In fact, one study showed that calcium intakes over 800 mg/day *increased* fracture risk (242). A recent French study showed that calcium given together with low-dose vitamin D was effective in preventing bone loss and decreasing fracture rates (243). Given the variable results with calcium, large-scale studies will be needed before it can be used in place of better-documented therapies.

Calcium is probably the most commonly prescribed agent for postmenopausal women (232,244), but it has appeared to be among the least effective based on both peripheral BMD and spine BMD. There is no association between calcium intake and postmenopausal bone loss (245–247). Calcium appears to have its greatest influence during growth (233,237). Supplementation during growth may accelerate attainment of peak mass, but there is no evidence that it increases the peak level achieved. After growth terminates in late adolescence, there is remarkably little influence of calcium supplementation. There appears to be a small effect on femoral BMD in older women, particularly in women with calcium intakes < 400 mg/day (220,240,243). However, most trials show no effect of calcium supplements, perhaps because many of these trials do not provide concomitant vitamin D to ensure absorption. Moreover, there appears to be no association between hip fracture and calcium intake (241). One epidemiologic study in the U.S. suggested a small (but nonsignificant and inconsistent) effect (248). It may be that some variable associated with calcium intake, such as muscle strength or postural stability, is responsible for the occasional associations of low intake with increased risk.

Calcium continues to attract the attention of nutritionists and clinical researchers. The Second International Symposium on Nutritional Aspects of Osteoporosis was held in Switzerland in May 1994; calcium was a major factor. The NIH Consensus Conference on Optimal Calcium Intake was held in Washington, D.C., in June of the same year. As expected, the calcium advocates again called for widespread supplementation of children, adults, and the elderly. Probably no agent has been more extensively used in relation to bone status than calcium, and probably none has produced such small and divergent results. As a consequence, some see calcium as a "good placebo," while others consider it at least partially effective in a substantial minority, if not a majority, of elderly subjects.

Epidemiologic studies evaluating the role of calcium in children have shown some effect, and longitudinal trials have shown that supplements accelerate bone growth. However, it is not clear that peak bone mass is increased; it may simply be attained earlier. The 1% annual increment in BMC achievable by supplementation is equivalent to only 2 months' acceleration of growth. A recent report showing that milk consumption during childhood was associated with adult BMD levels (249,250), supports the notion of an increased peak bone mass; however, Scandinavian countries with very high calcium intakes show identical BMD values to the U.S. and the rest of Europe. The effect of current calcium intake in normal adults is very small. Usually there is a very low correlation ($r < .2$) between calcium intakes and skeletal status. Small-scale studies ($n < 100$) sometimes show an association of calcium intake and BMD (251), but the larger the study, the less the effect. Major studies in thousands of subjects have shown no positive effect of dietary calcium intake on the rate of bone loss with aging (245–247,252). There appears to be no positive effect of calcium intake on rate of hip fracture (248). In fact, two recent studies showed increased risk of hip fracture with high dietary calcium intakes (253,254). This included a 10-year prospective trial in 76,000 women (254). An earlier study by Kreiger et al. (255) in Canadian women showed a doubling of both hip and wrist fracture with high-calcium intake. Hip fracture is elevated in northern Europe, an area with calcium intakes > 1,000 mg, and even within the U.S. the areas with high intakes of calcium have the highest rates of hip fracture. The diversity of subjects and their sources of dietary calcium, however, makes such studies difficult to interpret. Small effects can be readily offset by other factors, such as caffeine (256–258). Certainly the value of supplements, particularly in subjects with low intakes, cannot be assessed by epidemiologic studies.

Calcium supplementation seems to have its major effects in growing children and in the very elderly, with almost no effect between 20 and 60 years. Even in these groups, calcium only has an effect on those with low intakes (> 400 mg/day). Detailed longitudinal trials have generally found little effect of calcium at the menopause (225,259). The few positive studies typically show a decrease of bone loss, but not a maintenance or increase of bone as occurs with estrogen, bisphosphonates, and other skeletally active agents. For example, a recent 3-year study by Aloia et al. (260) reported that the loss of total body and femoral neck BMD was halved by supplementing with ~ 1,200 mg/day of elemental calcium (−1% versus −2%/year). Loss of spine and radius BMD was not significantly affected. One complication of calcium supplementation studies has been the varying forms in which it is given and variation in bioavailability (261). Some calcium supplements are insoluble, while others are readily absorbed. Another complication is the skeletal site measured; some sites (femur) seem more responsive than others (spine/radius).

Perhaps the clearest evidence for a calcium effect in adults is in older patients with a nutritional deficiency. Studies in the U.S. (220), France (243,262), and New Zealand (240) have demonstrated that calcium supplementation can reduce the extent of bone loss, at least form the proximal femur. This is particularly true in those with the lowest calcium intake (< 400 mg/day) or with low vitamin D levels. Moreover, calcium supplementation given with vitamin D can reduce the rate of both hip fracture and nonvertebral fractures by 30% (243,262). In one study, calcium supplements without vitamin D had no effect on hip fracture (241); calcium alone does not prevent spine fractures (263), but vitamin D does.

The possible effect of calcium on compact bone in older subjects may be because mild secondary hyperparathyroidism plays a role in femoral bone loss. Given the deficiencies of calcium in the elderly, and the low levels of vitamin D, calcium supplements should be accompanied by a safe dose of vitamin D (400 IU) to assume proper absorption. Supplements also are required in patients with defects of vitamin D metabolism, lactose intolerance, and/or celiac disease (264,265). Some calcium supplements contain lead and/or aluminum, which give rise to safety concerns with chronic use (266), particularly for children. Safety is not a problem for refined calcium carbonate or chelates but is a concern with "oyster shell" calcium, dolomite, and bone meal. Excessive calcium intake (> 2,000 mg/day) is to be avoided; elderly subjects may find difficulties with flatulence and constipation as intakes exceed 1,500 mg/day. High intakes depress vitamin D and double urinary calcium. The real danger of calcium, however, is the increased fracture rates seen in older subjects at intakes above 1,000 mg/day.

E. Miscellaneous Considerations

Studies continue to show that use of GnRH and LHRH agonists are very effective in endometriosis. However, nearly every study to date has shown that these agents reduce estrogen levels dramatically, and cause a rapid loss of bone (267–270).

Spinal and femoral loss within 6 months may be about 5%. The loss from the radius typically is about 1–2% over the same time period. Total body BMD increases by about 3%. In most subjects, this loss appears to be reversible, but in some patients the bone is not regained even one year after therapy has been discontinued (271).

Scharla et al. (272) showed that the magnitude of the loss appears related to initial biochemical state. Urinary calcium is increased, as is serum osteocalcin, but serum 1,25-D_3 levels are reduced. The serum 1,25-D_3 level was the only biochemical variable associated with lumbar BMD during GnRH treatment; changes in 1,25-D_3 levels were correlated with pretreatment 1,25-D_3. High pretreatment levels of serum 1,25-D_3 were associated with greater loss of bone mass with GnRH agonists treatment. This is because the higher the initial level of 1,25-D_3, the greater the decrease with the GnRH agonist. The greater the decrease, the greater the loss of lumbar BMD. Scharla et al. concluded that women with low dietary calcium intake, and consequently elevated 1,25-D_3 concentrations, are probably at higher risk to develop accelerated bone loss after the onset of estrogen deficiency.

This bone loss apparently can be prevented. Riis et al. (273) show that administration of 400 μg of intranasal nafarelin combined with ½ mg of norethisterone did not produce bone loss. In the group treated with nafarelin plus norethisterone, bone resorption, as indicated by urinary hydroxyproline, was unchanged and bone formation (osteocalcin) was only modestly increased. This useful study needs to be verified with regard to other GnRH and LHRH agonists. Another study has shown that growth hormone has similar inhibitory effects (274). These studies suggest that the bone loss associated with these antiestrogens is not inevitable, so that they may eventually be used without compromising skeletal integrity.

F. Which Drugs Affect Fracture of the Proximal Femur?

Most of the studies that have been done over the past decade have focused on spine fracture as an end point for efficacy. However, public health officials and leading researchers recognize that hip fracture is more important. Only estrogens have been widely recognized as being effective; estrogens are believed to halve the rate of hip fracture. A new retrospective study by Kanis et al. (241) addresses this issue. A total of 2,086 women with hip fracture and 3,532 women matched for age were included in a study done at 14 centers in six countries in southern Europe. The study was sponsored by the World Health Organization. The study investigated the background of which drugs the women were taking for osteoporosis. However, the case control study was retrospective, and used a questionnaire, an approach that is open to uncertainties. The relative risk for hip fracture was unaffected by vitamin D and related compounds, and by calcium. Calcitonin and anabolic steroids both had a lower relative risk (24% and 35%), though not as great as that achieved by estrogens (55%). These results also were adjusted for age, body mass index, and previous fragility factors; however, the validity of such adjustments is unclear. The fundamental results show that only estrogens significantly decreased the risk of hip fracture. Sodium fluoride, which is widely used in some countries for treatment of spinal osteopenia, was associated with a higher risk (1.86) of hip fracture. This may be due to the greater cortical porosity associated with high-dose immediate-release fluoride that seems to be used in Europe. It is surprising that this study missed the dramatic effect of vitamin D supplements on hip fracture. Several large-scale studies, including the recent report of French researchers (243), have shown that vitamin D, with or without calcium, can reduce hip fracture risk as much as estrogen. Calcium supplements, the most common "treatment" given to women with risk of osteoporosis, had no significant effect. A recent Canadian study showed that calcium intakes over 800 mg/day doubled the risk for fractures of the proximal femur and/or distal forearm (255).

G. Calcitonin

Calcitonin is widely used in some countries for treatment of established osteoporosis (275–278). The known analgesic effects of calcitonin make its use desirable immediately after a fracture. There has been less emphasis on using calcitonin in the immediate postmenopausal period (115). A recent study by Danish investigators (279) confirmed calcitonin's efficacy in stabilizing spinal BMD, as shown earlier by Reginster (280), but suggested that peripheral bone could not be maintained with nasal calcitonin (100 IU). Mazzouli et al. (284) have shown that salmon calcitonin (100 IU injected every other day) can prevent bone loss from the radius in the first year following ovariectomy. A higher dose (200 IU) may be needed with intranasal administration to maintain peripheral bone. Calcitonin has a particular effect on lowering bone turnover and may be especially appropriate to use in the postmenopausal period if estrogen is not desired, or is not a therapeutic alternative.

Calcitonin continues to be widely used for treatment of osteoporosis, particularly in the immediate months following a fracture when its analgesic action is desirable (285). Calcitonin is used more in southern Europe and Japan than elsewhere in the world. In the U.S., calcitonin has been approved for prevention of osteoporosis since 1981. Recently the FDA reviewed the phase IV fracture-prevention trial of women treated with Calcimar (Rhone-Poulenc Rorer). That study was not able to provide evidence for fracture efficacy, which led to some uncertainty with regard to labeling for the drug.

Evidence is accumulating that nasal calcitonin is as effective as injectable calcitonin (286); a suppository form is also under investigation. Long-term calcitonin therapy seems effective in stopping bone loss (287). Reginster amplified his earlier 1-year study (280); he found that patients maintained spine BMD for 3 years on 50 IU of nasal calcitonin while controls lost bone. Other studies continue to show a positive effect of calcitonin on postmenopausal bone loss (281–283). Calcitonin, similar to bisphosphonate, seems most effective in patients with high turnover (275,277).

There is increasing evidence that calcitonin prevents bone loss in corticosteroid osteoporosis (288–291). It is unclear why calcitonin, an antiresorptive agent, reduces bone loss, since corticosteroids depress bone formation rather than stimulate bone resorption.

Calcitonin is widely used in Europe for treatment of symptomatic osteoporosis in older women in part because of its analgesic effect (276–278,285,292,293). However, calcitonin deficiency is not a factor in the etiology of osteoporosis (294). Calcitonin also appears to be effective in the immediate postmenopausal period, when bone turnover is high (275,279,295,296). Gennari et al. (297) recently confirmed that the administration of intranasal salmon calcitonin prevented early postmenopausal spinal bone loss in high-turnover cases. Calcitonin (200 IU) administration reduced all indicators of elevated bone turnover that were apparent in the control group. While calcitonin is generally effective in high-turnover states, it appears to have only a short-term and variable effect on serum calcium in primary hyperparathyroidism (298,299).

Calcitonin is widely used for short-term amelioration of pain associated with osteoporotic fracture (300). For the last decade there has been debate regarding the long-term effectiveness of calcitonin in osteoporosis. Although several studies indicated that bone density of the axial skeleton was maintained, there were few studies on fracture. An international symposium on calcitonin containing 10 articles was published in the March 1992 issue of *Bone and Mineral* (301). Newer studies show that calcitonin is effective in reducing fracture rates, even though it has a modest influence on spine BMD (1–2% increase per year) and almost no influence on peripheral BMD (275,302). Overgaard et al. (279) gave nasal calcitonin at 50, 100, and 200 IU over 2 years. Calcitonin decreased signs of turnover, including osteocalcin, alkaline phosphatase, and urinary hydroxyproline. Spine BMD increased by 2–3% over this period. However, BMC of the distal forearm decreased by about 1% after 2 years in all groups. In spite of these modest skeletal changes, the spine deformation rate reportedly was decreased to one-quarter that in the placebo group (relative risk 0.23). Rico et al. (303) reported that new fractures were reduced by calcitonin treatment in women with established osteoporosis. These studies will help reassure physicians disturbed by the findings of the phase IV study of Miacalcin (Rorer). In that study, which experts consider to be flawed, fracture rate in the calcitonin-treated patients doubled compared to controls. That observation was a major concern at a recent FDA meeting.

In general, calcitonin, like bisphosphonates, appears to be most successful in high-turnover disease. However, a recent report suggested that intermittent calcitonin with phosphate could be used to treat low-turnover osteoporosis resulting from prolonged reserpine therapy (304).

Calcitonin is widely used in Italy and Japan for short-term amelioration of pain associated with fracture (285,292). Long-term use of calcitonin appears to be quite safe; this has been confirmed in a study of mostly pagetic patients followed for a median duration of 6.5 years (305). Still, long-term use of calcitonin for osteoporosis is not well accepted because of the high cost of the drug, because antibodies develop over time, which may lessen efficacy, and because the injectable formulation is not desirable. The latter difficulty is being overcome as nasal calcitonin becomes more available (279,286,306,307). Nasal calcitonin at 100 IU/

day is effective in older women but does not stop bone loss at the menopause (279,286). Fioretti et al. (308) recently confirmed that continuous and cyclical nasal calcitonin at a higher dose (200 IU/day) stopped bone loss in oophorectomized women over 2 years, but calcium supplements at 500 mg/day did not. These studies suggest that nasal calcitonin can minimize spinal bone loss during the high-turnover period at the menopause or in older patients with elevated turnover. It is unclear if there will be a positive effect on compact bone. No effect on hip fracture is expected based on a recent large-scale epidemiological study (241).

Calcitonin is probably one of the most widely used agents for treatment of established osteoporosis. However, it is unclear if there is any significant effect on osteoporotic fractures (241,309), and some studies even show no effect on BMD (310). Recent studies continue to suggest that both nasal and injectable calcitonin have limitations in the prevention of postmenopausal bone loss (311,312), at least in comparison to estrogen. Calcitonin also has no effect in the prevention of bone loss in young women associated with GnRH agonists (313) or primary amenorrhea (314), but it reportedly increased BMD slightly in amenorrheic athletes (315). Contrary to early reports, calcitonin also appears ineffective in preventing immobilization bone loss (316). However, most investigators believe it is a safe agent. Calcitonin, because of the requirement that it be injected, has not proven to be popular for long-term use in most countries, but it is widely used in many countries for analgesic relief at the time of fracture. Alternative forms (suppository, patch, and even oral) are being investigated (317–319), in addition to nasal spray, in order to overcome objections to injections.

Perhaps the major finding over the past few years is that nasal spray calcitonin, which many felt would be a useful agent, has not been effective in doses of 100 or 200 IU in the early postmenopausal years (311). At these doses, there is at least some short-term antiresorptive activity (320), but not enough to inhibit bone loss. This makes it unlikely that calcitonin will be approved for prevention in women without fractures. In fact, there has been some unwarranted speculation that existing approvals for use in established osteoporosis may be withdrawn. While regulatory authorities are taking a harder stance on approvals for all osteoporosis drugs, and even reportedly have reexamined the indications for calcitonin use, most experts believe that approvals for calcitonin will not be withdrawn since in many countries it is the only alternative to estrogen.

Calcitonin is widely used for short-term amelioration of pain of osteoporotic fracture in Europe and Asia. There has been hope that it could be used long-term for prevention of bone loss, particularly in high-turnover states (321). However, calcitonin has been ineffective in stopping high-turnover bone loss in the immediate postmenopausal period (311,312), and there are questions about its long-term use in older women. For example, there appear to be neutralizing antibodies against calcitonin which develop with long-term treatment. Antibody formation is most common after treatment with salmon calcitonin, but is rare after treatment with human calcitonin (322). There also appears to be receptor down-regulation so that resistance occurs after 12–18 months. Intermittent treatment may delay onset of such resistance. Reginster et al. (323) reported low-dose (50 IU), intermittent treatment of women within a few years of the menopause over 3 years. The same group has shown there was no difference in spine BMD in treated women with and without antibodies (324), so factors other than antibody differences may be responsible for such unusual positive results.

The rationale for use of calcitonin is unclear, since there does not appear to be a calcitonin deficiency in osteoporosis (325). Most efforts with calcitonin today are focused on the intranasal form, which appears to be as effective as the injectable calcitonin, and much more acceptable to patients for long-term treatment. However, the effect on spine and femur BMD has been difficult to demonstrate, particularly at lower doses (179,310,326). Positive studies have come from one Danish research group (276); cautious researchers are awaiting independent confirmation from ongoing large-scale studies. There are questionable effects of calcitonin, if any, on fracture rates (309). Calcitonin could be used short-term to reverse the rapid increase of resorption that follows fracture (327,328) or rheumatoid arthritis (306), as well as for hypercalcemia and Paget's disease.

Calcitonin is experiencing increasing competition from bisphosphonates in both hypercalcemia and Paget's disease. Calcitonin also has experienced declining acceptance by osteoporosis experts as new antiresorptives become available.

Calcitonin has been widely used in both Asia and southern Europe for treatment of osteoporosis (321,329). It has been difficult to demonstrate that either injectable or intranasal calcitonin inhibits bone loss in the immediate postmenopausal period (311,312), though one small study using suppositories has been successful (330). Calcitonin has been effective for treatment of established osteoporosis in some studies (323,324,331) but not in others (179,310); it has been difficult to demonstrate fracture efficacy (309). The effects of calcitonin may be subtle, and the actions limited to a selected minority of patients, for example, those with high bone turnover. Studies have not specifically targeted high-turnover patients. Presumably a separate analysis of the subgroup will become available with the results of clinical trials currently in progress.

Injectable calcitonin has been widely used over the past decade to inhibit bone resorption in Paget's disease. It also has been used to prevent bone loss in osteoporosis (331,332), despite lingering questions about its long-term efficacy on bone and fracture. Nearly all experts agree it is safe. Studies with the intranasal formulation have confirmed a positive effect on bone loss and fractures in the elderly (333). A medical advisory panel of the U.S. FDA voted for registration of nasal calcitonin for treatment of osteoporosis in November 1994. However, there is no significant effect in the immediate postmenopausal period at the doses used (334–336). Intranasal administration provides only about half the effect of an injectable form (337). Thus, the injectable dose of 200 IU which may be used in the elderly requires 400 IU in intranasal form. In postmenopausal women, however, 200 IU, and even 400 IU, decreased bone turnover without producing a significant effect on BMD (334–336). In order to have a bone effect in early postmenopausal women, 400 IU of injectable calcitonin might have to be used, and the intranasal form might require a dose of 800 IU. Unfortunately, the clinical trials of intranasal calcitonin concentrated on much lower doses, in part based on a study by Reginster et al. (338) showing efficacy at low doses (50 IU). Calcitonin also does not appear to be effective in primary biliary cirrhosis (339) or corticosteroid-induced osteoporosis (340).

III. THERAPIES THAT INHIBIT RESORPTION

A. Estrogen

Estrogen therapy has been used extensively in the U.S. for prevention of osteoporosis, stroke, and cardiovascular diseases in estrogen-deficient, oophorectomized, or postmenopausal women, but is used less in Europe and Asia. All parts of the skeleton have a positive response to estrogen, and both axial and peripheral fractures are prevented in all stages of postmenopausal life. Part of the effect may come from progesterone, which is often taken concurrently. Although this hormone was previously assumed to have no effect on bones, it may in fact positively influence bone formation (365).

The negative effects of estrogen are increased risks of breast cancer (383), fatal ovarian cancer (384), and other cancers as well as periodic bleeding (which can be controlled by continuous combined therapy with progesterone (420) or other agents such as tibolone (521). Since these possible consequences can be a strong deterrent to estrogen use, the American College of Physicians published guidelines in 1992 to aid in counseling postmenopausal women about hormone therapy (413).

Although estrogen positively affects BMD both in the early postmenopausal period and beyond, there are two schools of thought on the timing of treatment. Some patients are started on estrogen in early menopause because 5–10% of peripheral bone (488) and up to 15% of axial bone (489) are lost within the first 5 years. Yet recent studies suggest that several years of therapy at the time of menopause may not reduce the risk of fractures later in life, especially in the proximal femur (459,460). Furthermore, changes in BMD vary greatly in women treated with estrogen at menopause, but a uniform BMD increase is seen in women over 65 (and those with a low initial BMD) (462).

Older patients receiving estrogen have more rapid increases in bone structure, and even osteoporotic women can reach normal BMD if therapy is started later in life (482,483). The advantage of this is that the length of exposure can be reduced, lessening the elevation of cancer risk. Furthermore, one study has demonstrated that by age 75 the BMD of treated versus untreated controls is about the same (460).

Many patients do not get positive results with standard doses, however, and up to 50% can show a decrease in spinal or femoral BMD (462). It has thus been hypothesized that estrogen therapy should be tailored to the individual patient. For example, while smokers might require a higher dose, obese women may need lower amounts.

Results continue to show that estrogens in a variety of forms and routes of administration (oral, transdermal, percutaneous) are effective in stopping bone loss and preventing fractures. These same studies are showing that chronic administration of estrogen reduces lipids, particularly the LDL fraction resulting in a positive HDL/LDL ratio. This presumably is associated with reduction in cardiovascular risk, though some argue the estrogens act directly on microvasculature. The rationale for chronic estrogen therapy is therefore high (341).

However, gynecologists will not administer estrogen without a concomitant progestin in women having a uterus, and in the U.S., the FDA mandates combined therapy. Since most gynecologists administer the drug cyclically, this results in periodic bleeding, which is unsatisfactory for most postmenopausal women. Now several studies have indicated that continuous estrogen/progestin therapy can be given, eliminating the periodic bleeding within several months of initiation (342–346). If the progestin is given at a low dose (for example, 2.5 mg medroxy progesterone), then lipids are unaffected, and presumably the cardiovascular risks remain low. Combined estrogen/progestin therapy is effective in reducing bone loss (347–350).

Recent studies have focused on a subsegment of the population that may lose bone at conventional doses, a fact that was obscured by the overall positive response seen in the treated groups. A multicenter study (351) showed that 20% of patients lost spinal density at conventional doses, and 30–50% lost from the femur. This suggests that higher doses of estrogens may be necessary in some individuals, or that concomitant therapy with other agents may be indicated. With regard to older patients, an important paper has appeared confirming results from several cross-sectional studies (352,353) showing that older women can respond positively to estrogens.

Lindsay and Tohme (116) demonstrated in a prospective 2-year study that estrogen increased vertebral bone by 10.6% and femoral BMD by 5.5% in an older group of women with osteoporosis. A calcium-treated group lost 3% from the spine and femur over the 2-year period. At the end of 2 years, the treatment-control difference was 14% for the spine and 8% for the femur. This new study shows that estrogen can be effective even in the older women with substantial bone loss. It appeared that bone gain stabilized in the last 6 months of the study. Consequently, clinicians still must focus on preventing loss, since it is unlikely that there would be full restoration. Still, bone maintenance is sufficient to cause at least a 50% reduction in fracture rate.

The spine increase in these patients was about 0.06 g/cm^2, which is comparable in absolute magnitude to the changes seen with treatment in the immediate postmenopausal period. This is the same absolute spine increase that can be obtained with calcitonin or bisphosphonates. All these agents increase spine BMD by about 5% and femur BMD by about 3% during the first years of therapy; peripheral density is simply maintained.

These new studies suggest that patients who are approaching a spine fracture threshold of 1.0 g/cm^2 or a femoral fracture threshold of 0.70 g/cm^2 should be considered for treatment as rapidly as possible, regardless of age. Continuous estrogen/progestin therapy may prove acceptable for many patients.

Conjugated estrogens have dominated the U.S. market for estrogen replacement therapy (ERT) over the past 15 years. The 15% of postmenopausal women who receive ERT do so chiefly for symptomatic relief of menopausal symptoms and often stop therapy within a year or so of initiation. In fact, 30% of women who agreed to start ERT failed to fill their prescription (354,355). Another 30% take estrogen intermittently or stop within several months. Of the remaining 40% who receive prescriptions, about half stop within 2 years. Since ERT could be beneficial for both bones and cardiovascular risk, this failure of "uptake" and compliance is extraordinary. It is particularly difficult to understand, given strong epidemiologic support for ERT and the advocacy by gynecologists who often state, "All my postmenopausal patients get estrogens."

Focus groups have shown that women do not wish to take estrogens for general "health" purposes because of perceived risks of breast or endometrial cancer, and the inconvenience of menstruation and of side effects, like edema. These objections can be overcome by showing that the risk of cancer is small (354). Also, the new mode of continuous estrogen administration, together with a continuous low-dose progestin 1. minimizes the risk of endometrial cancer; 2. does not compromise positive lipid changes; and 3. eliminates periodic bleeding. Effatic bleeding, which is nearly always asymptomatic, can occur in 30–50% of patients during the first few months of continuous estrogen/progestin therapy. Still women need a positive reason to start and continue ERT. One major reason for continuation of ERT in long-term users is the risk of osteoporosis. A recent advertisement for Premarin recognized this in a particularly clear way (Fig. 1; reprinted here with permission from Wyeth-Ayerst). The ad also noted the failure of conventional nostrums, increased calcium intake and exercise, in stopping bone loss.

Bone densitometry has been suggested by many as one means to identify those at greatest risk. The lowest third of women at menopause are definite candidates for therapy, including ERT, bisphosphonates, and calcitonin. The middle third can be reviewed later while the upper third can view ERT as an option for reasons other than osteoporosis. Bone densitometry also can be used to monitor the efficacy of treatment (356). Recent studies suggest that 20% of long-term patients lose bone from the spine on conventional estrogen doses, and as many as 30–50% lose bone from the femoral neck. The subgroups of bone losers may require increased levels of estrogen and/or supplemental therapies.

Studies continue to show that estrogens are effective in preventing bone loss in both the spine and proximal femur, even in elderly patients. A recent study by Christiansen and Riis (357) shows that continuous 17β-estradiol and norethisterone stabilized compact bone and increased spine BMD by 8%. An earlier study showed the same therapy was effective in the immediate postmenopausal period (348). Lindsay and Tohme (116) also showed the effectiveness of estrogens in the elderly. For estrogen to be accepted in older women it cannot be given cyclically with a progestin, as this produces periodic bleeding. However, several studies have shown estrogen with a continuous low-dose progestin is equally effective (349,350). Continuous therapy is now considered to be the most acceptable because women are more likely to utilize it long-term given the absence of periodic bleeding. Cyclical therapy is most useful for short-term amelioration of postmenopausal symptoms. There has been some concern about the effect of a low-dose progestin on lipid profiles and coronary heart disease. Newer evidence suggests that the addition of low-dose progestin does not have adverse effects, and there may be no difference between combined therapy and unopposed estrogen for risk of coronary heart disease.

Studies over the past 20 years have demonstrated conclusively that estrogen therapy during the first decade after the postmenopause preserves both compact and trabecular bone in both the peripheral and axial skeleton (358–360). New evidence suggests that hormonal therapy actually increases spinal BMD, and even femoral BMD, as measured by DPA or DEXA (116,361). Part of the effectiveness of hormonal therapy may be due to the progestogen that is often given together with estrogen. The skeletal influence of progestogen alone is less clear, but studies have shown a decrease of resorption, particularly for compact bone (362–364). Progestogens also may influence bone formation positively; a recent study by Grecu et al. (365) showed that medroxyprogesterone increased the depressed osteocalcin in corticosteroid osteoporosis. Estrogen therapy alone apparently stabilizes, but does not increase, trabecular bone as measured by spine QCT. Gallagher et al. (366) showed that medroxyprogesterone (20 mg/day), like estrogen, reduced loss of compact bone throughout the skeleton. Trabecular loss measured by spine QCT was identical to that in controls (4–5%/year) while integral bone mass was maintained with both estrogen and progestogen. Norethisterone may increase trabecular bone, whereas medroxyprogesterone seems to have little effect. A recent study by Riis et al. (273) showed that norethisterone maintained spine and radius BMD in endometriosis patients treated with an osteopenia-inducing LHRH agonist.

There is now reason to question the assumption that progestogens do not have a bone effect. There is also good reason to examine compounds like tamoxifen, or like OD 14 (367), that have both mild estrogenic and progestogenic properties.

Estrogens continue to be the major therapy for osteoporosis in the U.S., although calcitonin is widely used in Europe and vitamin D in Japan. Estrogen replacement therapy (ERT) is effective in preserving bone in the immediate postmenopausal period (359). Further, it is now clear that spinal bone loss is actually reversed in older women (116). Established products, like conjugated estrogens and estradiol, are being utilized more. Most experts believe that continuous ERT, with a continuous low-dose progestin, is effective and eliminates the bleeding problem that stops women from adopting chronic ERT. Even wider use of ERT may result from 1. the expected approvals of an osteoporosis indication for transdermal (patch) estrogens, and 2. eventual introduction of combined estrogen-progestin patches. Also, it is now recognized that estrogen decreases overall mortality, especially cardiovascular mortality (368,369).

New compounds with weak estrogenic properties and less side effects, such as Org OD 14, are being studied in Europe. Several research groups have found that this compound produces a slight increase in spine BMD in longitudinal studies (367,370,371). The advantage of Org OD 14 is that it does not cause appreciable endometrial stimulation, which minimizes the need for a progestational agent. Several recent studies have also indicated that progestins may have an independent effect on bone. Gallagher et al. (366) showed that medroxyprogesterone preserved compact bone, but not spinal BMD. Grecu et al. (365) showed that medroxyprogesterone was effective in reversing the decreases of skeletal turnover induced by corticosteroids. Tremollieres et al. (372) reported that a 19-nor progesterone derivative preserved bone in postmenopausal women and acted as a bone cell mitogen.

Estrogens continue to be a mainstay for prevention of bone loss, at least in the United States (373,374). In the past 5 years, studies have confirmed estrogens have a positive effect on spine and femoral BMD in older women, including osteoporotics (116). Contrary to popular belief, the skeletal effect is better, and side effects lesser (375) in older women. The exceptions are that estrogen therapy is particularly effective after oophorectomy (376), or in premenopausal women with estrogen deficiency (377). In the latter group, spine BMD can be increased by 40% from osteoporotic to normal levels in 2 years.

There is no doubt about the efficacy of estrogen in preserving and increasing spine BMD. It also appears that density of the proximal femur is maintained, at least in many subjects. However, spine BMD may decrease in 20% of treated patients (378), and femoral BMD may decrease in 50%, at conventional doses. Consequently, both spine BMD and femoral BMD should be measured. If only one can be measured, the femur may be preferable because if femur BMD is maintained, then spine BMD will be preserved whereas the reverse is not the case. Dose may need to be adjusted to maintain femoral density.

Studies continue to show that estrogens decrease lipid levels, diminish atherosclerosis, and reduce cardiovascular mortality (368,379,380,381,425). Estrogen replacement therapy does not increase risk of coagulation problems and thrombosis (381,382); doses are effectively 5× lower than those used for oral contraception. Stampfer et al. (380) point out that except for hospital case control studies, which show increased risk, studies show a halving of risk. Also estrogen apparently increases the risk of breast cancer by 35% (383). There appears to be no influence of progestins on breast cancer (385). Most women would prefer to take a glass of red wine or some other lipid-lowering modality rather than estrogens if estrogen in fact increases the risk of breast cancer. Combining estrogens with periodic administration of tamoxifen may be one route of avoiding breast cancer that has not been explored.

In spite of substantial benefits compared to risks (386), many women do not accept estrogen, and even after starting, become noncompliant. Estrogens are often taken for symptoms, like hot flashes, and avoided because of perceived risks (387). Periodic bleeding is one problem (388). Continuous estrogen with a continuous low-dose progestin eliminates the periodic bleeding that has made estrogen therapy unacceptable to most women, and in particular older women (389). Coupling estrogen with an agent that protects against breast cancer, such as tamoxifen, may be another strategy for wider acceptance. An FDA advisory committee recently indicated that clinical trials (i.e., research) of estrogen in women with breast cancer were justified. However, estrogen therapy for patients with breast cancer is not recommended, although women who have had endometrial cancer remain candidates under some circumstances (390).

Estrogen continues to be the mainstay of osteoporosis prevention in the United States (391,392). It is much less common in the U.K. and rarely used in Asia. The principal drug has been oral conjugated estrogens (Premarin from Wyeth Ayerst) for the past 20 years, but estrogen patches, such as Estroderm (Ciba), are beginning to compete. Forest Laboratories will be introducing an estradiol transdermal patch in the U.S., and other companies are working on combined estrogen/progestogen patches.

The principal problem with estrogen has been poor compliance. One factor is the fear of both endometrial and breast cancer. The former can be prevented by giving a progestogen, preferably in a continuous low dose such as 2.5 mg/day of medroxyprogesterone. Several meta-analyses have failed to demonstrate an increase in relative risk of breast cancer (393), but a major study by Colditz et al. (383) showed a 30% increase in risk. In those with a family history of breast cancer or benign breast disease there certainly is an increased risk. Various strategies, including education, have been used to improve compliance (394). One of the best ways of doing this, however, is by providing the patient feedback on maintenance and increases of their bone density (395,396). While it is important for the physician to monitor the femur, the site of morbidity in osteoporosis, the patient can get greater feedback from total body scans where a compelling image can be provided; BMD of the total spine can be derived from total body scans and can show increases.

New studies confirm that estrogen dramatically decreases risk of fracture, even though bone density is only maintained or slightly increased (397). There is evidence that estrogen not only prevents bone resorption but has a weak effect on stimulating formation, though it is unclear how this acts. The only other agent known to both stimulate formation and prevent resorption is prostaglandin E2 (398).

There continues to be confirmation that estrogens given to older women (i.e., after age 60) not only stabilize BMD, but increase spinal BMD by 5–10%. Recently, Savvas et al. (399) showed that implantation of percutaneous estradiol and testosterone (75 mg and 100 mg, respectively, implanted at 6-month intervals) increased spine and femur density by 5% over 1 year in women who had previously been on oral therapy for many years. Testosterone was given for libido and to avoid depression but had no effect on bone. Oral therapy, which kept estradiol well below premenopausal levels, maintained bone density over the same period. The implants increased serum estradiol to premenopausal levels. This suggests that a higher dose of estrogen in older women increases BMD (400). Lufkin et al. (401) reported that serum estradiol levels reached premenopausal levels in 65-year-old osteoporotic women using transdermal estrogen. Spine BMD increased by 5% and fracture rate decreased. Even 0.625 mg/day of conjugated estrogens increased spine BMD (5%/year) almost as much as fluoride (7%/year) in older women (59). In contrast, Reginster et al. (402) found that increasing doses of estrogen had little incremental effect on reducing urinary calcium or hydroxyproline, but they used women only 5 years postmenopause and did not examine spine BMD. Anabolic steroids combined with estrogens also do not give an improved response (403).

Estrogen is the main therapy for preventing osteoporosis in North America, but it is less widely used in Europe and Asia (386,404–406). Estrogen, in a variety of forms and application modes (oral, transdermal patch, percutaneous creams), is effective in stabilizing both axial and appendicular bone. All areas of the skeleton (spine, femur, radius, and os calcis) respond positively to estrogen therapy, not only in the immediate postmenopausal period (407–409), but 10–20 years later (59,399–402). Estrogen also prevents the bone loss associated with GnRH in young women (410). Estrogen, unlike some other therapies, does not change the composition of strength of bone (411). The positive effect on bone prevents all types of osteoporotic fractures—i.e., not only spine, but hip fractures (397). Other agents, such as bisphosphonates, seem to have a positive effect on spine fracture but have no effect, or perhaps even a negative effect (as with fluoride), on hip fracture. Many studies show that estrogen therapy can prevent cardiovasular disease and prolong life in postmenopausal women. New evidence confirms a protective effect on risk of stroke (412). A major review commissioned by the

American College of Physicians has summarized and synthesized these studies (413). Basically, estrogens decreased morbidity and increased life expectancy for all women, especially those at risk of coronary disease or osteoporosis (415). On the basis of this review, guidelines were developed counseling postmenopausal women about preventive hormone therapy (416). However, many women will not even attempt therapy because of the increased risk of breast cancer (30%) and endometrial cancer (383,393,417,418). The inconvenience of periodic bleeding is another negative factor (388,394,419), although this can often be eliminated by continuous combined therapy (420). New transdermal patches that contain both estrogen and a progestational agent provide easy continuous therapy (421). Bone densitometry can influence women to begin taking estrogens (396,575), but it may not be sufficient to foster long-term compliance (575). Physicians may need to provide both bone and lipid results in order to demonstrate the positive value of estrogen for the individual patient.

Estrogen use worldwide is increasing by at least 20% annually. Estrogen continues to be the prime focus for treatment of osteoporosis in the United States and certain parts of Europe, but only a small minority of postmenopausal women are treated with estrogens, and most is used for short-term symptomatic relief. The trend for increased use over long periods is most evident in healthier women (422–424) with knowledge of the benefits for lipids and heart disease (425). There continue to be both patient and physician concerns about the risk of breast and endometrial cancer (418,426–429), as well as about menses or episodic bleeding. There are confounding variables, however. Women who take estrogen tend to be healthier, smoke less, and exercise more. While gynecologists are uniform in approval, other physicians are often negative. Perhaps 20% of women discontinue ERT because of physician advice, and most others stop out of fear or because of inconvenience of side effects. A recent meta-analysis of 31 epidemiologic studies by Colditz et al. (428) suggests there is an increased risk in current users but not in past users. Many physicians, particularly gynecologists, consider this an acceptable risk if heart disease is halved, but women fear cancer more than heart disease.

Estrogens are, of course, useful in preserving bone at the menopause (430) and even for increasing bone density by about 1%/year in older women and osteoporotic patients (431,432). Even a progestin alone can help preserve bone in the postmenopausal period (366,433).

Unlike humans, rats do not increase bone in response to estrogen (434). Rats may not be a good experimental model. Treatment of oophorectomized rats with estrogen of bisphosphonates depressed bone turnover and protected against loss (435).

New therapeutic approaches, such as transdermal estradiol, appear equally effective as conjugated equine estrogens (436,437). Daily continuous estrogen with a low-dose progestin (438,439) continues to gain favor as the preferred long-term modality because it provides a eutrophic endometrium without compromising lipids, eliminates bleeding, and fosters compliance. A new alternative (440) could be continuous estrogen with alternating 3-day cycles of a progestin (i.e., 3 days on followed by 3 days off). A new concept, that is as yet not well accepted, is that estrogen therapy may have to be adjusted to the individual patient. About 30% of women lose bone at conventional doses of estrogen, yet might maintain bone, particularly femoral BMD, at higher doses. Smokers may need a higher dose of estrogen (441,442), while overweight women may require a much lower dose (443).

Great interest has been aroused in raloxifene following initial presentations at the Hong Kong meeting in April 1993. Several papers have since suggested this new agent has potentially beneficial effects (104,444–446).

Estrogen treatment continues to get positive reviews for its cardioprotective effects in the postmenopausal woman (414,415,447–452). It is the choice for preventing bone loss in postmenopausal women (453,454), as new studies continue to show (414,455,456). There still remain a few doubters (457). More opposition to estrogen may develop since the risks of breast cancer have been underestimated (428,458) and the benefits to bone have been overestimated. There is increasing realization that several years of estrogen treatment at the menopause cannot provide long-term protection against fracture later in life, particularly fracture of the proximal femur (459). A major study by Felson et al. (460) in older women (mean 76 years) showed past estrogen use was not protective against hip fractures that occurred 10–20 years after treatment was terminated; only use of estrogen for more than 7 years was protective. Most women in this study took estrogen for a few years at the menopause, and even those few (under 10%) who had taken it long-term had terminated by age 65. This suggests that estrogen must be used later in life rather than at the menopause (461). Moreover, many of the women who received estrogen at the menopause eventually show bone loss even with continued use. Rozenberg et al. (462) showed that about half of women (age 55) treated with estrogen increased spine BMD, but 20% had significant loss. Over 50% of subjects with high initial BMD lost bone, but women with low initial BMD uniformly gained at a high rate. Apparently an even higher percentage of women (50%) show loss of femoral BMD on conventional estrogen doses. On the other hand, estrogens given to older women (> 65 years), who already have somewhat diminished BMD, produces almost uniformly increased BMD.

These new studies suggest that the current practice of treating at the menopause may be inadequate. Estrogen treatment for osteoporosis could begin at age 60 to 70 years, rather than at the menopause, especially for those women with normal BMD. Another way of expressing the same concept is that estrogen therapy should be initiated on the basis of BMD (for example, spine BMD 2 SD below young normal) rather than on the basis of age. If estrogen is started 10 or 20 years postmenopause, it becomes even more essential that the regimen be acceptable for long-term compliance. Since bleeding is a major reason for patients' rejection of estrogen (463), the continuous combined estrogen-progestin program will be essential.

Estrogen appears to be effective in stopping bone loss associated with corticosteroids in rheumatoid arthritis (464) and inflammatory bowel disease (465), but bisphosphonates may be preferred to avoid side effects. Estrogen seems to be less effective for loss induced by GnRH agonists (466).

Estrogen therapy at the time of the menopause is increasingly advocated by physicians (447,467–473). The health benefits of estrogen, primarily a reduction in cardiovascular risk, overweigh shortcomings due to increased risk of breast and/or endometrial cancer (447,470–475). However, most women choose not to take estrogen because of the fear of breast cancer and the inconvenience of periodic bleeding.

With regard to the first issue, there is a 40% increased risk of breast cancer with current estrogen use (428). In fact, a new Canadian study shows that risk increases by 7% for each year of estrogen use (474), so use for 5–10 years would increase risk by 35–70% and longer use could double the already high risk of breast cancer. Fortunately the termination of therapy reduces the risk of cancer (428).

With regard to the second objection, which is particularly important in elderly women, therapy must produce either amenorrhea or controllable cycles. Continuous estrogen combined with a low-dose progestin (2.5 or 5 mg of medroxyprogesterone) produces effective amenorrhea in many women within 6 months. A recent multicenter study in 1724 women over 1 year (476) showed that sequential administration with progesterone provided regular cycles and little irregular bleeding. Continuous combined therapy produced amenorrhea in 60–70% of women, but breakthrough bleeding was a problem.

Many women feel that the potential advantages of estrogen for them may not be great enough to warrant long-term treatment, even though 30% may use estrogen as a palliative in the immediate postmenopausal period. The average lifetime is increased by only 2 years for long-term estrogen users (467) due to the difficulties of extending an already prolonged lifespan in modern societies. The real advantage of estrogen, therefore, may be in quality improvement, not life extension. Education and counseling are needed since the long-term use of replacement therapy is a complex, individual decision (469). Reducing the risk of osteoporosis appears to be an important factor in this decision, and bone density results can affect decision making. A recent study in France confirmed the impact of fear of osteoporosis on estrogen use (477).

Studies continue to demonstrate that estrogen in all forms has a positive effect on BMD, both in the immediate postmenopausal period and later in life (456,478–488). Some believe that it is important to intervene early because 5–10% of appendicular bone (both compact and trabecular portions) (489), and 12–15% of axial bone is lost in the first 5 years after the menopause (490). An early menopause (490,491), or a high frequency of sweating (492), is associated with greater bone loss. Oligomenorrhea in perimenopausal women is associated with decreased estradiol, increased FSH, and some bone loss (493). There are virtually no nonresponders in the early postmenopausal period (479); however, bone is stabilized or increases by only a few percent annually. Estrogen therapy given to older women increases axial bone much more rapidly (5–10%/year) so that normal levels can be achieved after a few years, even in osteoporotic patients (482,483). Some experts have suggested that treatment need not be initiated until later in life, when it has its greatest effect. This lowers cancer risk by decreasing the length of drug exposure; it also lowers cost. Felson et al. (460) demonstrated that there was virtually no advantage to treating women from the menopause onward, because by age 75, treated women showed no BMD advantage compared to untreated controls. The bone increase induced by estrogen endures for al least 3–4 years and may decline thereafter. Nielsen et al. (484) recently showed bone decreases occurred after 4 years of therapy in early postmenopausal women. One alternative to continuous treatment after the menopause might be to initiate therapy at age 65–70 years (depending on BMD) and to continue it for 5–10 years.

Estrogen therapy is moderately, but not completely, effective in the state of amenorrheic premenopausal women (494–496). Low-dose contraceptives can be helpful in perimenopausal women (497). A large-scale study in Finland showed only a minor effect of previous use of oral antiresorptives in 3,222 perimenopausal women (498). It must be noted that estrogen in perimenopausal women dramatically increases the risk of breast cancer (even though that risk is smaller than in older women).

There is increasing evidence that subclinical PTH increases with aging are associated with bone loss. PTH increases at the menopause; estrogen reduces PTH secretion by 30% (499). Estrogen decreases the PTH increase due to hypocalcemia (500) and increased PTH suppression produced by hypercalcemia (501). Estrogen therapy is effective in postmenopausal women with mild primary hyperparathyroidism, but not as effective as in normal women (485).

Estrogen replacement therapy in postmenopausal women continues to be in favor with many U.S. and European clinicians because of its cardioprotective effects (502–509). However, some believe at least part of this effect is due to a selection bias. For example, Posthuma et al. (510) found that while cardiovascular disease was reduced by estrogens, so was cancer. This suggested a cohort effect; i.e., healthier women take estrogen, or perhaps those at risk of cardiovascular disease avoid it. Presuming there is a real effect, it can be shown that ERT is cost-effective even without considering potential benefits for osteoporosis (511). On the other hand, half an aspirin daily, or a glass of red wine, is equally cardioprotective without risks of breast cancer and without costs of gynecological care associated with ERT. Most women do not choose estrogen for cardiovascular benefits, but rather for its known positive effect on bone maintenance and fracture prevention (512–515). The mechanisms underlying the effect of estrogen continue to be elucidated (516–520). The major new clinical finding is that estrogen appears especially effective in treating older (> 65 years) women (201,521). Bone turnover is reduced by estrogen in these older women as in younger women (522). One objection in older women is the resumption of menstrual cycles. This can be minimized by using a continuous estrogen-progestin regime (523) or by alternatives such as tibolone (524).

A more controversial proposal has been the suggestion that ERT be provided for breast cancer survivors (525). Most nongynecologist physicians are cautious because of the evidence from large studies showing that ERT can increase risk of breast cancer by 3–10% or more (428,474). There is certainly contrary evidence showing little increased risk, however. The combination of estrogen with tamoxifen, or another antiestrogen, is a possible solution. However, many physicians still question the rationale for using ERT in view of both patient concerns and the availability of risk-free alternatives for bone maintenance and cardiovascular health.

B. Growth Hormone, Ipriflavone, Exercise

1. Growth Hormone

While GH has been studied as a therapy for osteoporosis over the last decade, its effectiveness has not been demonstrated. Decreased levels of insulinlike growth factors are seen in aging and osteoporosis, implying that lower GH levels may be a factor in this disease (531,532). However, while osteoporotics do show a normal osteoblast response to GH, since the hormone also increases resorption of bone, the net effect is insignificant (537). Furthermore, the high cost and serious side effects tend to limit its applications for clinical use.

A recent study by Rudman et al. (526) indicated that growth hormone given to older males for 6 months increased BMD of the spine, and stabilized femoral BMD versus controls. The 1.6% increase in spine BMD was smaller than the usual precision error (about 2%) of dual-photon absorptiometry and could be due to osteophyte proliferation. Most peculiarly, the femoral neck BMD and radius BMD in the control group declined at annual rates of 9% and 13%, respectively. These rates are over twice those seen in chemically or surgically oophorectomized women and indicate problems in the bone measurements. Cross-sectional data on normal males (527,528) show only a small annual loss rate (0.5%). The skeletal influences of growth hormone must await more precise evaluation. Growth hormone apparently inhibits bone loss associated with GnRH agonists (274).

Over the past 10 years, interest has increased for use of growth hormone (GH) as an osteoporosis treatment, but there has been little evidence of efficacy (526,529–533). Osteopenia is evident in GH-deficient adults (534), but the GH excess of acromegaly fails to protect against axial osteopenia. GH stimulates osteoblasts and remodeling (535,537); GH decreases with aging could be responsible for the low turnover seen in osteoporosis. This decrease is demonstrated by lower plasma levels of insulinlike growth factor in aging and osteoporosis (531,535). Osteoblast responsiveness to GH in osteoporotic is normal (538). The net skeletal effect of GH treatment may be minimal (537), since GH also stimulates bone resorption. Prospective trials have shown no effect of GH treatment on bone over a 6- to 12-month period in osteoporotic adults. Even GH treatment of hypopituitary adults has no short-term skeletal effect, although turnover is increased (539); over 30 months, however, there was a 5% increase of spine BMD in one study (540).

GH may have a role in short-term fracture repair (541) rather than long-term treatment of osteoporosis. However, GH does have a high cost and significant side effects, so even limited clinical application may be problematic.

There continues to be active investigation of the effects of insulinlike growth factor (IGF) and GH, which regulates circulatory levels of IGF, on bone (531,532, 542–545). Both GH and IGF stimulate bone and muscle metabolism, and they each increase bone and muscle mass in young animals (546,547). The extreme case is acromegaly (548,549). With normal aging, both GH and IGF decrease, and IGF is definitely lower in osteoporosis (535,536). Replacement therapy could have an anabolic effect (533), but this is difficult to demonstrate in adults, even in cases of clear deficiency. GH deficiency in children, including that induced by treatment for leukemia, results in low bone density. This osteopenia is due, in part, to small skeletal size but remains significant even after correction for height or expression of results as volumetric density (552). Provision of GH to deficient children increases muscle and bone mass (553,554). Even adult-onset GH deficiency causes bone loss (534,555), though not as great as that occurring during childhood. GH supplementation to hypopituitary adults decreases fat and increases both muscle mass (550,551) and bone turnover, but bone density may not increase (539,556–558). One study (540) showed an initial decrease of bone density, possibly related to expansion of remodeling space, with subsequent return to baseline values after 1 year (i.e., no significant net gain). Another study (559) showed about a 4% increase in both spine and radius over 1 year. Similarly, treatment of healthy older patients with either recombinant human GH or IGF decreased fat mass and increased bone turnover (537,560). The earlier study by Rudman et al. (526) is flawed; GH had an apparent effect over 6 months but only because the control group showed an impossibly large decrease of bone (> 5%). One limitation of GH or IGF treatment is a potential adverse effect on HDL cholesterol (537). There may be particular use for growth hormone to stimulate osteoblastic activity in corticosteroid-treated patients, who tend to have reduced bone turnover (561,562).

2. *Ipriflavone*

Ipriflavone, developed in Hungary, has been suggested to have a positive effect on bone. Initial reports have implied that ipriflavone may inhibit turnover of bone and maintain bone density, but clinical benefits such as fewer fractures or increased BMD have yet to be demonstrated. This may be because the drug is poorly absorbed and the low serum levels are much less than those needed for a biologic effect on osteoclastic resorption in vitro (587). The value of ipriflavone is still very much in question.

Many U.S. and European researchers heard little about ipriflavone, a natural isoflavone derivative, until the Osteoporosis Congress in Copenhagen in 1990. At that time, several reports were given on the mechanism of action and preliminary clinical work (566). Subsequently, a satellite symposium was held at the ICCRH in Florence in April 1992. The proceedings of that symposium were published as a supplement to *Bone and Mineral*, edited by C. Gennari and M.L. Brandi (567–573). Another symposium was held in Yokohama in January 1992, and the proceedings appeared as a supplement to *Calcified Tissue International* (574–580).

In general, large doses of ipriflavone are needed because absorption is very low. There may be wide individual variability in response because of the differences in absorption. Ipriflavone apparently has direct effects on both osteoblasts and osteoclasts, but it is unclear if concentrations in vivo reach the levels needed to produce these effects. Still, in humans, preliminary studies suggest ipriflavone may decrease bone turnover and possibly maintain bone density. No large-scale trials, however, have demonstrated efficacy in terms of either increased bone density or decreased fracture risk.

Ipriflavone was first developed by the Hungarian drug company Chinoin and was subsequently licensed in Italy and Japan. Most of the research has been done in these two countries (581–586). In Japan there is a growing market for the drug Osten, developed by Takeda; in Italy, ipriflavone is being developed by Chiesi and Takeda Italia.

Ipriflavone, which was developed in Hungary, is currently registered in Italy and Japan for use in osteoporosis. Some preliminary trials suggested it may have an effect on bone. However, substantial questions have been raised by leading experts around the world about whether ipriflavone has any effect at all at the doses delivered. The typical treatment is 600 mg/day of which only a small fracture is absorbed; very low blood levels are achieved. Significant biological effects of ipriflavone have been shown in vitro only at levels 1,000-fold higher than those achieved in vivo. A recent study by Azria et al. (587) demonstrated that ipriflavone had no effects on osteoclast motility and bone resorption at levels 100× higher than those achieved in vivo. Melis et al. (588) have demonstrated that there is no effect of ipriflavone on biochemical indices of bone resorption in post-menopausal women. Other studies also failed to show effects on known markers of bone turnover. These results have caused researchers to question the results of the small clinical studies of ipriflavone. Most experts today believe that ipriflavone has not been proven to have a significant skeletal effect. Additional studies will be needed to define the mechanisms of action and the effects on bone density and fracture.

3. *Exercise*

While lack of physical activity leads to disuse osteoporosis, strenuous exercise can stimulate hypertrophy of the bone, especially during the years of growth and development. Most research on the effects of exercise and skeleton structure indicates that the only positive effect comes from weight-bearing exercise, and prevention of bone loss occurs only in the loaded bones. Clinically, elderly people who are routinely physically active have been shown to have decreased bone loss (735), but extensive exercise regimens may not be feasible in many cases.

C. Parathyroid Hormone (PTH)

Paradoxically, low doses of PTH often cause both increased formation of trabecular bone and increased resorption of compact bone. Elevated serum calcium and 1,25-D_3 may also be factors in this mechanism. For the treatment of osteoporosis, concurrent administration of an antiresorptive agent decreases the catabolism of compact bone but has little effect on the increase of bone formation by PTH. For example, the combination of PTH and estrogen allows a significant increase of spinal BMD without significant adverse effects on the femoral neck (608).

Parathyroid hormone is well recognized as a bone-stimulating agent. Experimentally it increases trabecular bone density in rats (589–597), but at the expense of compact bone. Histologically there is a thickening of existing trabecular structures, particularly at quiescent surfaces (598–600). In fact, some have suggested that PTH is more effective than antiresorptives, like estrogen or bisphosphonates, and gives increases as large as those induced by other osteoblast stimulators, like fluoride. Part of the anabolic effect of PTH may be mediated by 1,25-D_3, since PTH increases the activity of renal 1,α-hydroxylase; presumably 1,25-D_3 both stimulates oteoblasts and increases calcium absorption. In addition, certain portions of the peptide may be useful for inhibiting bone resorption (601).

It is well known that hyperparathyroidism protects trabecular bone, even though it results in loss of compact bone. There were early attempts to use PTH, chiefly the 1-34 fragment, for treatment for osteoporosis (602,603). However, until recently there was little evidence that this could be a useful modality, as there have been persistent concerns that compact bone would be compromised. Initial studies in women showed increased trabecular bone density, but there was a decrease of compact bone similar to that seen in hyperparathyroidism. Newer agents and better treatment plans, including use of a concomitant antiresorptive agent, may mitigate this effect. A recent study shows that PTH injected in rats actually increased mechanical strength and thickness of cortical bone (604). Intermittent treatment of PTH with calcitonin did not appear promising, although it stopped the loss of compact bone (598). Combination with estrogen has been more promising in rats (604) and humans (605–607). Lindsay et al. reported on a recent clinical trial (608) in which the 1,34 fragment of PTH injected daily over 18 months had a positive effect in women with established osteoporosis who had already had their bone stabilized by prior estrogen therapy. Spine BMD increased by 10% at 18 months but was stable in the estrogen-treated controls. Both groups showed some loss of femoral neck BMD. Apparently PTH can be used effectively to increase spine BMD provided it is given together with estrogen without adverse effects on the femur.

It is unclear if PTH treatment will always require concomitant treatment with estrogen or if vitamin D can be used. Alteration of the PTH–vitamin D axis can result in mineralization defects, for example, in renal disease, and is one potential problem. Vitamin D, like estrogen, has positive effects on compact bone. In North America, PTH is being jointly developed by Allelix, a Canadian company, and Glaxo.

Low doses of PTH stimulate osteoblasts and formation of trabecular bone but may cause loss of compact bone. The latter effect reportedly can be minimized by concomitant use of an antiresoprtive agent (bisphosphonate, estrogen, calcitonin); the latter agents do *not* block anabolic effects. The anabolic action of PTH has been reviewed recently by Dempster et al (609). The paradoxical effects of PTH on bone are explained by dose; continuous high-dose infusion, simulating hyperparathyroidism, causes loss while intermittent low-dose administration stimulates formation. Increased 1,25-D_3 and serum calcium may be important in the mechanism of action. For example, increased PTH secondary to chelation with EDTA, which reduces serum calcium, does not increase markers of bone formation, but rather increases bone resorption (610). This suggests that an elevated serum calcium may be one factor in the anabolic action of PTH. Administration of PTH fragments invariably increases serum calcium (611).

Combining PTH with estrogen may be the first practical treatment regimen (607), but combination with 1,25-D_3 and bisphosphonates has also been proposed (589). More convenient and cheaper therapies, like fluoride and promethazine, seem to have a similar, or greater, additive effect with estrogen (612) and may compete with PTH for clinical acceptance. Riggs (613) has suggested that intermittent PTH therapy should be examined and that the effect on fracture risk needs to be tested.

Parathyroid hormone continues to be of interest as a potential bone stimulator (609). There is growing evidence that PTH fragments stimulate bone and increase its strength (614–619) as well as stimulate osteoclastic resorption (620). Clinical trials using PTH will be started during this year. Researchers remain concerned that the site of action is limited to the spine and that there are potential negative effects elsewhere in the skeleton. However, proponents of PTH therapy feel these objections can be overcome with concomitant therapies or cyclical treatment. It will be critical to have measurements of total body BMD in such clinical trials in order to demonstrate a systematic positive effect throughout the skeleton.

D. Vitamin D

Vitamin D serves many functions, such as inhibition of PTH, increased calcium absorption in the intestine, and stimulation of osteoblast activity and hence bone formation. Calcium absorption deficiency has been shown to be a common problem in patients with very low axial and peripheral BMD compared to matched controls (640).

Vitamin D precursors have been given to elderly and osteoporotic patients because they often have low serum levels (689). At menopause, there is an indirect relationship between serum vitamin D levels and bone turnover (and loss) (677). Even more important may be the vitamin D levels in bone, which have been shown to be significantly lower in patients with hip fracture than in controls (678). Yet only recently has vitamin D been investigated outside of Japan for clinical usage.

While vitamin D may not increase BMD as much as other therapies, it has been shown to stabilize bone mass and reduce the incidence of both hip and vertebral fracture in the elderly, often by rates of 50–75% (263,622,650,709,710). It is especially beneficial to patients with low bone turnover. This positive effect is interesting in that the rate of fracture prevention exceeds that which would be expected from the degree of inhibition of bone loss that is observed, perhaps affecting the collagen matrix as well as the BMD.

A relatively recent treatment is the use of active vitamin D analogs (such as 1,25-D_3 and 1αD_3). Clinically, these analogs have been shown to prevent corticosteroid-induced osteoporosis (896) and postmenopausal bone loss (680, 685–687) as well as significantly reduce the rate of fracture (263,622). Furthermore, these compounds have a short half-life, preventing accumulation in soft tissues and adverse long-term effects.

Even doses of 0.5 μg/day of 1,25-D_3 have been shown to be effective (263). Doses of 1.0 μg/day of 1αD_3 have similar positive effects (622,680) as it is converted to 1,25-D_3 in vivo. One concern is that patients with a Western diet have a relatively high calcium intake (500–1,000 mg/day), and vitamin D therapy has resulted in hypercalciuria in a significant percentage of individuals.

Vitamin D in various forms is often used for renal bone disease (621). It is well known that osteoporotic patients, like corticosteroid-treated patients, have decreased calcium absorption, decreased numbers of vitamin D receptors, and decreased production of vitamin D. There are also decreased levels of vitamin D in the bone of patients who actually go on to fracture. One would expect more frequent use of vitamin D in senile and corticosteroid osteoporosis.

Actually, vitamin D analogs are probably the most common treatment for established osteoporosis on a worldwide basis. They are used principally in countries with low calcium intake, where side effects due to "calcium hyper-absorption" are small. In Japan, over 1 million women are treated with 1,α-D_3 and 1,25-D_3; there are few side effects, and a high efficacy in terms of a decreased fracture rate (622,623). The use of these active analogues in the U.S. and Europe is limited because of occasional hypercalcuria and hypercalcemia at moderate doses (0.5– 1.0 μg/day). Studies over the past 15 years have shown that treatment with doses of 1 μg was effective in correcting absorptive defects and increasing bone mass (624–626), but the efficacy of lower, safer doses has not been as clear. A multicenter study of calcitriol showed that it increased bone mass at modest doses (0.7–0.8 μg/day) (627,628). One center, however, provided an average dose of only 0.4 μg/day, which was not effective in reducing bone loss (629). A reanalysis of data from that center has indicated that patients who tolerated doses above 0.5 μg/day did in fact respond positively (630). A dose of 0.5 μg/day of 1-α-D_3 stops bone loss in corticosteroid-treated patients (631). These studies suggest that moderate doses can be at least partially effective.

It is important to remember that the endogenous production of calcitriol is roughly 1 μg/day. Oral administration of calcitriol probably delivers only half of the drug to the bloodstream. It is remarkable that the small amount available for stimulation of bone has such dramatic effects. Fracture rates are reduced by 50–75% (622,626,632,633). These new data, together with the prospective trial showing fracture reduction by Tilyard, will bring new consideration of vitamin D analogs in the therapy of established osteoporosis.

Vitamin D has been of research interest in relation to metabolic bone disease because it strongly influences both intestinal absorption of calcium and bone metabolism. The therapeutic effects of vitamin D in calcium malabsorption and osteomalacia are obvious, but its role in osteoporosis remains unclear. A supplement to *Metabolism* (Vol 39 No 4 Suppl 1, 1990) contained 12 articles reviewing this area. Alfacalcidol (1, (OH)-D_3) is the most widely used therapy for established osteoporosis on a worldwide basis. Numerous studies over the past 20 years have demonstrated that either calcitriol (1,25(OH)-D_3) or alfacalcidol can be modestly effective at doses comparable to basal physiological production (= 1 μg/day). However, even at these doses, episodic hypercalciuria occurs in 30% of patients on U.S. and European calcium intakes (800 mg/day). Consequently, studies of calcitriol have concentrated on subphysiological doses (0.5–1.0 μg). A study by Gallagher (634,635) has confirmed the results of Aloia et al. (628,636), using an average calcitriol dose in the range of 0.6–0.8 μg/day. This dose was sufficient to increase spinal BMD by 3% in treated patients, while there was a 3% loss in the calcium-treated controls. Total body BMD was maintained over the 2-year period in the treated patients, while there was a 2% loss in the controls. These two studies were part of a multicenter trial in which the calcitriol dose was adjusted based on urinary calcium. The third center (S. Ott and C. Chesnut) did not obtain a significant effect over 2 years at an average dose of 0.4 μg/day (629). The latter results have been reevaluated in a poster at the ASBMR (630). These results confirmed that patients treated with < 0.5 μg/day had no skeletal effects; however, those receiving 0.5–0.6 μg/day exhibited stablized BMD, and those receiving > 0.6 μg/day increased BMD (+2% total body and +10% spine). Results from the three centers show BMD increased when calcitriol dose over 0.6 μg/day was achieved.

Recent studies of established osteoporosis by M. Tilyard have shown that low-dose calcitriol (0.5 μg/day) was sufficient to halve fracture rate compared to calcium-treated controls (633,637). Moreover, this dose reduced fractures by 80% in calcium malabsorbers. An earlier study in the U.S. had shown that calcitriol halved vertebral fracture rate (632). Similar effects on fracturing have been observed in Japan (622,638) and Italy (626). These studies also demonstrated stabilization of compact bone and increases of axial bone, together with decreases of serum alkaline phosphatase and urinary hydroxyproline. Calcitriol and alfacalcidol now are being considered alternative therapies for established osteoporosis, particularly where calcium absorption is compromised (639). However, clinical monitoring may be needed to prevent hypercalciuria. New metabolites that have less side effects are under development in several countries.

There is often a vitamin D deficiency in elderly individuals that becomes extreme in osteoporosis. This poor calcium absorption in osteoporosis probably does not cause the bone deficit, which seems more associated with a low calcitriol level relative to the elevated PTH. A recent study by Nuti et al. (640) demonstrated that deficiency of calcium absorption was a distinguishing feature in 160 osteoporotic patients whose total body and spine BMDs were 15–20% below age-matched females. Correction of the absorptive deficit by calcium supplementation has not been demonstrated to stop bone loss. Vitamin D itself may be necessary, perhaps because vitamin D has a direct stimulatory effect on bone as well as inhibiting PTH. A recent study from the University of Heidelberg (641) showed that 1,25-D_3 had a direct effect on new bone formation in both intact and parathyroidectomized rats. Many studies have shown that vitamin D stimulates osteoblasts in cell culture. It does increase the depressed osteocalcin that is observed in postmenopausal and corticosteroid-induced osteoporosis (642,645). The Ferman study was unique in that it examined implants of demineralized bone matrix; 1,25-D_3 increased implant mineralization, whereas calcium supplements decreased it.

Studies continue to show a vitamin D deficiency in elderly subjects and in patients with osteoporosis, and vitamin D analogs seem effective in minimizing fractures (646), but the reasons are unclear. Vitamin D could play a role due to substrate deficiency of precursor, defective hydroxylation, or even receptor resistance (647). One biochemical finding that suggests a therapeutic role for vitamin D is its consistent stimulatory effect on osteoblasts and bone formation (648,649). Recent studies in Italy (640,642,650) show not only low serum levels of vitamin D, but a defect of intestinal calcium absorption in osteoporotic women. Studies from New Zealand (650) show that even low doses (0.5 g/day) of 1,25-D_3 are especially effective in stopping fractures in "poor absorbers" (those with urinary calcium < 150 mg/day). Poor calcium absorption and/or low excretion could be markers for low turnover.

New analogs of vitamin D are under investigation to inhibit PTH, to stimulate osteoblasts, and to promote absorption. These agents may be especially effective in low-turnover patients, while antiresorptive therapy would be appropriate for high turnover.

Vitamin D analogs, particularly 1-α,-D_3, have been widely used in Japan over the past 10 years for treatment of established osteoporosis (651). Researchers continue to look at new analogs (652–656). There is continued interest in fundamental aspects of vitamin D in the U.S., as evidenced by a series of eight reviews in the recent *Journal of Cell Biochemistry* (657–662). However, there has been less clinical interest since calcitriol at effective doses ($>$ 0.6–1.0 μg/day), the active form available in the U.S., has side effects (slight hypercalciuria) in 80% of patients on U.S. calcium intakes of 500–1,000 mg/day. The recent report by Tilyard et al. (263) showed that even subphysiological doses (0.5 μg/day) of calcitriol, with rare side effects, could have a very positive effect on fracture rates, especially in patients with poor calcium absorption. The mechanism of action remains unclear since low-dose calcitriol does not increase spine BMD greatly. There has been speculation that vitamin D analogs act to strengthen compact bone as well as improve trabecular density (655,656).

Vitamin D analogs have been used mostly for patients with established osteoporosis, with the idea that they would enhance depressed calcium absorption and stimulate bone formation. Newer studies show that both 1-α,-D_3 and 1,25-D_3 preserve bone in oophorectomized rats (663). A recent report from Tokyo Geriatric Hospital (664) showed that 1-α,-D_3 at 0.25 μg/day prevented bone loss in women immediately after oophorectomy, but was effective in stopping bone loss when begun 3 years postoperation only at 0.75 μg/day. These studies suggest that vitamin D analogs may be useful in prevention as well as for therapy in established disease.

Certainly there is a need for vitamin D in patients who have poor exposure to the sun or intake, but "deficiency" is more complex to define for normal subjects (665,666). Several recent studies have shown the elderly have low vitamin D levels, even in sunny climates (667), and supplements maintain femoral BMD and reduce the rate of hip fracture.

About 20 years ago the active form of vitamin D, 1,25$(OH)_2D_3$, was isolated and identified from chicken intestines. The original paper by Holick et al. (668) has been republished as a landmark research paper in the *Journal of NIH Research*, along with comments by Mike Holick, Hector DeLuca, and Ragiv Kumar. New studies continue to show vitamin D has a profound effect not only on intestinal absorption, but bone formation, skeletal muscle, skin, and the immune system. In the elderly decreased vitamin D levels (due to decreased intakes and sunlight exposure) are accompanied by altered receptor concentrations and responsiveness (669). Both bone formation and calcium absorption may be blunted. Osteoporotic women also show reduced responsiveness to D_3 in lymphocytes (670). There also is a complex interaction with other hormones in the elderly, particularly PTH; the mild secondary hyperparathyroidism of aging is suppressible by vitamin D (671). Vitamin D has been effective in reducing fracture rate in the elderly (263,622,672,673).

A recent report in the *New England Journal of Medicine* by French researchers from INSERM in Lyons (243) examined 3,270 elderly women (84 ± 6 years) of whom half received 20 μg (800 IU) of vitamin D_3 plus calcium in the from of tricalcium phosphate for 18 months. Hip fractures were halved in the treated group, and nonvertebral fractures were 32% lower. Vitamin D treatment reduced serum PTH and increased serum 25(OH)D. Femoral neck BMD increased by 2.7% in the treated group and decreased by 4.6% in the controls. The 7% difference of BMD between the two groups is compatible with a 100% difference (i.e., a halving) of the fracture rate. A 10% difference of femoral neck BMD in population studies is associated with a tripling of fracture risk. There were no significant side effects (hypercalcemia or renal stones) due to the vitamin D_3 treatment. Vitamin D is the only drug other than estrogen that has a demonstrated effect on decreasing both spine and hip fractures.

Vitamin D is recognized to be of critical importance to calcium absorption and to osteoblast function. Several recent reviews (674–676) deal with mechanism of action, new analogs, and new functions in relation to cancer, immune systems, diabetes, and psoriasis.

Dietary intake of vitamin D and serum levels inversely correlate with PTH, bone turnover, and bone loss at the menopause (677). Low levels of serum vitamin D are usually found in osteoporotic patients, particularly those with hip fracture. Bone levels of vitamin D may be of even greater importance. The recent report by Lidor et al. (678) showed that bone levels of 1,25-D_3 were extremely low in hip fracture patients (5 vs. 27 pg/g), but 25 (OH)D content of bone was identical. Serum 1,25-D_3 was somewhat reduced (27 vs. 34 pg/ml) in the fracture patients, as is usually the case. In spite of this evidence for a deficit, vitamin D agents are not widely used outside of Japan for treatment of osteoporosis. However, new studies are showing vitamin D can be effective. Research done during the 1980s in the U.S. and Italy showed that 1,25-D_3 given at levels above 0.5 μg/day increased spine density in osteoporotic patients (626,635). Even at 0.5 μg/day Tuktard et al. (263) reported a dramatic reduction in spine fracture and height loss. The drug 1α-D_3, which is commonly used in Japan, is rapidly metabolized to 1,25-D_3 in vivo. It must be given at 1 μg/day to simulate the effect of 1,25-D_3 itself. However, serum levels of 1,25-D_3 may not increase after treatment with 1α-D_3 (679). Studies in Japan have shown that a dose of 1 μg/day of 1α-D_3 stabilizes bone and prevents fracture (622). A new study from France confirms that 1 μg/day of 1α-D_3 stabilizes spine BMD over 2 years (680). During a third year, significant bone loss occurred after withdrawal of treatment, but bone mass remained stable in a subgroup of patients who underwent continued treatment. In French women, unlike Japanese, who have a lower calcium intake, there was significant biochemical changes due to the increased absorption. Urinary calcium increased significantly; one-third of patients developed hypercalciuria, although serum calcium and creatinine levels did not change. This was a reason for concern, although there were no pathological changes. Safer analogs, with a lower calciuric effect, may make vitamin D more acceptable.

Vitamin D continues to be a fascinating topic for skeletal metabolism because so many cellular responses are modulated by it. There appear to be receptors in most organs and in bone cells, particularly osteoblasts. Moreover, there appears to be heterogeneity in the phenotypic response of osteoblasts (681).

Active vitamin D compounds have potent effects on osteoblasts, the kidney, and the gut. This makes them useful for dealing with secondary hyperparathyroidism, for example, in chronic renal failure (682). They can also be used in relation to corticosteroids, which have negative effects on both osteoblasts and gut absorption (340,683). In the latter condition, bisphosphonates and calcitonin seem less effective (340,683).

Most studies of vitamin D and osteoporosis have concentrated on established disease in older patients (622,684–688). In these patients PTH may be elevated, calcium absorption is compromised, and bone formation is seriously depressed. Low doses of both 1,25-D_3 (0.5 μg/day) have been shown to dramatically reduce fracture rates (263,622), even though these doses do not have a substantial effect on spine BMD. These doses prevent bone loss from the spine but do not cause the increases of several percent normally seen with antiresorptives. Instead, there is an increase of compact bone. In fact, 1α-D_3 and 1,25-D_3 are the only agents known to increase compact bone and total body BMD by about 1%/year (684,685,687). Even ordinary vitamin D_3 (cholecalciferol at 800 IU/day) maintains femur neck BMD and prevents hip fractures in elderly women (243).

Surprisingly, two studies (from Japan [688] and France [680]) have now shown that 1α-D_3 can help can help maintain BMD in the early postmenopausal years. In the Japanese study, low-dose 1α-D_3 was used in oophorectomized women. This only partially inhibited the bone loss, but larger doses (1–2 μg/day) undoubtedly were called for. In the French study, a dose of 1 μg/day was given over 3 years; spine BMD was preserved in women 2–5 years postmenopausal. These studies suggest the need for further investigation of modest doses in the immediate postmenopausal period.

Vitamin D supplementation has been considered useful in the elderly and osteoporotic, both male and female, because these groups invariably have low circulatory levels of 25(OH)D and poor calcium absorption (689–692). Vitamin D levels are particularly low during the winter in areas of low sunlight (690,691) and in vegetarians (692). Treatment with ordinary vitamin D precursors corrects these problems, stabilizes bone, and prevents hip fracture (243). Much recent research, however, has focused on active analogs (1,25-D_3 and 1α-D_3) because their shorter half-life prevents soft-tissue accumulation, and problems of long-term toxicity.

The active vitamin D analogs stimulate osteoblasts and bone formation. There are additional effects on intestinal absorption of calcium, the kidney, and PTH. The active analogs have been effective in preventing both postmenopausal bone loss (686,687,693) and corticosteroid osteopenia (340,622,694). More importantly, they produce a greater reduction in fracture rate (89,263) than any other osteoporosis agents. This profound effect on fractures suggests that vitamin D may have preferential effects on bone strength, perhaps through the collagen matrix, as well as effects on bone density. Vitamin D can be combined with fluoride to produce even greater effects (695). Vitamin D analogs are being developed for use in psoriasis and cancer as well as bone disease (696).

A recent report by Australian researchers demonstrated a strong genetic influence of the vitamin D receptor gene on BMD. This may explain low vitamin D levels in osteoporosis and the generally positive, but heterogeneous, response to therapy.

Vitamin D continues to gain recognition as an important factor in the maintenance of bone mass and prevention of osteoporosis (697,698). In Japan, where vitamin D analogs are used to treat osteoporosis, both fundamental and clinical research is strong. Interest by clinical researchers outside of Japan, however, has abated since no major clinical trials with vitamin D analogs have been undertaken recently. Vitamin D also has important roles for other areas of metabolic bone disease—for example, the osteopenia induced by corticosteroids (340) and by anticonvulsant drugs (699). Both the latter interfere with vitamin D metabolism and calcium absorption, so vitamin D could have a major role. In addition, vitamin D analogs are used in renal disease to control PTH (700–702). Unrelated uses in psoriases and as an antitumor agent derive from antiproliferative and immunosuppressive activity (703–706).

A recent study by Australian researchers showed a strong influence of a gene for the vitamin D receptor on BMD (696). This association needs to be verified in other populations (707). Investigators at Indiana University have not confirmed this. Despite the conflicting conclusions, these studies have renewed interest for vitamin D therapy of osteoporosis.

Studies have shown that vitamin D supplementation inhibits bone loss and prevents both spine and hip fractures in the elderly (243,263,708–710). The antifracture efficacy is the best achieved with any osteoporosis therapy and is puzzling because it exceeds the effect expected from stabilization of bone mass.

Many of the elderly, particularly those who are institutionalized, are subject to at least seasonal vitamin D deficiencies in 25(OH)D that may, but do not necessarily, affect 1,25-D_3 levels (691,711–713). There is good evidence of PTH increases with age and of end-organ resistance to vitamin D (intestinal and bone). Episodic treatment with vitamin D can correct the deficiencies and correct secondary hyperparathyroidism (243,713,714).

Long-term treatment with the active hormone 1,25-D_3 has been observed to decrease creatinine clearance. This appears to have been associated with hypercalcemia, and creatinine normalizes with return to normocalcemia. There are no persistent changes in glomerular filtration rate. Corresponding creatinine changes are rarely seen with long-term administrations of other vitamin D analogs (1α-D_3, 1α-D_2), even when episodic hypercalcemia occurs (715,716).

Several active vitamin D analogs, such as ED71, 1α-D_2, EB1089, and others, may provide effective alternatives to 1,25-D_3 with much less calcemic potential (716,717). These analogs, because of their antiproliferative and immunosuppressive activity, also may be used as antitumor agents.

There has been increasing interest in vitamin D over the past year due to: 1. extensive evidence that there is vitamin D deficiency, indicative of mild secondary hyperparathyroidism, in a large proportion of the elderly (718); 2. studies showing that vitamin D receptor alleles are associated with bone mineral density (696); and 3. studies showing that vitamin D supplementation stops loss of femoral BMD in the elderly and decreases the rate of both vertebral and hip fracture (262,263,723).

There is a well-known decrease of both vitamin D levels and calcium absorption with aging that is exaggerated in osteoporotic patients. Defective absorption appears to be associated with a reduced intestinal responsiveness to vitamin D as well as lower blood and bone levels of vitamin D and a mildly elevated PTH. This is analogous to the pattern of secondary hyperparathyroidism. The problem can appear seasonally in elderly women in northern climates (719) and may be responsible for the small seasonal shifts of BMD that have been observed. There is an association between low BMD and low 25-hydroxyvitamin D levels in older women (720); 1,25-D_3 levels also are lower but may not correlate as well with BMD. Interestingly, there appears to be a similar pattern of vitamin D deficiency, elevated PTH, and osteopenia in multiple sclerosis (721). The elevated PTH (+40%) in elderly women is reversible by administration of vitamin D (722,723). This same subgroup of vitamin D–deficient women have excretion of pyridinolines threefold greater than controls (724). Elderly patients with fractures also have generally low 25-OHD levels and elevated PTH. PTH levels may fall after surgery (725); this may mask the underlying secondary hyperparathyroidism rather than indicating that the PTH elevation at time of fracture is due to injury or surgery. There is increasing recognition that treatment of elderly patients with parent or active vitamin D, even without calcium supplementation, can be effective in preventing both hip and spine fracture in the elderly (685–687,726).

E. Vitamin K

Neither vitamin K nor warfarin, a vitamin K antagonist, has significant effects on BMD (732). However, this vitamin may be important in the risk of fracture. One common indicator of bone turnover is osteocalcin, a vitamin K–dependent, γ-carboxylated protein. While osteocalcin has been shown to be at normal levels in elderly women with hip fractures, the uncarboxylated fraction was higher in these patients (730). Therefore vitamin K may play a role in bone fracture, perhaps via collagen matrix rather than BMD. Only recently have studies begun to emerge that suggest that vitamin K may have antiresorptive activity and can thus be an effective treatment for osteoporosis (733).

It is widely thought that bone turnover decreases with aging (after the initial 5 years of postmenopausal loss) and that it is especially decreased in osteoporotic women. This is shown by osteocalcin, a vitamin K–dependent, γ-carboxylated protein, that is commonly used as a marker of bone turnover. Both osteocalcin, and circulatory levels of vitamin K_1 and K_2, are reduced in women with spine and hip fracture compared to age-matched controls (727–729). However, vitamin K levels can decrease within an hour of a fracture, so the interpretation of these data is unclear. In a prospective trial of 195 elderly women, the osteocalcin level was normal in hip fracture cases, but the undercarboxylated fraction of osteocalcin was increased (730). Carboxylation was influenced by both vitamins D and K. This suggested a role for possible vitamin K or vitamin D deficiency in fracture.

Studies from Japan suggest that vitamin K is an antiresorptive that can be used to treat osteoporosis (733). It has only a minor effect, if any, on spine BMD, but apparently preserves compact bone (734). These minor effects on bone, however, could disguise a potentially major effect on fracture risk if, like vitamin D, it affects bone matrix.

Researchers have used the warfarin model, as well as induced deficiency, to examine vitamin K. Warfarin is a vitamin K antagonist that inhibits γ-carboxylation of osteocalcin, decreases osteocalcin, and decreases bone turnover resulting in osteopenia (731). It is noteworthy that patients receiving warfarin anticoagulant therapy long-term (5–10 years) have equal (732), or only slightly lower, BMD compared to controls. Moreover, vitamin K does not correlate with BMD (732). The apparent effect of vitamin K (and vitamin D) on fracture could be through the collagen matrix rather than bone density.

REFERENCES

1. Heaney RP, Baylink DJ, Johnston CC, et al. Fluoride therapy for the vertebral crush fracture syndrome. Ann Intern Med 1989; 111:678–680.
2. Pak CY, Sakhaee K, Zerwekh JE, et al. Safe and effective treatment of osteoporosis with intermittent slow release sodium fluoride: augmentation of vertebral bone mass and inhibition of fractures. J Clin Endocrinol Metab 1989; 68:150–159.

3. Pak CY. Fluoride and osteoporosis. Proc Soc Exp Biol Med 1989; 191(3):278–286.
4. Brown EM. Fluoride and the therapy of osteoporosis. J Clin Endocrinol Metab 1989; 69(5):929–931.
5. Duursma SA, Glerum JH, Dijk AV, et al. Responders and non-responders after fluoride therapy in osteoporosis. Bone 1987; 18:131–136.
6. Baylink DJ, Vose GP, Dotter WE, Hurxthal LM. Two new methods for the study of osteoporosis and other metabolic bone diseases. II. Radiographic densitometry. Lahey Clin Bull 1964; 13:217–227.
7. Briancon D, Meunier PJ. Treatment of osteoporosis with fluoride, calcium and vitamin D. Ortho Clin North Am 1981; 12:629–648.
8. Riggs BL, Hodgson SF, O'Fallon WM, et al. Effect of fluoride treatment on the fracture rate in postmenopausal women with osteoporosis. N Engl J Med 1990; 22: 802–809.
9. Proceedings from the International Workshop on Fluoride and Bone. J Bone Miner Res 1990; 5(suppl 1):19.
10. Hedlund LR, Gallagher JC. Increased incidence of hip fracture in osteoporotic women treated with sodium fluoride. J Bone Min Res 1989; 4(2):223–225.
11. Riggs BL, Baylink DJ, Kleerekoper M, et al. Incidence of hip fractures in osteoporotic women treated with sodium fluoride. J Bone Miner Res 1987; 2(2):123–126.
12. Kragstrup J, Shijie Z, Mosekilde LE, Melsen F. Effects of sodium fluoride, vitamin D, and calcium on cortical bone remodeling in osteoporotic patients. Calcif Tissue Int 1989; 45:337–341.
13. Courvoisier B, Baud C, Very J, et al. Etude multi-disciplinaire du traitement prolonge de l'osteoporose d'involution par le fluorure de sodium, avec calcium, phosphate et vitamine D. Schweiz Med Wschr 1985; 115:922–931.
14. Farley S, Libanati C, Odvina C, et al. Efficacy of long-term fluoride and calcium therapy in correcting the deficit of spinal bone density in osteoporosis. J Clin Epidemiol 1989; 42:1067–1074.
15. Hansson TH, Roos BO. The effect of fluoride and calcium on spinal bone mineral content: a controlled prospective (3 years) study. Calcif Tissue Int 1987; 40:315–317.
16. Hodsman AB, Drost DJ. The response of vertebral bone mineral response of vertebral bone mineral density during the treatment of osteoporosis with sodium fluoride. J Clin Endocrinol Metab 1989; 69:932–938.
17. Mamelle N, Meunier PJ, Dusan R. Risk-benefit ratio of sodium fluoride treatment in primary vertebral osteoporosis. Lancet 1988; 13:361–365.
18. Nagant de Deuxchaisnes C, Devogelaer JP, Stein F. Comparison of the bioavailability of the NaF enteric-coated tablets commercially available in Europe. (Abstract.) J Bone Miner Res 1990; 5:2251.
19. Pak CYC, Sakhaee K, Parcel C. Fluoride bioavailability from slow-release sodium fluoride given with calcium citrate. J Bone Miner Res 1990; 5:857–862.
20. Pouilles HM, Tremollieres F, Causse E, Louvet JP, Ribot C. Fluoride therapy in postmenopausal osteopenic women: effect on vertebral and femoral bone density and prediction of bone response. Osteoporos Int 1991; 1:103–109.
21. Hodsman AB, Drost DJ, Goldenberg J. Reduced vertebral fracture rates in osteoporotic patients responding to fluoride treatment with an increasing vertebral bone

mineral density. In: Christiansen C, Overgaard K, eds. Osteoporosis. Copenhagen: Osteopress APS, 1990:1484–1485.

22. Einhorn TA, Wakley G, Linkhart S, et al. A test of the hypothesis that sodium fluoride alters the mechanical properties of bone. In: Christiansen C, Overgaard K, eds. Osteoporosis. Copenhagen: Osteopress APS, 1990:1471–1473.
23. Vesterby A, Gundersen HJG, Melsen F, Mosekilde L. Marrow space star volume in the iliac crest decreases in osteoporotic patients after continuous treatment with fluoride, calcium, and vitamin D_2 for five years. Bone 1991; 12:33–37.
24. Lundy MW, Wergedal JE, Teubner E, Burnell J, Sherrard D, Baylink D. The effect of prolonged fluoride therapy for osteoporosis: bone composition and histology. Bone 1989; 10:321–327.
25. Gutteridge DH, Boivin G, Meunier PJ. Fluoride in postmenopausal osteoporosis: selective increase in external cortical porosity correlates with cancellous volume increase without change in cortical bone volume. In: Christiansen C, Overgaard K, eds. Osteoporosis. Copenhagen: Osteopress APS, 1990:718–720.
26. Ringe JD, Maurer H. Fracture incidence does not increase during long-term fluoride/ calcium therapy of primary osteoporosis. In: Christiansen C, Overgaard K, eds. Osteoporosis. Copenhagen: Osteopress APS, 1990:1341–1343.
27. Sowers MR, Clark MK, Jannausch ML, Wallace RB. A prospective study of bone mineral content and fracture in communities with differential fluoride exposure. Am J Epidemiol 1991; 133:649–659.
28. Gruber HE, Baylink DJ. The effects of fluoride on bone. Clin Orthop 1991; 267: 264–277.
29. Kleerekoper M, Balena R: Fluorides and osteoporosis. Annu Rev Nutr 1991; 11: 309–324.
30. Kleerekoper M, Peterson EL, Nelson DA, et al. A randomized trial of sodium fluoride as a treatment for postmenopausal osteoporosis. Osteoporosis Int 1991; 1:155–161.
31. Vesterby A, Mosekilde Li, Gundersen HJG, et al. Biologically meaningful determinants of the in vitro strength of lumbar vertebra. Bone 1991; 12:219–224.
32. Raymakers JA, Boereboom FJL, Buursma SA. Fluoride for osteoporosis with and without antiresorptive therapy with estrogen or pamidronate. J Bone Miner Res 1991; 6(suppl 1):278.
33. Conrozier T, Meunier PJ. Traitement de l'osteoporose cortisonique par le fluorure de sodium. Effets cliniques et donnees histomorphometriques. Ann Endocrinol 1985; 46:2369–370.
34. Rico H, Cabranes JA, Hernandez ER, Barabash A, Romero P. Reversion of the steroid-induced decrease of serum osteocalcin with sodium fluoride. Clin Rheumatol 1991; 10:10–12.
35. Meunier PJ. Fluoride therapy for vertebral osteoporosis. In: Munro H, Schliert G, eds. Nutrition in the Elderly. Nestle Nutrition Workshop Series. New York: Vevy/ Raven Press, 1992; 29:177–184.
36. Chavassieux P, Pastoureau P, Boivin G, et al. Fluoride-induced bone changes in lambs during and after exposure to sodium fluoride. Osteoporosis Int 1991; 2: 26–33.

37. Lundy MW, Russell JE, Avery J, Wergedal JE, Baylink DJ. Effect of sodium fluoride on bone density in chickens. Calcif Tissue Int 1992; 50:420–426.
38. Gordon SL, Corbin SB. Summary of workshop on drinking water fluoride influence on hip fracture on bone health. Osteoporosis Int 1992; 2:109–117.
39. Fioravanti N, Asti SS, Filgueira MLA, Negri AL, Zanchetti JR. Treatment of involutional osteoporosis with monofluorophosphate (MFP): a pilot study. Bone Miner 1992; 17(suppl 1):28.
40. Riggs B, O'Fallon W, Hodgson S, et al. Clinical trial of fluoride in osteoporotic women: extended observation and additional analyses. Bone Miner 1992; 17(suppl 1):74.
41. Lindsay R. Fluoride and bone: quantity versus quality. [Editorial.] N Engl J Med 1990; 322:845–846.
42. Aaron JE, deVernejoul MC, Kanis JA. Bone hypertrophy and trabecular generation in Paget's disease and in fluoride-treated osteoporosis. Bone Miner 1992; 17: 399–413.
43. Zerwekh JE, Antich PP, Sakhaee K, et al. Lack of deleterious effect of slow-release sodium fluoride treatment on cortical bone histology and quality in osteoporotic patients. Bone Miner 1992; 18:65–76.
44. Einhorn TA, Wakley GK, Linkhart S, et al. Incorporation of sodium fluoride into cortical bone does not impair the mechanical properties of the appendicular skeleton in rats. Calcif Tissue Int 1992; 51:127–131.
45. Farley Sm, Wergedal JE, Farley JR, et al. Spinal fractures during fluoride therapy for osteoporosis: relationship to spinal bone density. Osteoporos Int 1992; 2:213–218.
46. Guanabens N, Pares A, del Rio L, et al. Sodium fluoride prevents bone loss in primary biliary cirrhosis. J Hepatol 1992; 15:345–349.
47. Chavassieux P, Chenu C, Valentin-Opran A, et al. In vitro exposure to sodium fluoride does not modify activity or proliferation of human osteoblastic cells in primary cultures. J Bone Miner Res 1993; 8:37–44.
48. Turner CH, Boivin G, Meunier PJ. A mathematical model for fluoride uptake by the skeleton. Calcif Tissue Int 1993; 52:130–138.
49. Kleerekoper M, Mendlovic DB. Sodium fluoride therapy of postmenopausal osteoporosis. Endocrinol Rev 1993; 14:312–323.
50. Boivin G, Dupuis J, Meunier PJ. Fluoride and osteoporosis. In: Simopoulos AP, Galli C, eds. Osteoporosis: Nutritional Aspects. World Rev Nutr Diet. 1993; 73: 80–103.
51. Marie PJ, deVernejoul MC, Lomri A. Stimulation of bone formation in osteoporosis patients treated with fluoride associated with increased DNA synthesis by osteoblastic cells in vitro. J Bone Miner Res 1992; 7:103–113.
52. Chavassieux P, Boivin G, Serre CM, Meunier PJ. Fluoride increases rat osteoblast function and population after in vivo administration but not after in vitro exposure. Bone 1993; 14:721–720.
53. Resch H, Libanati C, Farley S, et al. Evidence that fluoride therapy increases trabecular bone density in a peripheral skeletal site. J Clin Endocrinol Metab 1993; 76:1622–1624.

54. Dambacher MA, Ittner J, Ruegsegger P. Long-term fluoride therapy of post-menopausal osteoporosis. Bone 1986; 7:199–205.
55. Boivin G, Duriez J, Chapuy M-C, et al. Relationship between bone fluoride content and histological evidence of calcification defects in osteoporotic women treated long term with sodium fluoride. Osteoporos Int 1993; 3:204–208.
56. Meunier PJ, Boivin G. Fluoride salts for vertebral osteoporosis: the benefit-to-risk ratio depends on the cumulative dose reaching bone. Osteoporos Int 1993; 3(suppl 1):211–214.
57. Gutteridge DH, Kent GN, Prince RL, et al. Fluoride treatment of osteoporosis: cyclical non-blinded or continuous blinded studies? Osteoporos Int 1993; 3(suppl 1):215–217.
58. Severt JL, Richard P, Mennecier I, Bisset JP, Loeb G. A double-blind study with a combined therapy (monofluorophosphate and calcium) in marked osteopenia without vertebral fracture. J Bone Miner Res 1993; 8(suppl 1):205.
59. Marx CW, Dailey GE, Cheney C, Vint VC, Muchmore DB. Do estrogens improve bone mineral density in osteoporotic women over age 65? J Bone Miner Res 1992; 7:1275–1279.
60. Meys E, Terreaux-Duvert F, Beaume-Six T, Dureau G, Meunier PJ. Bone loss after cardiac transplantation: effects of calcium, calcidiol and monofluorophosphate. Osteoporos Int 1993; 3:322–329.
61. Resch H, Libanati C, Talbot J, et al. Pharmacokinetic profile of a new fluoride preparation: sustained-release monofluorophosphoate. Calcif Tissue Int 1994; 54: 7–11.
62. Kanis JA. Treatment of symptomatic osteoporosis with fluoride. Am J Med 1993; 95(suppl 5A):535–615.
63. Kassem M, Mosekilde L, Eriksen EF. 1,20-Dihydroxyvitamin D_3 potentiates fluoride-stimulated collagen type 1 production in cultures of human bone marrow stromal osteoblast-like cells. J Bone Miner Res 1993; 8:1453–1458.
64. Riggs BL, O'Fallon WM, Lane A. Clinical trial of fluoride therapy in post-menopausal osteoporotic women: extended observations and additional analysis. J Bone Miner Res 1994; 9:265–275.
65. Richards A, Mosekilde Li, Sogaard CH. Normal age-related changes in fluoride content of vertebral trabecular bone—relation to bone quality. Bone 1994; 15: 21–26.
66. Sogaard CH, Mosekilde Li, Richards A, Mosekilde L, et al. Marked decrease in trabecualr bone quality after five years of sodium fluoride therapy—assessed by biomechanical testing of iliac crest bone biopsies in osteoporotic patients. Bone 1994; 15:393–399.
67. Mamelle N, Meunier PJ, Netter P. Fluoride and vertebral fractures. Lancet 1990; 336:243–246.
68. Pak CYC, Sakhaeee K, Piziak V, et al. Slow-release sodium fluoride in the management of postmenopausal osteoporosis. Ann Intern Med 1994; 120:620–632.
69. Heaney RP. Fluoride and osteoporosis. Ann Intern Med 1994; 120:689–690.
70. Thiebaud D, Burckhardt P, Melchior J, et al. Two years' effectiveness of intravenous

pamidronate (APD) versus oral fluoride for osteoporosis occurring in the post-menopause. Osteoporos Int 1994; 4:76–83.
71. Jackson R, Kelly S, Noblitt T, et al. The effect of fluoride therapy on blood chemistry parameters in osteoporotic females. Bone Miner 1994; 27:13–23.
72. Zerwekh JE, Hagler HK, et al. Effect of slow-release sodium fluoride on cancellous bone histology and connectivity in osteoporosis. Bone 1994; 15:691–699.
73. Thomsen JS, Mosekilde L, Boyce RW, Mosekilde E. Stochastic simulation of vertebral trabecular bone remodeling. Bone 1994; 15:655–666.
74. Fratzl P, Roschger P, Eschberger J, et al. Abnormal bone mineralization after fluoride treatment in osteoporosis: a small-angle X-ray-scattering study. J Bone Miner Res 1994; 9:1541–1549.
75. Kroger H, Alhava E, Honkanen R, et al. The effect of fluoridated drinking water on axial bone mineral density—a population-based study. Bone Miner 1994; 27: 33–41.
76. Sogaard CH, Mosekilde LI, Schwartz W, et al. Effects of fluoride on rat vertebral body biomechanical competence and bone mass. Bone 1995; 16:163–169.
77. Lafage MH, Balena R, Battle MA, et al. Comparison of alendronate and sodium fluoride effects on cancellous and cortical bone in minipigs. J Clin Invest 1995; 95:2127–2133.
78. Ringe JD, Meunier PJ. What is the future for fluoride in treatment of osteoporosis? Osteoporos Int 1995; 5:71–74.
79. Chlebowski RW, Butler J, Nelson A, Lillington L. Breast cancer chemoprevention. Tamoxifen: current issues and future prospective. Cancer 1993; 72:1032–1037.
80. Gray R. Tamoxifen: how boldly to go where no women have gone before. (Editorial.) J Natl Cancer Inst 1993; 85:1358–1360.
81. Neven P. Tamoxifen and endometrial lesions. Lancet 1993; 342:452–453.
82. O'Connell G, Arnold A. Tamoxifen and cancer of the endometrium. Can Med Assoc J 1993; 148:2113–2114.
83. Early Breast Cancer Trialists' Collaborative Group. Systemic treatment of early breast cancer by hormonal, cytotoxic, or immune therapy: 133 randomized trials involving 31,000 occurrences and 24,000 deaths among 75,000 women. Lancet 1992; 339:1–15, 71–85.
84. Rutqvist LE, Mattsson A. Cardiac and thromboembolic morbidity among post-menopausal women with early-stage breast cancer in a randomized trial of adjuvant tamoxifen. J Natl Cancer Inst 1993; 85:1398–1406.
85. Love RR, Mazess RB, Barden HS, et al. Effects of tamoxifen on bone mineral density in postmenopausal women with breast cancer. N Engl J Med 1992; 326: 852–856.
86. Love RR, Barden HS, Mazess RB, et al. Effect of tamoxifen on lumbar spine bone mineral density in postmenopausal women after five years. (In press.)
87. Ward RL, Morgan G, Dalley D, Kelly PJ. Tamoxifen reduces bone turnover and prevents lumbar spine and proximal femoral bone loss in early postmenopausal women. Bone Miner 1993; 22:87–94.
88. Plowman PN. Tamoxifen as adjuvant therapy in breast cancer. Drugs 1993; 46: 819–833.

89. Neven P, Shepherd JH, Lowe DG. Tamoxifen and the gynaecologist. Br J Obstet Gynecol 1993; 100:893–897.
90. Jordan VA. A current view of tamoxifen for the treatment and prevention of breast cancer. Br J Pharmacol 1993; 110:507–517.
91. Love RR, Koroltchouk V. Tamoxifen therapy in breast cancer control worldwide. Bull World Health Organ 1993; 71(6):795–803.
92. Gallagher A, Chambers TJ, Tobias JH. The estrogen antagonist ICI 182,780 reduces cancellous bone volume in female rats. Endocrinology 1993; 133:2787–2791.
93. Neal AJ, Evans K, Hoskin PJ. Does long-term administration of tamoxifen affect bone mineral density? Eur J Cancer 1993; 29A:1971–1973.
94. Wright CDP, Garrahan NJ, Stanton M, et al. Effect of long-term tamoxifen therapy on cancellous bone remodling and structure in women with breast cancer. J Bone Miner Res 1994; 9:153–159.
95. Thangaraju M, Kumar K, Gandhirajan R, Sachdanandam P: Effect of tamoxifen on plasma lipids and lipoproteins in postmenopausal women with breast cancer. Cancer 1994; 73:659–663.
96. Gold E, Stapley S, Goulding A. Tamoxifen and norethisterone: effects on plasma cholesterol and total body calcium content in the estrogen-deficient rat. Horm Metab Res 1994; 26:100–103.
97. Shewmon DA, Stock JL, Abusamra LC, et al. Tamoxifen decreases lipoprotein (a) in patients with breast cancer. Metabolism 1994; 43:531–532.
98. Kedar RP, Bourne TH, Powles TJ, et al. Effects of tamoxifen on uterus and ovaries of postmenopausal women in a randomized breast cancer prevention trial. Lancet 1994; 343:1318–1321.
99. Neven P, DeMuylder X, VanBelle Y, Campo R, Vanderick G. Tamoxifen and the uterus. Br Med J 1994; 309:1313–1314.
100. Van Leeuwen FE, Benraadt J, Coebergh JWW, Kiemeney LALM, et al. Risk of endometrial cancer after tamoxifen treatment of breast cancer. Lancet 1994; 343: 448–452.
101. Seachrist L. Restating the risks of tamoxifen. Science 1994; 263:910–911.
102. Williams GM. Safety of tamoxifen. Br Med J 1994; 308:534.
103. Black LJ, Sato M, Rowley ER, et al. Raloxifene (LY139481 HCl) prevents bone loss and reduces serum cholesterol without causing uterine hypertrophy in ovariectomized rats. J Clin Invest 1994; 93:63–69.
104. Sato M, McClintock C, Kim J, et al. Dual-energy X-ray absorptiometry of ralloxifene effects on the lumbar vertebrae and femora of ovariectomized rats. J Bone Miner Res 1994; 9:715–724.
105. Bijvoet OLM, Valkema R, Lowik CWGM, Papapoulos SE. The use of bisphosphonate in osteoporosis. In: DeLuca HF, Mazess RB, eds. Osteoporosis Physiological Basis, Assessment, and Treatment. New York: Elsevier, 1990:331–338.
106. Storm T, Thamsborg G, Steiniche T, et al. Effect of intermittent cyclical etidronate therapy on bone mass and fracture rate in women with postmenopausal osteoporosis. N Engl J Med 1990; 322:1265–1271.
107. Watts N, Harris ST, Genant H, et al. Intermittent cyclical etidronate treatment of postmenopausal osteoporosis. N Engl J Med 1990; 323:73–79.

108. Jowsey J, Riggs BL, Kelly PJ, et al. The treatment of osteoporosis with disodium enthane-1-hydroxy-1, 1-diphosphonate. J Lab Clin Med 1971; 78:574–584.
109. Mautalen C, Gonzalez D, Blumenfeld EL, et al. Spontaneous fractures of uninvolved bones in patients with Paget's disease during unduly prolonged treatment with disodium etidronate (EHDP). Clin Orthop Rel Res 1986; 207:150–155.
110. Johnston C, Altman R, Canfield R, et al. Review of fracture experience during treatment of Paget's disease of bone with etidronate disodium (EHDP). Clin Orthop 1983; 172:186–194.
111. Hodsman AB. Effects of cyclical therapy for osteoporosis using an oral regimen of inorganic phospphate and sodium etidronate: a clinical and bone histomorphometric study. Bone Miner 1989; 5:201–212.
112. Devogelaer JP, Nagant de Deuxchaisnes C. Treatment of involutional osteoporosis with the bisphosphonate APD (disodium pamidronate): non-linear increase of lumbar bone mineral density. J Bone Miner Res 1990; 5(suppl 2):201.
113. Valkema R, Vismans JFE, Papapoulos SE, et al. Maintained improvement in calcium balance and bone mineral content in patients with osteoporosis treated with the bisphosphonate APD. Bone Miner 1989; 5:183–192.
114. Reginster JY, Deroisy R, Denis D, et al. Prevention of postmenopausal bone loss by tiludronate. Lancet 1989; 30:1469–1471.
115. Reginster JY, Deroisy R, Lecart MP, et al. Calcitonin and postmenopausal bone loss. Exp Gerontol 1990; 24:349.
116. Lindsay R, Tohme JF. Estrogen treatment of patients with established postmenopausal osteoporosis. Obstet Gynecol 1990; 72(2):290–295.
117. Riggs BL. A new option for treating osteoporosis. (Letter to the Editor.) N Engl J Med 1990; 323:124.
118. Siris ES, Sherman WH, Baquiran DC, et al. Effects of dichloromethylene diphosphonate on skeletal mobilization of calcium in multiple myeloma. N Engl J Med 1980; 302:310–315.
119. Movsowitz C, Epstein S, Fallon M, et al. The bisphosphonate 2-PEBP inhibits cyclosporin A induced high-turnover osteopenia in the rat. J Lab Clin Med 1990; 115:62–68.
120. Lidor C, Meyer MS, Wasserman RH, Edelstein S. The effect of disodium thane-a-hydroxy-1, 1-diphosphonate on the metabolism of calcitriol in chicks. Biochem J 1987; 243:75–78.
121. Papapoulos SE, Bijvoet OLM, Valkema R, et al. New bisphosphonates in the treatment of osteoporosis. In: Christiansen C, Overgaard K, eds. Osteoporosis 1990. Copenhagen: Osteopress APS, 1990:1294–1300.
122. Wronski TJ, Yen CF, Scott KS. Estrogen and diphosphonate treatment provide long-term protection against osteopenia in ovariectomized rats. J Bone Miner Res 1991; 6:387–394.
123. Seedor JG, Quartuccio HA, Thompson DD. The bisphosphonate alendronate (MK-217) inhibits bone loss due to ovariectomy in rats. J Bone Miner Res 1991; 6: 339–346.
124. Thompson DD, Seeder JG, Solomon H, et al. Alendronate prevents bone loss in

estrogen deficient baboons. In: Christiansen C, Overgaard K, eds. Osteoporosis 1990. Copenhagen: Osteopress APS, 1990:1015–1017.

125. Chappard D, Petitjean M, Alexandre C, et al. Cortical osteoclasts are less sensitive to etidronate than trabecular osteoclasts. J Bone Miner Res 1991; 6:673–680.
126. Fromm GA, Vega E, Plantalech L, et al. Differential action of pamidronate on trabecular and cortical bone in women with involutional osteoporosis. Osteoporos Int 1991; 1:129–133.
127. Miller PD, Neal BJ, McIntyre DO, et al. Effect of cyclical therapy with phosphorus and etidronate on axial bone mineral density in postmenopausal osteoporotic women. Osteoporos Int 1991; 1:171–176.
128. Toolan BC, Shea M, Myers ER, et al. The effect of long-term alendronate treatment on vertebral strength in ovariectomized baboons and rats. J Bone Miner Res 1991; 4(suppl 1):248.
129. Ferretti JL, Mondelo N, Vazquez S, et al. Mineral density and structural properties of male and female rat femora as affected by dimethyl pamidronate. J Bone Miner Res 1991; 6(suppl 1):128.
130. Barbier A, Bonjour JP, Geusens P, et al. Tiludronate: a bisphosphonate with a positive effect on bone quality in experimental models. J Bone Miner Res 1991; 6(suppl 1):217.
131. Thamsborg G, Kollerup G, et al. Five years of intermittent, cyclical etidronate therapy increases bone mass and reduces vertebral fracture rate in postmenopausal osteoporosis. Bone Miner 1992; 17(suppl 1):124.
132. Kasting GB, Francis MD. Retention of etidronate in human, dog, and rat. J Bone Miner Res 1992; 7:513–522.
133. Grynpas MD, Acito A, Dimitriu M, et al. Changes in bone mineralization, architecture and mechanical properties due to long-term (1 year) administration of pamidronate (APD) to adult dogs. Osteoporos Int 1992; 2:74–81.
134. O'Doherty DP, Gertz BJ, Tindale W, et al. Effects of five daily 1 h infusions of alendronate in Paget's disease of bone. J Bone Miner Res 1992; 7:81–87.
135. Reginster JY, Colson F, Morlock G, et al. Evaluation of the efficacy and safety of oral tiludronate in Pafet's disease of bone. Arthritis Rheum 1992; 35:967–974.
136. Reginster JYL: Oral tiludronate: pharmacological properties and potential usefulness in Paget's disease of bone and osteoporosis. Bone 1992; 13:351–354.
137. Fleisch H. Bisphosphonates—pharmacology and use in the treatment of tumor-induced hypercalcaemic and metastatic bone disease. Drugs 1991; 42:919–944.
138. Abe T, Chow JWM, Lean JM, Chambers TJ. The anabolic action of 17β-estradiol (E_2) on rat trabecular bone is suppressed by (3-amino-1-hydroxy-propylidene)-1-bisphosphonate (AHPrBP). Bone Miner 1992; 19:21–29.
139. Tang LY, Jee WSS, Ke HZ, Kimmel DB. Restoring and maintaining bone in osteopenic female rat skeleton: 1. Changes in bone mass and structure. J Bone Miner Res 1992; 7:1093–1104.
140. Papapoulos SE, Landman JO, Bijvoet OLM, et al. The use of bisphosphonates in the treatment of osteoporosis. Bone 1992; 13:S41–49.
141. Sansoni P, Passeri G, Snelli G, et al. Diphosphonates suppress the immune function

by a selective inhibition on antigen presenting cells. J Bone Miner Res 1992; 7(suppl 1):890.
142. Reid IR, King AR, Alexander CJ, Ibbertson HK. Prevention of steroid-induced osteoporosis with (3-amino-1-hydroxypropylidene)-1, 1-bisphosphonate (APD). Lancet 1988; 1:143–146.
143. Gallacher Sj, Fenner JAK, Anderson K, et al. Intravenous pamidronate in the treatment of osteoporosis associated with corticosteroid dependent lung disease: an open pilot study. Thorax 1992; 47:932–936.
144. Storm T, Steiniche T, Thamsborg G, Melsen F. Changes in bone histomorphometry after long-term treatment with intermittent, cyclic etidronate for postmenopausal osteoporosis. J Bone Miner Res 1993; 8:199–208.
145. Price RI, Gutteridge DH, Stuckey BGA, et al. Rapid, divergent changes in spinal and forearm bone density following short-term intravenous treatment of Paget's disease with pamidronate disodium. J Bone Miner Res 1993; 8:209–217.
146. Fleisch H. Prospective use of bisphosphonates in osteoporosis. (Editorial.) J Clin Endocrinol Metab 1993; 76:1397–1398.
147. Fleisch H. New bisphosphonates in osteoporosis. Osteoporos Int 1993; 3(suppl 2): 15–22.
148. Kanis JA, McCloskey EV, Sirtori P, et al. Rationale for the use of clodronate in osteoporosis. Osteoporos Int 1993; 3(suppl 2):S23–28.
149. Hamdy NAT. Role of bisphosphonates in metabolic bone diseases. Trends Endocrinol Metab 1993; 4:19–20.
150. Bijvoet OLM, Valkema R, Lowik CWGM, Papapoulos SE. Bisphosphonates in osteoporosis? Osteoporosis Int 1993; 3(suppl 1):230–236.
151. Sahni M, Guenther HL, Fleisch H, et al. Bisphosphonates act on rat bone resorption through the mediation of osteoblasts. J Clin Invest 1993; 91:2004–2011.
152. Wimalawansa SJ, Gunasekera RD. Pamidronate is effective for Paget's disease of bone refractory to conventional therapy. Calcif Tissue Int 1993; 53:237–241.
153. Rosen HN, Moses AC, Gundberg C, et al. Therapy with parenteral pamidronate prevents thyroid hormone-induced bone turnover in humans. J Clin Endocrinol Metab 1993; 77:664–669.
154. Rosen HN, Sullivan EK, Middlebrooks VL, et al. Parenteral pamidronate prevents thyroid hormone-induced bone loss in rats. J Bone Miner Res 1993; 8:1205–1261.
155. Yamamoto M, Markatos A, Seedor JG, et al. The effects of the aminobisphosphonates alendronate on thyroid hormone-induced osteopenia in rats. Calcif Tissue Int 1993; 53:278–282.
156. Surrey ES, Fournet N, Voigt B, Judd HL. Effects of sodium etidronate in combination with low-dose norethindrone in patients administered a long-acting GnRH agonist: a preliminary report. Obstet Gynecol 1993; 81:581–586.
157. Selby PL, Rehman MT, Economou G, et al. Cyclical etidronate therapy has a preferential effect on the axial skeleton in osteoporosis whatever the cause. Presented at Bone and Tooth Society Summer Meeting, Oxford, UK, 1993.
158. Adachi JD, Bensen WG, Bianchi F, et al. Intermittent cyclic etidronate therapy (ICT) prevents corticosteroid-induced bone loss. J Bone Miner Res 1993; 8(suppl 1):320.

159. Giannini S, D'Angelo A, Malvasi L, et al. Effects of one-year cyclical treatment with clodronate on postmenopausal bone loss. Bone 1993; 14:137–141.
160. Evans RA, Somers NM, Dunstan CR, et al. The effect of low-dose cyclical etidronate and calcium on bone mass in early postmenopausal women. Osteoporos Int 1993; 3:71–75.
161. Licata AA, Chesnut CH III, Genant HK, et al. Effects of 2 years' follow-up cyclical etidronate treatment in postmenopausal osteoporotic women. J Bone Miner Res 1993; 8(suppl 1):141.
162. Cosman F, Nieves J, Lindsay R. Comparative effects of cyclical etidronate and continuous estrogen on bone mass. J Bone Miner Res 1993; 8(suppl 1):S260.
163. Wasnich RD, Rodd PD, Genant HK, et al. Cyclical etidronate therapy increases bone mass and reduces fracture incidence: a 4-year prospective study. Presented at Fourth International Symposium on Ostoeporosis, Hong Kong, 1993:134.
164. Rajan KT, Evans WD, Blacker M. Bisphosphonates in osteoporosis. J Bone Miner Res 1993; 8(suppl 1):135.
165. Harris ST, Gertz BJ, Genant HK, et al. The effect of short term treatment with alendronate on vertebral density and biochemical markers of bone remodeling in early postmenopausal women. J Clin Endocrinol Metab 1993; 76:1399–1406.
166. McClung MR, Yates AJ: Alendronate prevents or reverses bone loss at the spine and hip in recently menopausal women. J Bone Miner Res 1993; 8(suppl 1):141.
167. Santora AC, Bell NH, Chesnut CH, et al. Oral alendronate treatment of bone loss in postmenopausal osteopenic women. J Bone Miner Res 1993; 8(suppl 1):131.
168. Lauritzen DB, Balena R, Shea M, et al. Effects of combined prostaglandin and alendronate treatment on the histomorphometry and biochemical properties of bone in ovariectomized rats. J Bone Miner Res 1993; 8:871–879.
169. Guy JA, Shea M, Balena R, et al. The bisphosphonate alendronate preserves both the mechanical properties and bone mineral density in the aging estrogen-deficient rat. J Bone Miner Res 1993; 8(suppl 1):134.
170. Guy JA, Shea M, Peter CP, et al. Continuous alendronate treatment throughout growth, maturation, and aging in the rat results in increases in bone mass and mechanical properties. Calcif Tissue Int 1993; 53:283–288.
171. Black DM, Reiss TR, Karpf DB, et al. The Fracture Intervention Trial Research Group: Fracture intervention trial: design and interim recruitment results. J Bone Miner Res 1993; 8(suppl 1):209.
172. Bilezikian JP. Clinical review 51: management of hypercalcemia. J Clin Endocrinol Metab 1993; 77:1445–1449.
173. Lombardi A, Santora AC. Clinical trials with bisphosphonates. Bone Miner 1993; 22(suppl 1):59–70.
174. Ott SM. Clinical effects of bisphosphonates in involutional osteoporosis. J Bone Miner Res 1993; 8(suppl 2):597–606.
175. Fleisch H. Bisphosphonates in bone disease. Privately printed, Switzerland, 1993.
176. Black DM, Reiss TF, Nevitt MC, et al. Design of the fracture intevention trial. Osteoporosis Int 1993; 3(suppl 3):29–39.
177. Harris ST, Watts NB, Jackson TD, et al. Four-year study of intermittent cyclic

etidronate treatment of postmenopausal osteoporosis: three years of blinded therapy followed by one year of open therapy. Am J Med 1993; 95:557–567.

178. Marcus R. Cyclic etidronate: has the rose lost its bloom? Am J Med 1993; 95: 555–556.
179. Adami S, Baroni MC, Broggini M, et al. Treatment of postmenopausal osteoporosis with continuous daily oral alendronate in comparison with either placebo or intranasal salmon calcitonin. Osteoporos Int 1993; 3(suppl 3):21–27.
180. Rodan GA, Seedor JG, Balena R. Preclinical pharmacology of alendronate. Osteoporos Int 1993; 3(suppl 3):7–12.
181. Gertz BJ, Holland SD, Kline WF, et al. Clinical pharmacology of alendronate sodium. Osteoporos Int 1993; 3(suppl 3):13–16.
182. Chesnut CH III, Harris ST. Short-term effect of alendronate on bone mass and bone remodeling in postmenopausal women. Osteoporos Int 1993; 3(suppl 3):17–19.
183. Anderson DC. Alendronate: some remaining paradoxes. Osteoporos Int 1993; 3(suppl 3):41–42.
184. Kanis JA, Gertz BJ, Singer F, Ortolani S. Rationale for the use of alendronate in osteoporosis. Osteoporos Int 1995; 5:1–13.
185. Lafage MH, Balena R, Battle MA, et al. Comparison of alendronate and sodium fluoride effects on cancellous and cortical bone in minipigs. J Clin Invest 1995; 95:2127–2133.
186. Seeman E, Nagant de Deuxchaisnes C, Meunier P, Santora AC. Treatment of postmenopausal osteoporosis with oral alendronate. Bone 1995; 16(suppl 1):120.
187. Ammann P, Rizzoli R, Caverzasio J, et al. Effects of the bisphosphonate tiludronate on bone resorption, calcium balance, and bone mineral density. J Bone Miner Res 1993; 8:1491–1498.
188. Ammann P, Rizzoli R, Muller K, et al. IGF-1 and pamidronate increase bone mineral density in ovariectomized adult rats. Am J Physiol 1993; 265:E770–776.
189. Monier-Faugere MC, Friedler RM, Bauss F, Malluche HH. A new bisphosphonate, BM 21.0955, prevents bone loss associated with cessation of ovarian function in experimental dogs. J Bone Miner Res 1993; 8:1345–1355.
190. Passeri M, Baroni MC, Pedrazzoni M, Vescovi PP. Protocols of treatment of chronic back pain in involutional osteoporosis. Bone Miner 1993; 22(suppl):23–52.
191. Lacy ME, Bevan JA, Boyce RW, Geddes AD. Antiresorptive drugs and trabecular bone turnover: validation and testing of a computer model. Calcif Tissue Int 1994; 54:179–185.
192. Ongphiphadhanakul B, Jenis LG, Braverman LE, et al. Etidronate inhibits the thyroid hormone-induced bone loss in rats assessed by bone mineral density and messenger ribonucleic acid markers of osteoblast and osteoclast function. Endocrinology 1993; 133:2002–2007.
193. Balena R, Toolan BC, Shea M, et al. The effects of 2-year treatment with the aminobisphosphonate alendronate on bone metabolism, bone histomorphometry, and bone strength in ovariectomized nonhuman primates. J Clin Invest 1993; 92: 2077–2086.
194. Roux C, Ravaud P, Cohen-Solal M, et al. Biologic, histologic and densitometric

effects of oral risedroante on bone in patients with multiple myeloma. Bone 1994; 15:41–49.

195. Kanis JA. What constitutes evidence for drug efficacy in osteoporosis? Drugs Aging 1993; 3:391–399.
196. Ott SM, Woodson GC, Huffer WE, et al. Bone histomorphometric changes after cyclic therapy with phosphate and etidronate disodium in women with postmenopausal osteoporosis. J Clin Endocrinol Metab 1994; 78:968–972.
197. Compston JE. The therapeutic use of bisphosphonates. Br Med J 1994; 309: 711–715.
198. Tovey FI, Hall ML, Ell PJ, Hobsley M. Cyclical etidronate therapy and postgastrectomy osteoporosis. Br J Surg 1994; 81:1168–1169.
199. Selby PL, Davies M, Rehman MTE, Adams JE. Cyclical etidronate therapy benefits the spine but not overall calcium balance. J Bone Miner Res 1994; 9(suppl 1):398.
200. Geusens P, Nijs J, Eben K, et al. Cyclic etidronate and calcium in male osteoporosis. J Bone Miner Res 1994; 9(suppl 1):397.
201. Hasling C, Charles P, Jensen FT, Mosekilde L. A comparison of the effects of oestrogen/progestogen, high-dose oral calcium, intermittent cyclic etidronate and an ADFR regime on calcium kinetics and bone mass in postmenopausal women with spinal osteoporosis. Osteoporos Int 1994; 4:191–203.
202. Orme SM, Simpson M, Stewart SP, et al. Comparison of changes in bone mineral in idiopathic and secondary osteoporosis following therapy with cyclical disodium etidronate and high dose calcium supplementation. Clin Endocrinol 1994; 41:245–200.
203. Rajan KT, Evans WD. Intermittent cyclical etidronate for treatment of osteoporosis. J Bone Miner Res 1994; 9(suppl 1):269.
204. Weinsein RS, Bone H, Tucci J, et al. Alendronate treatment of osteoporosis in elderly women. J Bone Miner Res 1994; 9(suppl 1):144.
205. Axelrod DW, Teitelbaum SL. Results of long-term cyclical etidronate therapy: bone histomorphometry and clinical correlates. J Bone Miner Res 1994; 9(suppl 1):136.
206. Lin BY, Jee WSS, Ma YF, et al. Effects of prostaglandin E_2 and risedronate administration on cancellous bone in older female rats. Bone 1994; 15:489–496.
207. Khan SA, McCloskey EV, Orgee J, et al. Comparative effects of alendronate and etidronate in postmenopausal osteoporosis. J Bone Miner Res 1994; 9(suppl 1):396.
208. Heaney RP. The bone-remodeling transient: implications for the interpretation of clinical studies of bone mass change. J Bone Miner Res 1994; 9:1515–1523.
209. Worth H, Stammen D, Keck E. Therapy of steroid-induced bone loss in adult asthmatics with calcium, vitamin D, and a diphosphonate. Am J Respir Crit Care Med 1994; 150:394–397.
210. Adachi JD, Cranney A, Goldsmith CH, et al. Intermittent cyclic therapy with etidronate in the prevention of corticosteroid induced bone loss. J Rheumatol 1994; 21:1922–1926.
211. LoCascio V, Braga V, Bertoldo F, et al. Effect of bisphosphonate therapy and parathyroidectomy on the urinary excretion of galactosylhydroxylysine in primary hyperparathyroidism. Clin Endocrinol 1994; 41:47–51.

212. Samuel R, Katz K, Papapoulos SE, et al. Aminohydroxypropylidene bisphosphonate (APD) treatment improves the clinical skeletal manifestations of Gaucher's disease. Pediatrics 1994; 94:385–389.
213. Shaw NJ, White CP, Fraser WD, Rosenbloom L. Osteopenia in cerebral palsy. Arch Dis Child 1994; 71:235–238.
214. Nordin BEC, Heaney RP. Calcium supplementation of the diet: justified by present evidence. Br Med J 1990; 300:1056–1060.
215. Heaney RP. Estrogen-calcium interactions in the postmenopause: a quantitative description. Bone Miner 1990; 11:67–84.
216. Hasling C, Charles P, Jenson FT, Mosekilde L. Calcium metabolism in postmenopausal osteoporosis: the influence of dietary calcium and net absorbed calcium. J Bone Miner Res 1990; 5:939–946.
217. Heaney RP, Recker RR, Saville PD. Calcium balance and calcium requirements in middle-aged women. Am J Clin Nutr 1977; 30:1603–1611.
218. Baran D, Sorensen A, Grimes J, et al. Dietary modification with dairy products for preventing vertebral bone loss in premenopausal women: a three-year prospective study. J Clin Endocrinol Metab 1990; 70:264–270.
219. Fujita T, Fukase M, Miyamoto H, et al. Increase of bone mineral density by calcium supplement with oyster shell electrolysate. Bone Miner 1990; 11:85–91.
220. Dawson-Hughes B, Dallal G, Krall E, et al. A controlled trial of the effect of calcium supplementation on bone density in postmenopausal women. N Engl J Med 1990; 323:878–883.
221. Matkovic V, Fontant D, Tominac C, et al. Factors that influence peak bone mass formation: a study of calcium balance and the inheritance of bone mass in adolescent females. Am J Clin Nutr 1990; 52:878–888.
222. Anderson JJB, Reed JA, Tylavsky RA, et al. Lack of an effect of dietary calcium in preventing the loss of radial bone mass in high-calcium consuming elderly white women. In: Christiansen C, Overgaard K, eds. Osteoporosis 1990. Copenhagen: Osteopress APS, 1990:981–984.
223. Kanis JA. The nutritional requirements for calcium derived from balance studies; fact or artefact. In: Christiansen C, Overgaard K, eds. Osteoporosis 1990. Copenhagen: Osteopress APS, 1990:341–342.
224. Heaney RP. Fecal calcium density: a measure of calcium compliance. J Bone Miner Res 1991; 6:469–471.
225. Dawson-Hughes B. Calcium supplementation and bone loss: a review of controlled clinical trials. Am J Clin Nutr 1991; 54:274–280.
226. Elders PJM, Netelenbos JC, Lips P, et al. Calcium supplementation reduces vertebral bone loss in perimenopausal women: a controlled trial in 248 women between 46 and 55 years of age. J Clin Endocrinol Metab 1991; 73:533–540.
227. Matkovic V. Calcium metabolism and calcium requirements during skeletal modeling and consolidation of bone mass. Am J Clin Nutr 1991; 54:245S-260S.
228. Peacock M. Calcium absorption efficiency and calcium requirements in children and adolescents. Am J Clin Nutr 1991; 54:261–265.
229. Reid IR, Ames R, Evans MC. Dietary calcium supplementation slows the decline in

total body bone mineral density in postmenopausal women. Bone Miner 1992; 17(suppl 1):73.
230. Elders PHM, Lips P, Netelenbos JC, et al. Calcium supplementation reduces lumbar bone loss in pre- and postmenopausal women, but not in early postmenopausal women. Bone Miner 1992; 17(suppl 1):163.
231. Villareal DT, Rupich RC, Pacifici R, et al. Effect of estrogen and calcitonin on vertebral bone density and vertebral height in osteoporotic women. Osteoporos Int 1992; 2:70–73.
232. Heaney RP. Calcium in the prevention and treatment of osteoporosis. J Intern Med 1992; 231:169–180.
233. Matkovic V. Calcium and peak bone mass. J Intern Med 1992; 231:151–160.
234. Mosekilde L. Minisymposium: osteoporosis and calcium. J Intern Med 1992; 231: 145–149.
235. Schaafsma G. The scientific basis of recommended dietary allowances for calcium. J Intern Med 1992; 231:187–194.
236. Toss G. Effect of calcium intake vs. other life-style factors on bone mass. J Intern Med 1992; 231:181–186.
237. Matkovic V, Heaney RP. Calcium balance during human growth: evidence for threshold behavior. Am J Clin Nutr 1992; 55:992–996.
238. Johnston CC, Miller JZ, Slemenda CW, et al. Calcium supplementation and increases in bone mineral density in children. N Engl J Med 1992; 327:82–87.
239. Chan GM, Hoffman K, McMurry M. Effects of dairy products on bone and body composition in pubertal girls. J Pediatr 1995; 126:551–556.
240. Reid IR, Ames RW, Evans MC, et al. Effect of calcium supplementation on bone loss in postmenopausal women. N Engl J Med 1993; 328:460–464.
241. Kanis JA, Johnell O, Gullberg B, et al. Evidence for efficacy of drugs affecting bone metabolism in preventing hip fracture. Br Med J 1992; 305:1124–1128.
242. Greiger N, Gross A, Hunger G, et al. Dietary factors and fracture in postmenopausal women: a case-control study. Int J Epidemiol 1992; 21(5):953–958.
243. Chapuy MC, Arlot ME, Duboeuf F, et al. Vitamin D_3 and calcium to prevent hip fractures in elderly women. N Engl J Med 1992; 327:1637–1642.
244. Heaney RP. Bone mass, nutrition, and other lifestyle factors. Am J Med 1993; 95(suppl 5A):29, 33.
245. Sowers MR, Clark MK, Jannausch ML, et al. Body size, estrogen use and thiazide diuretic use affect 5-year radial bone loss in postmenopausal women. Osteoporos Int 1993; 3:314–321.
246. Nordin BEC, Cleghorn DB, Chatterton BE, et al. A 5-year longitudinal study of forearm bone mass in 307 postmenopausal women. J Bone Miner Res 1993; 8:1427–1432.
247. Bauer DC, Browner WS, Cauley JA, et al. Factors associated with appendicular bone mass in older women. Ann Intern Med 1993; 118:657–665.
248. Looker AC, Hart TB. Dietary calcium and hip fracture risk: the NHANES I epidemiologic follow-up study. Osteoporos Int 1993; 3:177–184.
249. Murphy S, Khaw KT, May H, Compston JE. Milk consumption and bone mineral density in middle aged and elderly women. Br Med J 1994; 308:939–941.

250. Lindsay R, Nieves J. Milk and bones. You are what you drink. Br Med J 1994; 308: 930–931.
251. Ramsdale SJ, Bassey EJ, Pye DJ. Dietary calcium intake relates to bone mineral density in premenopausal women. Br J Nutr 1994; 71:77–84.
252. Reed JA, Anderson JJB, Tylavsky FA, Gallagher PN. Comparative changes in radial-bone density of elderly female lactoovovegetarians and monivores. Am J Clin Nutr 1993; 59(suppl):1197–1202.
253. Cumming RG, Klineberg RJ. Case-control study of dairy product consumption and risk of hip fracture. Am J Epidemiol 1994; 139:2–8.
254. Feskanich D, Colditz G, Stampfer M, Willett W. Dietary calcium and bone fractures in middle-aged women. Am J Epidemiol 1994; 139:55–62.
255. Kreiger N, Gross A, Hunter F. Dietary factors and fracture in postmenopausal women: a case-control study. Int J Epidemiol 1992; 21(5):953–958.
256. Barrett-Connor E, Chang JC, Edelstein SL. Coffee-associated osteoporosis offset by daily milk consumption. JAMA 1994; 271:280–283.
257. Massey LK. Perspectives: caffeine and bone: directions for research. J Bone Miner Res 1991; 11:1149–1151.
258. Barger-Lux MJ, Heaney RP. Caffeine and the calcium economy revisited. Osteoporos Int 1995; 5:97–102.
259. Nilas L. Calcium intake and osteoporosis. World Rev Nutr Diet. 1993; 73:1–26.
260. Aloia JF, Vaswani A, Yeh JK, et al. Calcium supplementation with and without hormone replacement therapy to prevent postmenopausal bone loss. Ann Intern Med 1994; 120:97–103.
261. Bronner F. Nutrient bioavailability, with special reference to calcium. J Nutr 1993; 123:797–802.
262. Chapuy MC, Arlot ME, Delmas PD, Meunier PJ. Effect of calcium and cholecalciferol treatment for three years on hip fractures in elderly women. Br Med J 1994; 308:1081–1082.
263. Tilyard MW, Spears GFS, Thomason J, Dovey S. Treatment of postmenopausal osteoporosis with calcitriol or calcium. N Engl J Med 1992; 326:357–362.
264. Corazza GR, Benati G, DiSario A, Tarozzi C, et al. Lactose intolerance and bone mass in postmenopausal Italian women. Br J Nutr 1995; 73:479–487.
265. Walters JRF. Bone mineral density in coeliac disease. Gut 1994; 35:150–151.
266. Whiting SJ. Safety of some calcium supplements questioned. Nutr Rev 1994; 52:95–97.
267. Cann CE, Henzl M, Burry K, et al. Reversible bone loss is produced by the GnRH agonist nafarelin. In Cohn DV, Martin TJ, Meunier PJ, eds. Calcium Regul Bone Metab 1987; 9:123–127.
268. Matta WH, Shaw RH, Hesp R, Evans R. Reversible trabecular bone density loss following induced hypoestrogenism with the GnRH analogue buserelin in premenopausal women. Clin Endocrinol 1988; 29:45–51.
269. Johansen JS, Riis BJ, Hassager C, et al. The effect of a gonadotropin-releasing hormone agonist analog (Nafarelin) on bone metabolism. J Clin Endocrinol Metab 1988; 67:701–706.
270. Waibel-Treber S, Minne HW, Scharla SH, et al. Reversible bone loss in women

treated with GnRH-agonists for endometriosis and uterine leiomyoma. Hum Reprod 1989; 4(4):384–388.
271. Stevenson JC, Lees B, Gardner R, Shaw RW. A comparison of the skeletal effects of Goserelin and Danazol in premenopausal women with endometriosis. Horm Res 1989; 32(suppl 1):161–164.
272. Scharla SH, Minne HW, Waibel-Treber S, et al. Bone mass reduction after estrogen deprivation by long-acting gonadotropin-releasing hormone agonists and its relation to pretreatment serum concentrations of 1,20-dihydroxyvitamin D_3. J Clin Endocrinol Metab 1990; 70:1055–1061.
273. Riis BJ, Christiansen C, Johansen JS, Jacobson J. It is possible to prevent bone loss in young women treated with luteinizing hormone–releasing hormone agonists? J Clin Endocrinol Metab 1990; 70:920–924.
274. Mann DR, Orr TE, Rudman CG, Gould KG. Effect of growth hormone supplements on bone loss in GnRH agonist-treated monkeys. J Bone Miner Res 1990; 5(suppl 2):139.
275. Civitelli R, Gonnelli S, Zacchei F, et al. Bone turnover in postmenopausal osteoporosis: effect of calcitonin treatment. J Clin Invest 1988; 82:1268–1274.
276. Overgaard K, Riis B, Christiansen C, et al. Nasal calcitonin for treatment of established osteoporosis. Clin Endocrinol 1989; 30:435–442.
277. Overgaard K, Hansen MA, Herss Nielsen VA, et al. Discontinuous calcitonin treatment of established osteoporosis—effects of withdrawal of treatment. Am J Med 1990; 89:1–6.
278. Ringe J. Behandlung der primaren Osteoporose mit Calcium and Lachscalcitonin. Dtsch Med Wochenschr 1990; 115:1176–1182.
279. Overgaard K, Riis BJ, Christiansen C, Hansen M. Effect of salcatonin given intranasally on early postmenopausal bone loss. Br J Med 1989; 299:477–479.
280. Reginster JY, Albert A, Lecart M, et al. 1-Year controlled randomized trial of prevention of early postmenopausal loss by intranasal calcitonin. Lancet 1987; 26:1481–1483.
281. Reginster JY, Deroisy R, Lecart MP, et al. A double-blind, placebo-controlled, dose-finding trial of intermittent nasal salmon calcitonin for prevention of postmenopausal lumbar spine bone loss. Am J Med 1995; 98:452–458.
282. Reginster JY, Jupsin I, Deroisy R, et al. Prevention of postmenopausal bone loss by rectal calcitonin. Calcif Tissue Int 1995; 56:539–542.
283. Rico H, Revilla M, Hernandez ER, Villa LF, Alvarez de Buergo M. Total and regional bone mineral content and fracture rate in postmenopausal osteoporosis treated with salmen calcitonin: a prospective study. Calcif Tissue Int 1995; 56: 181–185.
284. Mazzouli G, Tabolli S, Bigi F, et al. Effects of salmon calcitonin on the bone loss induced by ovariectomy. Calcif Tissue Int 1990; 47:209–214.
285. Gennari C, Agnusdei D, Camporeale A. Use of calcitonin in the treatment of bone pain associated with osteoporosis. Calcif Tissue Int 1991; 49(suppl 2):9–13.
286. Christiansen C. Use of nasally administered salmon calcitonin in preventing bone loss. Calcif Tissue Int 1991; 49(suppl 2):14–15.

287. Foti R, Martorana U, Broggini M. Long-term tolerability of nasal spray formulation of salmon calcitonin. Curr Ther Res 1995; 56:429–435.
288. Lukert BP, Raisz LG. Glucocorticoid-induced osteoporosis: pathogenesis and management. Ann Intern Med 1990; 112:352–364.
289. Ringe JD, Welzel D. Salmon calcitonin in the therapy of corticoid-induced osteoporosis. Eur J Clin Pharmacol 1987; 33:35–39.
290. Montemurro L, Schiraldi G, Fraioli P, et al. Prevention of corticosteroid-induced osteoporosis with salmon calcitonin in sarcoid patients. Calcif Tissue Int 1991; 49: 71–76.
291. Luengo M, Picado C, Del Rio L, et al. Treatment of steroid-induced osteopenia with calcitonin in corticosteroid-dependent asthma. Am Rev Respir Dis 1990; 142: 104–107.
292. Lyritis GP, Tsakalakos N, Magiasis B, et al. Analgesic effect of salmon calcitonin in osteoporotic vertebral fractures: a double-blind placebo-controlled clinical study. Calcif Tissue Int 1991; 49:369–372.
293. Resch H, Pietschmann P, Willvonseder R. Estimated long-term effect of calcitonin treatment in acute osteoporotic spine fractures. Calcif Tissue Int 1989; 45:209–213.
294. Reginster JY, Deroisy R, Bruwier M, Franchimont P. Calcitonin metabolism in senile (type II) osteoporosis. Osteoporos Int 1992; 2:141–145.
295. Avioli LV. Heterogeneity of osteoporotic syndromes and the response to calcitonin therapy. Calcif Tissue Int 1991; 49(suppl 2):16–19.
296. Reginster JY. Management of high turnover osteoporosis with calcitonin. Bone 1992; 13:S37–40.
297. Gennari C, Agnusdei D, Montagnani M, et al. An effective regimen of intranasal salmon calcitonin in early postmenopausal bone loss. Calcif Tissue Int 1992; 50: 381–383.
298. Stone MD, Marshall DH, Hosking DJ, et al. Comparison of low-dose intramuscular and intravenous calcitonin in the treatment of primary hyperparathyroidism. Bone 1992; 13:265–271.
299. Torring O, Bucht E, Sjostedt U, Sjoberg HE. Salmon calcitonin treatment by nasal spray in primary hyperparathyroidism. Bone 1991; 12:311–316.
300. Azria M. The Calcitonins. Physiology and Pharmacology. Basel: Karger Press, 1989.
301. Proceedings of the International Symposium Celebrating the 30th Anniversary of the Discovery of Calcitonin. Bone Miner 1992; 16(3):155–216.
302. Mazzuoli GF, Passeri M, Gennari C, et al. Effects of salmon calcitonin in postmenopausal osteoporosis: a controlled double-blind study. Calcif Tissue Int 1986; 38:3–8.
303. Rico H, Hernandez ER, Revilla M, et al. Salmon calcitonin reduces vertebral fracture rate in postmenopausal crush fracture syndrome. Bone Miner 1992; 16: 131–138.
304. Armamento-Villareal RC, Avioli LV. Successful treatment of low turnover osteoporosis resulting from prolonged reserpine therapy with intermittent calcitonin and phosphate therapy. Calcif Tissue Int 1992; 51:282–284.
305. Wimalawansa SJ. Long- and short-term side effects and safety of calcitonin in man: a prospective study. Calcif Tissue Int 1993; 52:90–93.

306. Sileghem A, Geusens P, Dequeker J. Intranasal calcitonin for the prevention of bone erosion and bone loss in rheumatoid arthritis. Ann Rheum Dis 1992; 51:761–764.
307. Perrone G, Galoppi P, Valente M, et al. Intranasal salmon calcitonin in postmenopausal osteoporosis: effect of different therapeutic regimens on vertebral and peripheral bone density. Gynecol Obstet Invest 1992; 33:168–171.
308. Fioretti P, Gambacciani M, Taponeco F, et al. Effects of continuous and cyclic nasal calcitonin administration in overiectomized women. Maturitas 1992; 15:220–232.
309. Burckhardt P, Burnand B. The effect of treatment with calcitonin on vertebral fracture rate in osteoporosis. Osteoporos Int 1993; 3:24–30.
310. Eriksson SA, Lindgren JU. Combined treatment with calcitonin and 1,20-dihydroxyvitamin D_3 for osteoporosis in women. Calcif Tissue Int 1993; 53:26–28.
311. Chesnut CH III, Campodarve J, Rencken M, et al. Lack of efficacy of nasal spray calcitonin in early postmenopausal women. J Bone Miner Res 1993; 8(suppl 1):249.
312. Meschia M, Brincat M, Barbacini P, et al. A clinical trial on the effects of a combination of elcatonin (carbocalcitonin) and conjugated estrogens on vertebral bone mass in early postmenopausal women. Calcif Tissue Int 1993; 53:17–20.
313. Roux CH, Pelissier C, Listrat V, et al. GnRH agonist-induced bone loss and use of nasal calcitonin. J Bone Miner Res 1993; 8(suppl 1):151.
314. Biberoglu K, Yildiz A, Kandemir O. Bone loss in young women with primary hypogonadism and its prevention with calcitonin. Gynecol Obstet Invest 1993; 36:114–118.
315. Drinkwater BL, Healy NL, Rencken ML, Chesbut CH. Effectiveness of nasal calcitonin in preventing bone loss in young amenorrheic women. J Bone Miner Res 1993; 8(suppl 1):264.
316. Skerry TM, Lanyon LE. Immobilization induced bone loss in the sheep is not modulated by calcitonin treatment. Bone 1993; 14:511–516.
317. Reginster JYL. Calcitonins: newer routes of delivery. Osteoporosis Int 1993; 3(suppl 2):3–7.
318. Devogelaer JP, Nagant de Deuxchaisnes C, Azria M, et al. Comparison of the acute biological action of injectable salmon calcitonin and an injectable and oral calcitonin analogue. J Bone Miner Res 1993; 8(suppl 1):234.
319. Devogelaer JP, Nagant de Deuxchaisnes C, Azria M, et al. Acute biological effects of an oral calcitonin analogue in Paget's disease. J Bone Miner Res 1993; 8(suppl 1):233.
320. Thamsborg G, Skousgaard SG, Daugaard H, et al. Acute effects of nasal salmon calcitonin on calcium and bone metabolism. Calcif Tissue Int 1993; 53:232–236.
321. Gennari C, Agnusdei D, Camporeale A. Long-term treatment with calcitonin in osteoporosis. Horm Metab Res 1993; 20:484–485.
322. Grauer A, Reinel HH, Ziegler R, Raue F. Neutralizing antibodies against calcitonin. Horm Metab Res 1993; 20:486–488.
323. Reginster JY, Denis D, Deroisy R, et al. Long-term (3 years) prevention of trabecular postmenopausal bone loss with low-dose intermittent nasal salmon calcitonin. J Bone Miner Res 1994; 9:69–73.
324. Reginster JY, Gaspar S, Deroisy R, et al. Prevention of osteoporosis with nasal salmon calcitonin: effect of anti-salmon calcitonin antibody formation. Osteoporos Int 1993; 3:261–264.

325. Body JJ. Calcitonin: from the determination of circulating levels in various physiological and pathological conditions to the demonstration of lymphocyte receptors. Horm Res 1993; 39:166–170.
326. Kolleerup G, Hermann AP, Brixen K, et al. Effects of salmon calcitonin suppositories on bone mass and turnover in established osteoporosis. Calcif Tissue Int 1994; 54:12–15.
327. Tsakalakos N, Magiasis B, Tsekoura M, Lytis G. The effect of short-term calcitonin administration on biochemical bone markers in patients with acute immobilization following hip fracture. Osteoporos Int 1993; 3:337–340.
328. Van der Wiel HE, Lips P, Nauta J, et al. Intranasal calcitonin suppresses increased bone resorption during short-term immobilization: a double-blind study of the effects of intranasal calcitonin on biochemical parameters of bone turnover. J Bone Miner Res 1993; 8:1459–1465.
329. Reginster JY. Calcitonin for prevention and treatment of osteoporosis. Am J Med 1993; 95(suppl 5A):44–47.
330. Polatti F, Perotti F, Angelini GP, et al. Effects of salmon calcitonin suppositories in the prevention of bone loss in oophorectomized women. Maturitas 1993; 18:73–76.
331. Kollerup G, Hermann AP, Brixen K, et al. Effects of salmon calcitonin suppositories on bone mass and turnover in established osteoporosis. Calcif Tissue Int 1994; 54:21.
332. Copp DH. Calcitonin: discovery, development, and clinical application. Clin Invest Med 1994; 17:268–277.
333. Overgaard K, Riis B. Nasal salmon calcitonin in osteoporosis. (Editorial.) Calcif Tissue Int 1994; 55:79–81.
334. Overgaard K. Effect of intranasal salmon calcitonin therapy on bone mass and bone turnover in early postmenopausal women: a dose-response study. Calcif Tissue Int 1994; 55:82–86.
335. Munk Nielsen N, von der Recke P, Hansen MA, et al. Estimation of the effect of salmon calcitonin in established osteoporosis by biochemical bone markers. Calcif Tissue Int 1994; 55:8–11.
336. Campodarve I, Drinkwater BL, Insogna KL, et al. Intranasal salmon calcitonin (INSC), 50–200 IU, does not prevent bone loss in early postmenopausal women. J Bone Miner Res 1994; 9(suppl 1):391.
337. Devogelaer JP, Azria M, Attinger M, et al. Comparison of the acute biological action of injectable salmon calcitonin and an injectable and oral calcitonin analogue. Calcif Tissue Int 1994; 55:71–73.
338. Reginster JY, Meurmans L, Deroisy R, et al. A 5-year controlled randomized study of prevention of postmenopausal trabecular bone loss with nasal salmon calcitonin and calcium. Eur J Clin Invest 1994; 24:565–569.
339. Camisasca M, Crosignani A, Battezzati PM, et al. Parenteral calcitonin for metabolic bone disease associated with primary biliary cirrhosis. Hepatology 1994; 20: 633–637.
340. Sambrook P, Birmingham J, Kelly P, et al. Prevention of corticosteroid osteoporosis. A comparison of calcium, calcitriol, and calcitonin. N Engl J Med 1993; 328:1747–1752.

341. Mack TM, Ross RK. A current perception of HRT risks and benefits. In: DeLuca HF, Mazess RB, eds. Osteoporosis Physiological Basis, Assessment, and Treatment. New York: Elsevier, 1990:161–178.
342. Sporrong T, Hellgren M, Sameioe G, Mattsson LA. Comparison of four continuously administered progestogen plus oestradiol combinations for climacteric complaints. Br J Obstet Gynaecol 1988; 95:1042–1048.
343. Sporrong T, Hellgren M, Sameioe G, Mattsson LA. Metabolic effects of continuous estradiol-progestin therapy in postmenopausal women. Obstet Gynecol 1989; 73: 754–758.
344. Bewtra C, Kable WT, Gallagher JC. Endometrial histology and bleeding patterns in menopausal women treated with estrogen and continuous or cyclic progestin. J Reprod Med 1988; 33:205–209.
345. Hovik P, Sundsbak HP, Gaasemyr M, Sandvik L. Comparison of continuous and sequential oestrogen-progestogen treatment in women with climacteric symptoms. Maturitas 1989; 11:75–82.
346. Williams SR, Frenchek B, Speroff T, Speroff L. A study of combined continuous ethinyl estradiol and norethindrone acetate for post-menopausal hormone replacement. Am J Obstet Gynecol 1990; 162:438–446.
347. Stevenson JC, Cust MP, Gangar KF, et al. Effects of transdermal versus oral hormone replacement therapy on bone density in spine and proximal femur in postmenopausal women. Lancet 1990; 335:265–269.
348. Riis BJ, Johansen J, Christiansen C. Continuous oestrogen-progestogen treatment and bone metabolism in postmenopausal women. Maturitas 1988; 10:51–58.
349. Ribot C, Tremollieres F, Pouilles HM, Louvet JP, Peyron R. Preventive effects of transdermal administration of 17β-estradiol on postmenopausal bone loss: a 2-year prospective study. Obstet Gynecol 1990; 75(4):42–46.
350. Munk-Jensen N, Pors Nielsen S, Obel EB, Bonne Eriksen P. Reversal of postmenopausal vertebral bone loss by oestrogen and progestogen; a double blind placebo controlled study. Br Med J 1988; 296:1150–1152.
351. Gallagher JC, Baylink D. Effect of estrone sulfate on bone mineral density of the femoral neck and spine. (Abstract.) J Bone Miner Res 1990; 5(suppl 2):275.
352. Kolb FO, Powell MR. Spine mineral content response to therapy of various osteopenic states, assessed by dual photon absorptiometry. In: Christiansen C, Nordin BEC, Parfitt AM, Peck WA, Riggs BL, eds. Osteoporosis. Copenhagen: Aalborg Stiftsbogtrykkeri, 1984:157–159.
353. Studd JWW, Savvas M, Garnett TJ. A comparison of oral and subcutaneous hormone replacement in the prevention of osteoporosis. In: Ring EFJ, ed. Current Research in Osteoporosis and Bone Mineral Measurement. London: British Institute of Radiology, 1990:95.
354. Nachtigall LE. Enhancing patient compliance with hormone replacement therapy at menopause. Obstet Gynecol 1990; 75(suppl 4):77–80.
355. Ravnikar VA. Compliance with hormone therapy. Am J Obstet Gynecol 1987; 156: 1332–1334.
356. Mazess RB, Gallagher JC, Notelovitz M, et al. Monitoring skeletal response to estrogen. Am J Obstet Gynecol 1989; 161:843–848.

357. Christiansen C, Riis BJ. 17β-estradiol and continuous norethisterone: a unique treatment for established osteoporosis in elderly women. J Clin Endocrinol Metab 1990; 71:836–841.
358. Lindsay R. Estrogen/progestogen therapy: prevention and treatment of postmenopausal osteoporosis. Proc Soc Exp Biol Med 1989; 191:275–277.
359. Christiansen C, Riis BJ. Hormonal replacement therapy and the skeletal system. Maturitas 1990; 12:247.
360. Barzel US. Estrogens in the prevention and treatment of postmenopausal osteoporosis: a review. Am J Med 1988; 85:847–850.
361. Studd J, Savvas M, Waston N, et al. The relationship between plasma estradiol and the increase in bone density in postmenopausal women after treatment with subcutaneous hormone implants. Am J Obstet Gynecol 1990; 163:1474–1479.
362. Schot LPC, Schuurs AHWM. Sex steroids and osteoporosis: effects of deficiencies and substitutive treatments. J Steroid Biochem Mol Biol 1990; 37:167–182.
363. Abdallah HI, McKay HD, Lindsay R, et al. Prevention of bone mineral loss in postmenopausal women by norethisterone. Obstet Gynecol 1985; 66:789–792.
364. Dequeker J, Demuylder E. Long-term progestogen treatment and bone remodling in postmenopausal women: a longitudinal study. Maturitas 1982; 4:309–313.
365. Grecu EO, Simmons R, Baylink DJ, et al. Effects of medroxyprogesterone acetate on some parameters of calcium metabolism in patients with glucocorticoid-induced osteoporosis. Bone Miner 1991; 13:153–161.
366. Gallagher JC, Kable WT, Goldgar D. Effect of progestin therapy on cortical and trabecular bone: comparison with estrogen. Am J Med 1991; 90:171–178.
367. Rymer J, Chapman M, Fogelman I. OD 14: bone protection with no endometrial stimulation. In: Christiansen C, Overgaard K, eds. Osteoporosis 1990. Copenhagen: Osteopress APS, 1990:1071–1074.
368. Stampfer MJ, Colditz GA, Willett WC, et al. Postmenopausal estrogen therapy and cardiovascular disease. N Engl J Med 1991; 320:756–762.
369. Henderson BE, Paganini-Hill A, Ross RK. Decreased mortality in users of estrogen replacement therapy. Arch Intern Med 1991; 151:75–78.
370. Netelenbos JC, Siregar-Emck MW, Schot LPC, et al. Short-term effects of Org OD 14 and 17β-oestradiol on bone and lipid metabolism in early postmenopausal women. Maturitas 1991; 13:137–149.
371. Geusens P, Dequeker J, Gielen J, Schot LPC. Non-linear increase in vertebral density induced by a synthetic steroid (Org OD 14) in women with established osteoporosis. Maturitas 1991; 13:155–162.
372. Tremollieres F, Mohan S, Strong D, et al. Promegestone (PM) prevents bone loss in postmenopausal patients in a double blind clinical trial and acts as a mitogen in normal human bone cells (HBC) in vitro. J Bone Miner Res 1991; 6(suppl 1):301.
373. Lindsay R. The effect of estrogens in prevention and treatment of osteoporosis. In: Munro H, Schlierf G, eds. Nutrition of the Elderly. Nestle Nutrition Workshop Series. New York: Vevy/Raven Press, 1992:29:161–167.
374. Christiansen C. Prevention and treatment of osteoporosis: a review of current modalities. Bone 1992; 13:35–39.
375. Bellantoni MF, Harman SM, Cullins VE, et al. Transdermal estradiol with oral

progestin: biological and clinical effects in younger and older postmenopausal women. J Gerontol 1991; 46:216–222.
376. Seimiya Y, Chen JT, Hirai Y, et al. Changes in bone mineral density and fracture prevalence in Japanese women after oophorectomy. Asia-Oceania J Obstet Gynaecol 1992; 18:89–94.
377. Holzer G, Metka M, Heytmanek G, et al. Knochendichte vor und nach Hormontherapie bei jungen Frauen mit hypergonadotroper hypogonader Amenorrhoe. Dtsch Med Wschr 1992; 117:283–286.
378. Rozenberg S, Gevers R, Peretz A, et al. Decrease of bone mineral density during estrogen substitution therapy. Bone Miner 1992; 17(suppl 1):288.
379. Bush TL. Extraskeletal effects of estrogen and the prevention of atherosclerosis. Osteoporos Int 1991; 2:5–11.
380. Stampfer MJ, Bechtel SD. Estrogen: what protection against heart disease? Contemp Ob/Gyn 1992; 13–30.
381. Lobo RA. Estrogen and the risk of coagulopathy. Am J Med 1992; 92:283–285.
382. Devor M, Barrett-Connor E, Renvall M, et al. Estrogen replacement therapy and the risk of venous thrombosis. Am J Med 1992; 92:275–282.
383. Colditz GA, Stampfer MJ, Willett WC, et al. Prospective study of estrogen replacement therapy and risk of breast cancer in postmenopausal women. JAMA 1990; 264:2648–2653.
384. Rodriguez C, Calle EE, Coates RJ, et al. Estrogen replacement therapy and fatal ovarian cancer. Am J Epidemiol 1995; 141:828–835.
385. Staff JA, Newschaffer CJ, Jones JK, et al. Progestins and breast cancer: an epidemiologic review. Fertil Steril 1992; 57:473–491.
386. Whitcroft SIJ, Stevenson JC. Hormone replacement therapy: risks and benefits. Clin Endocrinol 1992; 36:15–20.
387. Schmitt N, Gogate J, Rothert M, et al. Capturing and clustering women's judgement policies: the case of hormonal therapy for menopause. J Gerontol 1991; 46:92–101.
388. Ryan PJ, Harrison R, Blake GM, Fogelman I. Compliance with hormone replacement therapy (HRT) after screening for post menopausal osteoporosis. Br J Obstet Gynecol 1992; 99:320–328.
389. Plunkett ER, Wolfe BM. Prolonged effects of a novel, low-dosage continuous progestin–cyclic estrogen replacement program in postmenopausal women. Am J Obstet Gynecol 1991; 166:117–121.
390. Hutchinson-Williams KA, Gutmann JN. Estrogen replacement therapy (ERT) in high-risk cancer patients. Yale J Biol Med 1991; 64:607–626.
391. Riggs BL, Melton LH. The prevention and treatment of osteoporosis. N Engl J Med 1992; 327:620–627.
392. Dumesic CA. Clinical therapeutic conference—menopause and post-menopausal women. J Clin Pharmacol 1992; 32:774–778.
393. Henrich JB. The postmenopausal estrogen/breast cancer controversy. JAMA 1992; 268:1900–1902.
394. Coope J, Marsh J. Can we improve compliance with long-term HRT? Maturitas 1992; 15:151–158.
395. Garton MJ, Rennie EC, Togerson DJ, Reid DM. Osteoporosis, HRT and the meno-

pause, attitudes and experience of perimenopausal women attending for bone density screening. Presented at Joint Meeting of the Bone and Tooth Society and the British Connective Tissue Society Autumn Meeting, Aberdeen, UK, 1992.
396. Rubin SM, Cummings SR. Results of bone densitometry affect women's decisions about taking measures to prevent fractures. Ann Intern Med 1992; 116:990–995.
397. Spector TD, Brennan P, Harris PA, et al. Do current regimes of hormone replacement therapy protect against subsequent fractures? Osteoporos Int 1992; 2:219–224.
398. Ke HZ, Li M, Jee WSS. Prostaglandin E_2 prevents ovariectomy-induced cancellous bone loss in rats. Bone Miner 1992; 19:45–62.
399. Savvas M, Studd JWW, Norman S, et al. Increase in bone mass after one year of percutaneous oestradiol and testosterone implants in post-menopausal women who have previously received long-term oral oestrogens. Br J Obstet Gynecol 1992; 99: 757–760.
400. Garnett T, Studd J, Watson N, et al. The effects of plasma estradiol levels on increases in vertebral and femoral bone density following therapy with estradiol and estradiol with testosterone implants. Obstet Gynecol 1992; 79:968–972.
401. Lufkin EG, Wahner HW, O'Fallon WM, et al. Treatment of postmenopausal osteoporosis with transdermal estrogen. Ann Intern Med 1992; 117:1–9.
402. Reginster JY, Sarlet N, Deroisy R, et al. Minimal levels of serum estradiol prevent postmenopausal bone loss. Calcif Tissue Int 1992; 51:340–343.
403. Birkenhager JC, Erdtsieck RJ, Zeelenberg J, et al. Can nandrolone add to the effect of hormonal replacement therapy in postmenopausal osteoporosis? Bone Miner 1992; 18:201–265.
404. Jacobs JS, Loeffler FE. Postmenopausal hormone replacement therapy. Br Med J 1992; 305:1403–1408.
405. Oddens BJ, Boulet MJ, Lehert P, Visser AP. Has the climacteric been medicalized? A study on the use of medication for climacteric complaints in four countries. Maturitas 1992; 15:171–181.
406. Palferman TG. That oestrogen replacement for osteoporosis prevention should no longer be a bone of contention. Ann Rheum Dis 1993; 52:74–80.
407. Ribot C, Tremollieres F, Pouilles JM. Effect of 17β-oestradiol and norethisterone acetate on vertebral bone mass and lipid metabolism in early postmenopausal women. Maturitas 15:217–223.
408. Svendsen OL, Hassager C, Marslew U, Christiansen C. Changes in calcanean bone mineral occurring spontaneously and during hormone replacement therapy in early post-menopausal women. Scand J Clin Lab Invest 1992; 52:831–836.
409. Castelo-Branco C, Martines de Osaba MJ, Pons F, Conzalez-Merlo J. The effect of hormone replacement therapy on postmenopausal bone loss. Eur J Obstet Gynecol Reprod Biol 1992; 44:131–136.
410. Leather AT, Studd JWW, Watson NR, Holland EFN. The prevention of bone loss in young women treated with GnRH analogues with "add-back" estrogen therapy. Obstet Gynecol 1993; 81:104–107.
411. Danielsen CC, Mosekilde L, Svenstrup B. Cortical bone mass, composition, and mechanical properties in female rats in relation to age, long-term ovariectomy, and estrogen substitution. Calcif Tissue Int 1993; 52:26–33.

412. Finucane FF, Madans JH, Bush TL, et al. Decreased risk of stroke among postmenopausal hormone users. Arch Intern Med 1993; 153:73–79.
413. Grady D, Rubin SM, Petitti DB, et al. Hormone therapy to prevent disease and prolong life in postmenopausal women. Ann Intern Med 1992; 117:1016–1037.
414. Lufkin EG, Ory SJ. Postmenopausal estrogen therapy. Trends Endocrinol Metab 1995; 6:50–54.
415. Wolfe BM, Huff MW. Effects of continuous low-dosage hormonal replacement therapy on lipoprotein metabolism in postmenopausal women. Metabolism 1995; 44:410–417.
416. American College of Physicians. Guidelines for counseling postmenopausal women about preventive hormone therapy. Ann Intern Med 1992; 117:1038–1041.
417. Harris RE, Namboodiri KK, Wynder EL. Breast cancer risk: effects of estrogen replacement therapy and body mass. J Natl Cancer Inst 1992; 84:1575–1582.
418. Brinton LA, Hoover RN. Endometrial Cancer Collaborative Group. Estrogen replacement therapy and endometrial cancer risk: unresolved issues. Obstet Gynecol 1993; 81:265–271.
419. Hunskaar S, Backe B. Attitudes towards and level of information on perimenopausal and postmenopausal hormone replacement therapy among Norwegian women. Maturitas 1992; 15:183–194.
420. Session DR, Kelly A, Jewelwicz R. Current concepts in estrogen replacement therapy in the menopause. Fertil Steril 1993; 59:277–284.
421. Keller PH, Hotz E, Imthurn B. A transdermal regimen for continuous combined hormone replacement therapy in the menopause. Maturitas 1992; 15:195–198.
422. Derby CA, Hume AL, Barbour MM, et al. Correlates of postmenopausal estrogen use and trends through the 1980s in two southeastern New England communities. Am J Epidemiol 1993; 137:1120–1135.
423. Lindgren R, Berg G, Hammar M, Succon E. Hormonal replacement therapy in a population of Swedish postmenopausal women. Acta Obstet Gynecol Scand 1993; 72:292–297.
424. MacLennan AH, MacLennan A, Wilson D. The prevalence of oestrogen replacement therapy in South Australia. Maturitas 1993; 16:175–183.
425. Jensen J. Lipid and lipoprotein profiles in postmenopausal women. Effects of combined hormone replacement therapy. Acta Obstet Gynecol Scand 1993; 72: 500–502.
426. Fitzgerald CT, Elstein M, Mansel RE. Hormone replacement therapy and malignancy. Br J Obstet Gynecol 1993; 100:408–410.
427. Hemminki E, Topo P, Malin M, Kangas I. Physicians' views on hormone therapy around and after menopause. Maturitas 1993; 16:163–173.
428. Colditz GA, Egan KM, Stampfer MJ. Hormone replacement therapy and risk of breast cancer: results from epidemiologic studies. Am J Obstet Gynecol 1993; 168: 1473–1480.
429. Smellie WJB, Thomas JM. Hormone replacement therapy and breast cancer. Br J Obstet Gynecol 1993; 100:404–407.
430. Orimo H, Shiraki M, Inoue S. Estrogen and bone. Osteoporos Int 1993; 3(suppl 1): 153–156.

431. Lindsay R. Criteria for successful estrogen therapy in osteoporosis. Osteoporosis Int 1993; 3(suppl 2):9–13.
432. Naessen T, Persson I, Thor I, et al. Maintained bone density at advanced ages after long term treatment with low dose oestradiol implants. Br J Obstet Gynecol 1993; 100:454–459.
433. Tremollieres F, Pouilles JM, Ribot C. Effect of long-term administration of progestogen on post-menopausal bone loss: result of a two-year, controlled randomized study. Clin Endocrinol 1993; 38:627–631.
434. Abe T, Chow JWM, Lean JM, Chambers TJ. Estrogen does not restore bone loss after ovariectomy in the rat. J Bone Miner Res 1993; 8:831–838.
435. Wronski TJ, Dann LM, Qi H, Yen CF. Skeletal effects of withdrawal of estrogen and diphosphonate treatment in ovariectomized rats. Calcif Tissue Int 1993; 53: 210–216.
436. Mattsson LA, Samsioe G, von Schoultz B, et al. Transdermally administered oestradiol combined with oral medroxyprogesterone acetate: the effets on lipoprotein metabolism in postmenopausal women. Br J Obstet Gynecol 1993; 100: 450–453.
437. Reginster JY, Christiansen C, Dequinze B, et al. Effect of transdermal 17β-estradiol and oral conjugated equine estrogens on biochemical parameters of bone resorption in natural menopause. Calcif Tissue Int 1993; 53:13–16.
438. Fuleihan GEH, Brown EM, Curtis K, et al. Effect of sequential and daily continuous hormone replacement therapy on indexes of mineral metabolism. Arch Intern Med 1992; 152:1904–1909.
439. MacLennan AH, MacLennan A, Wenzel S, et al. Continuous low-dose oestrogen and progestogen hormone replacement therapy: a randomized trial. Med J Aust 1993; 159:102–106.
440. Casper F, Chapdelaine A. Estrogen and interrupted progestin: a new concept for menopausal hormone replacement therapy. Am J Obstet Gynecol 1993; 168:1188–1196.
441. Byyrjalsen I, Haarbo J, Christiansen C. Role of cigarette smoking on the postmenopausal endometrium during sequential estrogen and progestogen therapy. Obstet Gynecol 1993; 81:1016–1021.
442. Hollenbach KA, Barrett-Connor E, Edelstein SL, Holbrook T. Cigarette smoking and bone mineral density in older men and women. Am J Public Health 1993; 83: 1265–1270.
443. Tremollieres FA, Pouilles JM, Ribot C. Vertebral postmenopausal bone loss is reduced in overweight women: a longitudinal study in 155 early postmenopausal women. J Clin Endocrinol Metab 1993; 77:683–686.
444. Evans G, Bryant H, Sato M, Turner RT. Raloxifene is a tissue specific estrogen agonist. J Bone Miner Res 1993; 8(suppl 1):134.
445. Dodge JA, Stocksdale MG, Black LJ, et al. Effects of steroidal and non-steroidal anti-estrogens in the ovariectomized rat. J Bone Miner Res 1993; 8(suppl 1):278.
446. Sato M, McClintock G, Kim J, et al. DEXA analysis of raloxifene effects on the bones from ovariectomized rats. J Bone Miner Res 1993; 8(suppl 1):S355.
447. Ross D, Stevenson J. HRT and cardiovascular disease. Br J Sex Med 1993; 3:10–13.

448. Adami S, Rossinin M, Zamberlan N, et al. Long-term effects of transdermal and oral estrogens on serum lipids and lipoproteins in postmenopausal women. Maturitas 1993; 17:191–196.
449. Manolio TA, Furberg CD, Shemanski L, et al. Associations of postmenopausal estrogen use with cardiovascular disease and its risk factors in older women. Circulation 1993; 88:2163–2171.
450. Bush TL, Gambrell RD, Miller V. More reasons than ever for HRT. Patient Care 1993; Nov:103–132.
451. Ayalon D, Pines A. Cardiovascular disease and hormone replacement therapy: a review. Isr J Med Sci 1993; 29:660–663.
452. Subbiah MTR, Kessel B, Agrawal M, et al. Antioxidant potential of specific estrogens on lipid peroxidation. J Clin Endocrinol Metab 1993; 77:1095–1097.
453. Barrett-Connor E. Estrogen and estrogen-progestogen replacement: therapy and cardiovascular diseases. Am J Med 1993; 95(suppl 5A):40–43.
454. Lindsay R. Hormone replacement therapy for prevention and treatment of osteoporosis. Am J Med 1993; 95(suppl 5A):37–39.
455. Holland EFN, Leather AT, Studd JWW, Garnett TJ. The effect of a new sequential oestradiol valerate and levonorgestrel preparation on the bone mineral density of postmenopausal women. Br J Obstet Gynecol 1993; 100:966–967.
456. Holland EFN, Leather AT, Studd JWW. The effect of 20-mg percutaneous estradiol implants on the bone mass of postmenopausal women. Obstet Gynecol 1994; 83: 43–46.
457. Rosenberg L. Hormone replacement therapy: the need for reconsideration. Am J Public Health 1993; 83:1670–1673.
458. Hemminki E, Sihvo S. A review of postmenopausal hormone therapy recommendations: potential for selection bias. Obstet Gynecol 1993; 82:1021–1028.
459. Ettinger B, Grady D. The waning effect of postmenopausal estrogen therapy on osteoporosis. N Engl J Med 1993; 329:1192–1193.
460. Felson DT, Zhang Y, Hannan MT, et al. The effect of postmenopausal estrogen therapy on bone density in elderly women. N Engl J Med 1993; 329:1141–1146.
461. Prince RL, Geelhoed EA. When should postmenopausal women start taking oestrogen replacement therapy? Med J Australia 1995; 162:173–174.
462. Rozenberg S, Gevers R, Peretz A, et al. Decrease of bone mineral density during estrogen substitution therapy. Maturitas 1993; 17:205–210.
463. Barentsen R, Groeneveld FPMJ, Bareman FP, et al. Women's opinion on withdrawal bleeding with hormone replacement therapy. Eur J Obstet Gynecol Reprod Biol 1993; 51:203–207.
464. Hall GM, Daniels M, Wiltshire P, et al. The effects of estrogen replacement therapy (ERT) and calcium on bone loss in rheumatoid arthritis (RA): a 2 year prospective study. (Abstract.) Presented at 57th Annual Meeting of American college of Rheumatology, San Antonio, Tex, 1993:50.
465. Clements D, Compston JE, Evans WD, Rhodes J. Hormone replacement therapy prevents bone loss in patients with inflammatory bowel disease. Gut 1993; 34:1543–1546.
466. Sugimoto AK, Hodsman AB, Nisker JA. Long-term gonadotropin-releasing hor-

mone agonist with standard postmenopausal estrogen replacement failed to prevent vertebral bone loss in premenopausal woman. Fertil Steril 1993; 60:672–674.

467. Belchetz PE. Hormonal treatment of postmenopausal women. N Engl J Med 1994; 330:1062–1071.
468. Campagnoli C, Lesca L, Cantamessa C, Peris C. Long-term hormone replacement treatment in menopause: new choices, old apprehensions, recent findings. Maturitas 1993; 18:21–46.
469. Abernethy K. Counselling—the key to compliance with HRT. Br J Sex Med 1994; Jan/Feb:14–16.
470. Te Velde ER, van Leusden HAIM. Hormonal treatment for the climacteric: alleviation of symptoms and prevention of postmenopausal disease. Lancet 1994; 343: 654–658.
471. Gorsky RD, Koplan JP, Peterson HB, Thacker SB. Relative risks and benefits of long-term estrogen replacement therapy: a decision analysis. Obstet Gynecol 1994; 83:161–166.
472. Kim CJ, Jang HC, Cho DH, Min YK. Effects of hormone replacement therapy on lipoprotein (a) and lipids in postmenopausal women. Arterioscler Thromb 1994; 14: 275–281.
473. Lobo RA, Speroff L. International consensus conference on postmenopausal hormone therapy and the cardiovascular system. Fertil Steril 1994; 61:592–595.
474. Risch HA, Howe GR. Menopausal hormone usage and breast cancer in Saskatchewan: a record-linkage cohort study. Am J Epidemiol 1994; 139:670–683.
475. Bluming AZ. Hormone replacement therapy: benefits and risks for the general postmenopausal female population and for women with a history of previously treated breast cancer. Semin Oncol 1993; 20:662–674.
476. Archer DF, Pickar JH, Bottiglioni F. Bleeding patterns in postmenopausal women taking continuous combined or sequential regimens of conjugated estrogens with medroxyprogesterone acetate. Obstet Gynecol 1994; 83:686–692.
477. Ringa V, Ledesert B, Breart G. Determinants of hormone replacement therapy among postmenopausal women enrolled in the French GAZEL cohort. Osteoporos Int 1994; 4:16–20.
478. Erdsieck RJ, Pols HAP, Van Kuijk C, et al. Course of bone mass during and after hormonal replacement therapy with and without addition of nandrolone decanoate. J Bone Miner Res 1994; 9:277–283.
479. Hassager C, Jensen SB, Christiansen C. Non-responders to hormone replacement therapy for the prevention of postmenopausal bone loss: do they exist? Osteoporos Int 1994; 4:36–41.
480. Ryde SJS, Bowen-Simpkins K, Bowen-Simpkins P, et al. The effect of oestradiol implants on regional and total bone mass: a three-year longitudinal study. Clin Endocrinol 1994; 40:33–38.
481. Ringe JD, Meiss F. Vermeidung frühpostmenopausaler Knochensubstanzverluste durch transdermale Osteogensubstitution. Dtsch Med Wschr 1993; 118:769–774.
482. Holland EFN, Chow JWM, Studd JWW, et al. Histomorphometric changes in the skeleton of postmenopausal women with low bone mineral density treated with percutaneous estradiol implants. Obstet Gynecol 1994; 83:387–391.

483. Holland EFN, Studd JWW, Mansell JP, et al. Changes in collagen composition and cross-links in bone and skin of osteoporotic postmenopausal women treated with percutaneous estradiol implants. Obstet Gynecol 1994; 83:180–183.
484. Nielsen SP, Barenholdt O, Hermansen F, Munk-Jensen N. Magnitude and pattern of skeletal response to long term continuous and cyclic sequential oestrogen/progestin treatment. Br J Obstet Gynecol 1994; 101:319–324.
485. McDermott MT, Perloff JJ, Kidd GS. Effects of mild asymptomatic primary hyperparathyroidism on bone mass in women with and without estrogen replacement therapy. J Bone Miner Res 1994; 9:509–514.
486. MacDonald AG, Murphy EA, Capell HA, et al. Effects of hormone replacement therapy in rheumatoid arthritis: a double blind placebo-controlled study. Ann Rheum Dis 1994; 53:54–57.
487. Van den Brink HR, van Everdingen AA, van Wijk MJG, et al. Adjuvant oestrogen therapy does not improve disease activity in postmenopausal patients with rheumatoid arthritis. Ann Rheum Dis 1993; 52:862–865.
488. Grey AB, Cundy TF, Reid IR: Continuous combined oestrogen/progestin therapy is well tolerated and increases bone density at the hip and spine in postmenopausal osteoporosis. Clin Endocrinol 1994; 40:671–677.
489. Rico H, Hernandez ERD, Duran CS, et al. Quantitative peripheral computed tomodensitometric study of cortical and trabecular bone mass in relation wth menopause. Maturitas 1994; 18:183–189.
490. Gambacciani M, Spinetti A, De Simone L, et al. The relative contributions of menopause and aging to postmenopausal vertebral osteopenia. J Clin Endocrinol Metab 1993; 77:1148–1151.
491. Pouilles JM, Tremollieres F, Bonneu M, Ribot C. Influence of early age at menopause on vertebral bone mass. J Bone Miner Res 1994; 9:311–315.
492. Oldenhave A, Netelenbos C. Pathogenesis of climacteric complaints: ready for the change? Lancet 1994; 343:649–653.
493. Gambacciani M, Spinetti A, Taponeco F, et al. Bone loss in perimenopausal women: a longitudinal study. Maturitas 1994; 18:191–197.
494. Creatsas G, Arefetz N, Adamopoulos PN, et al. Transdermal estradiol plus oral medroxyprogesterone acetate replacement therapy in primary amenorrheic adolescents. Clinical, hormonal and metabolic aspects. Maturitas 1994; 18:105–114.
495. Constantini NW. Clinical consequences of athletic amenorrhoea. Sports Med 1994; 17:213–223.
496. Hoenggi W, Casez JP, Birkhaeuser MH, et al. Bone mineral density in young women with long-standing amenorrhea: limited effect of hormone replacement therapy with ethinylestradiol and desogestrel. Ossteoporos Int 1994; 4:99–103.
497. Gambacciana M, Spinetti A, Taponeco F, et al. Longitudinal evaluation of perimenopausal vertebral bone loss: effects of a low-dose oral contraceptive preparation on bone mineral density and metabolism. Obstet Gynecol 1994; 83:392–396.
498. Tuppurainen M, Kroger H, Saarikoski S, et al. The effect of previous oral contraceptive use on bone mineral density in perimenopausal women. Osteoporos Int 1994; 4:93–98.
499. Harms HM, Neubauer O, Kayser C, et al. Pulse amplitude and frequency modulation

of parathyroid hormone in early menopausal women before and on hormone replacement therapy. J Clin Endocrinol Metab 1994; 78:48–52.

500. Cosman F, Nieves J, Horton J, et al. Effects of estrogen on response to edetic acid infusion in postmenopausal osteoporotic women. J Clin Endocrinol Metab 1994;78: 939–943.
501. Zofkova I, Rojdmark S, Kancheva RL. Does estrogen replacement therapy influence parathyroid hormone responsiveness to exogenous hypercalcemia in postmenopausal women? J Endocrinol Invest 1994; 16:323–327.
502. Findlay I, Cunningham D, Dargie HJ. Coronary heart disease, the menopause, and hormone replacement therapy. Br Heart J 1994; 71:213–214.
503. Kafonek SD. Postmenopausal hormone replacement therapy and cardiovascular risk reduction. Drugs 1994; 47(suppl 2):16–24.
504. Rebar RW. Unanswered questions in hormonal replacement therapy. Exp Gerontol 1994; 29:447–461.
505. Seed M. Postmenopausal hormone replacement therapy, coronary heart disease and plasma lipoproteins. Drugs 1994; 47(suppl 2):20–34.
506. Stevenson JC, Crook D, Godsland IF, et al. Hormone replacement therapy and the cardiovascular system. Drugs 1994; 47(suppl 2):35–41.
507. Webber CE, Blake JM, Chambers LF, Roberts JG. Effects of 2 years of hormone replacement upon bone mass, serum lipids and lipoproteins. Maturitas 1994; 19:13–23.
508. Whitcroft SI, Crook D, Marsh MS, et al. Long-term effects of oral and transdermal hormone replacement therapies on serum lipid and lipoprotein concentrations. Obstet Cynecol 1994; 84:222–226.
509. Radford NB. Southwestern Internal Medicine Conference: Postmenopausal estrogen supplementation: a cardiologist's perspective. Am J Med Sci 1994; 308:63–73.
510. Posthuma WFM, Westendorp RGJ, Vandenbroucke JP. Cardioprotective effect of hormone replacement therapy in postmenopausal women: is the evidence biased? Br Med J 1994; 308:719–722.
511. Tosteson ANA. Hormone replacement therapy: benefit, risk and cost considerations. J Clin Pharmacol 1994; 34:719–722.
512. Lafferty FW, Fiske ME: Postmenopausal estrogen replacement: a long-term cohort study. Am J Med 1994; 97:66–77.
513. Marcus R, Greendale G, Blunt BA, et al. Correlates of bone mineral density in the postmenopausal estrogen/progestin interventions trial. J Bone Miner Res 1994; 9: 1467–1476.
514. Cicinelli E, Galantino P, Pepe V, et al. Bone metabolism changes after transdermal estradiol dose reduction during estrogen replacement therapy: a 1-year prospective study. Maturitas 1994; 19:133–139.
515. Studd JWW, Holland EFN, Leather AT, Smith RNJ. The dose-response of percutaneous oestradiol implants on the skeletons of postmenopausal women. Br J Obstet Gynecol 1994; 191:787–791.
516. Avioli LV. Impact of the menopause on skeletal metabolism and osteoporotic syndromes. Exp Gerontol 1994; 29:391–791.
517. Majeska RJ, Ryaby JT, Einhorn TA. Direct modulation of osteoblastic activity with estrogen. J Bone Joint Surg 1994; 76A:713–721.

518. Prince RL. Counterpoint: estrogen effects on calcitropic hormones and calcium homeostasis. Endocrinol Rev 1994; 15:301–309.
519. Schlemmer A, Hassager C, Delmas PD, Christiansen C. Urinary excretion of pyridinium cross-links in health women; the long-term effects of menopause and oestrogen/progesterone therapy. Clin Endocrinol 1994; 40:777–782.
520. Turner RT, Riggs BL, Spelsberg TC. Skeletal effects of estrogen. Endocrinol Rev 1994; 15:275–300.
521. Wimalawansa SJ. Is there a place for estrogen therapy for women over 70 years of age? J Bone Miner Res 1994; 9(suppl 1):326.
522. Prestwood KM, Pilbeam CC, Burleson JA, et al. The short term effects of conjugated estrogen on bone turnover in older women. J Clin Endocrinol Metab 1994; 79: 366–371.
523. Woodruff JD, Pickar JH. Incidence of endometrial hyperplasia in postmenopausal women taking conjugated estrogens (Premarin) with medroxyprogesterone acetate or conjugated estrogens alone. Am J Obstet Gynecol 1994; 170:1213–1223.
524. Rymer J, Fogelman I, Chapman MG. The incidence of vaginal bleeding with tibolone treatment. Br J Obstet Gynecol 1994; 101:53–56.
525. Cobleigh MA, Berris RF, Bush T, et al. Estrogen replacement therapy in breast cancer survivors. A time for change. JAMA 1994; 272:540–545.
526. Rudman D, Feller AG, Nagraj HS, et al. Effects of human growth hormone in men over 60 years old. N Engl J Med 1990; 323:1–6.
527. Mazess RB, Barden H, Drinka P, et al. Influence of age and body weight on spine and femur bone mineral density in U.S. white men. J Bone Miner Res 1990; 5(6):645–652.
528. Mazess R, Cameron J. Bone mineral content in normal US whites, In: Mazess RB, ed. International Conference Bone Mineral Measurements. Washington, DC: Dept Health Educ & Welfare Publ NIH 75-683, US Dept HEW. 1974:228–237.
529. Aloia JF, Vaswani A, Kapoor A, et al. Treatment of osteoporosis with calcitonin, with and without growth hormone. Metabolism 1984; 34:124–129.
530. Aloia JF, Vaswani A, Meunier PJ, et al. Coherence treatment of postmenopausal osteoporosis with growth hormone and calcitonin. Calcif Tissue Int 1987; 40: 203–209.
531. Rubin CD. Southwestern internal medicine conference: growth hormone—aging and osteoporosis. Am J Med Sci 1993; 305:120–129.
532. Wuster C. Growth hormone and br-metabolism. Acta Endocrinol 1993; 128(suppl 2):14–18.
533. Eriksen EF, Kassem M, Brixen K. Growth hormone and insulin-like growth factors as anabolic therapies for osteoporosis. Horm Res 1993; 40:95–98.
534. Rosen T, Hansson T, Granhed H, et al. Reduced bone mineral content in adult patients with growth hormone deficiency. Acta Endocrinol 1993; 129:201–206.
535. Wuster C, Blum WF, Schlemilch S, et al. Decreased serum levels of insulin-like growth factors and IGF binding protein 3 in osteoporosis. J Intern Med 1993; 234: 249.
536. Ravn P, Overgaard K, Spencer EM, Christiansen C. Insulin-like growth factors I and II in healthy women with and without established osteoporosis. Eur J Endocrinol 1995; 132:313–319.

537. Clemmesen B, Overgaard K, Riis B, Chrisen C. Human growth hormone and growth hormone releasing hormone: a double-masked, placebo-controlled study of their effects on bone metabolism in elderly women. Osteoporosis Int 1993; 3:330–336.
538. Kassem M, Brixen K, Mosekilde L, Eriksen EF. Human marrow stromal osteoblast-like cells do not show reduced responsiveness to in vitro stimulation with growth hormone in patients with postmenopausal osteoporosis. Calcif Tissue Int 1994; 54:1–6.
539. Thoren M, Soop M, Degerblad M, Saaf M. Preliminary study of the effects of growth hormone substitution therapy on bone mineral density and serum osteocalcin levels in adults with growth hormone deficiency. Acta Endocrinol 1993; 128(suppl 2): 41–43.
540. Vandeweghe M, Taelman P, Kaufman JM. Short and long-term effects of growth hormone treatment on bone turnover and bone mineral content in adult growth hormone-deficient males. Clin Endocrinol 1993; 39:409–415.
541. Bak B. Fracture healing and growth hormone. A biochemical study in the rat. Dan Med Bull 1993; 40:519–536.
542. Inzucchi SE, Robbins RJ. Effects of growth hormone on human bone biology. J Clin Endocrinol Metab 1994; 79:691–694.
543. Slootweg MC. Growth hormone and bone. Horm Metab Res 1993; 20:335–343.
544. Corpas E, Harman SM, Blackman MR. Human growth hormone and human aging. Endocrinol Rev 1993; 14:20–39.
545. Benedict MR, Adiyaman S, Ayers DC, et al. Dissociation of bone mineral density from age-related decreases in insulin-like growth factor-I and its binding proteins in the male rat. J Gerontol 1994; 49:224–230.
546. Denis I, Thomasset M, Pointillart A. Influence of exogenous porcine growth hormone on vitamin D metabolism and calcium and phosphorus absorption in intact pigs. Calcif Tissue Int 1994; 54:489–492.
547. Denis I, Zerath E, Pointillart A. Effects of exogenous growth hormone on bone mineralization and remodeling and on plasma calcitriol in intact pigs. Calcif Tissue Int 1994; 15:419–424.
548. O'Sullivan AJ, Kelly JJ, Hoffman DM, et al. Body composition and energy expenditure in acromegaly. J Clin Endocrinol Metab 1994; 78:381–386.
549. Hansen TB, Gram J, Bjerret P, et al. Body composition in active acromegaly during treatment with octreotide: a double-blind, placebo-controlled cross-over study. Clin Endocrinol 1994; 41:323–329.
550. Beshyah SA, Freemantle C, Thomas E, et al. Comparison of measurements of body composition by total body potassium, bioimpedance analysis, and dual-energy X-ray absorptiometry in hypopituitary adults before and during growth hormone treatment. Am J Clin Nutr 1995; 61:1186–1194.
551. Snel YEM, Brummer RJM, Doerga ME, Zelissen PMJ, et al. Adipose tissue assessed by magnetic resonance imaging in growth hormone replacement and a comparison with control subjects. Am J Clin Nutr 1995; 61:1290–1294.
552. DeBoer H, Blok GJ, VanLingen A, et al: Consequences of childhood-onset growth hormone deficiency for adult bone mass. J Bone Miner Res 1994; 9:1319–1326.
553. Nussey SS, Hyer SL, Brada M, Leiper AD. Bone mineralization after treatment of

growth hormone deficiency in survivors of childhood malignancy. Acta Paediatr Suppl 1994; 399:9–14.
554. Ogle GD, Moore B, Lu PW, et al. Changes in body composition and bone density after discontinuation of growth hormone therapy in adolescence: an interim report. Acta Paediatr Suppl 1994; 399:3–7.
555. Holmes SJ, Economou G, Whitehouse RW, et al. Reduced bone mineral density in patients with adult onset growth hormone deficiency. J Clin Endocrinol Metab 1994; 78:669–674.
556. Rosen T, Johannsson G, Bengtsson BA. Consequences of growth hormone deficiency in adults, and effects of growth hormone replacement therapy. Acta Paediatr Suppl 1994; 399:21–24.
557. Beshyah SA, Thomas E, Kyd P, et al. The effect of growth hormone replacement therapy in hypopituitary adults on calcium and bone metabolism. Clin Endocrinol 1994; 40:383–391.
558. Orme SM, Sebastian JP, Oldroyd B, et al. Comparison of measures of body composition in a trial of low dose growth hormone replacement therapy. Clin Endocrinol 1992; 37:453–459.
559. O'Halloran DJ, Tsatsouli A, Whitehouse RW, et al. Increased bone density after recombinant human growth hormone (GH) therapy in adults with isolated GH deficiency. J Clin Endocrinol Metab 1993; 76:1344–1348.
560. Kassem M, Brixen K, Blum WF, et al. Normal osteoclastic and osteoblastic responses to exogenous growth hormone in patients with postmenopausal spinal osteoporosis. J Bone Miner Res 1994; 9:1365–1370.
561. Giustina A, Bussi AR, Jacobello C, Wehrenberg WB. Effects of recombinant human growth hormone (GH) on bone and intermediary metabolism in patients receiving chronic glucocorticoid treatment with suppressed endogenous GH response to GH-releasing hormone. J Clin Endocrinol Metab 1995; 80:122–129.
562. Sanchez CP, Goodman WG, Brandli D, et al. Skeletal response to recombinant human growth hormone (rhGH) in children treated with long-term corticosteroids. J Bone Miner Res 1995; 10:2–6.
563. Ljunghall S, Lindh E, Johansson AG. Endocrine interactions of insulin-like growth factor 1 on bone. Acta Paediatr Suppl 1994; 399:178–179.
564. Ebeling PR, Jones JD, O'Fallon WM, et al. Short-term effects of recombinant human insulin-like growth factor 1 on bone turnover in normal women. J Clin Endocrinol Metab 1993; 77:1384–1387.
565. Holloway L, Butterfield G, Hintz RL, et al. Effects of recombinant human growth hormone on metabolic indices, body composition, and bone turnover in healthy elderly women. J Clin Endocrinol Metab 1994; 79:470–479.
566. Orimo H. Effect of ipriflavone in involutional osteoporosis. In: Christiansen C, Overgaard K, eds. Osteoporosis. Copenhagen: Osteopress APS, 1990:2156–2158.
567. Brandi ML. Flavonoids: biochemical effects and therapeutic applications. Bone Miner 1992; 19:3–14.
568. Bonucci E, Silvestrini G, Ballanti P, et al. Cytological and ultrastructural investigation on osteoblastic and preosteoclastic cells grown in vitro in the presence of ipriflavone: preliminary results. Bone Miner 1992; 19:15–26.

569. Mazzuoli G, Romagnoli E, Carnevale V, et al. Effects of ipriflavone on bone remodeling in promary hyperparathyroidism. Bone Miner 1992; 19:27–34.
570. Agnusdei D, Camporeale A, Gonnelli S, et al. Short-term treatment of Paget's disease of bone with ipriflavone. Bone Miner 1992; 19:35–42.
571. Agnusdei D, Adami S, Cervetti R, et al. Effects of ipriflavone on bone mass and calcium metabolism in postmenopausal osteoporosis. Bone Miner 1992; 19:43–48.
572. Melis GB, Peoletti AM, Bartolini R, et al. Ipriflavone and low doses of estrogens in the prevention of bone mineral loss in climacterium. Bone Miner 1992; 19:49–56.
573. Passeri M, Bionid M, Costi D, et al. Effect of ipriflavone on bone mass in elderly osteoporotic women. Bone Miner 1992; 19:57–62.
574. Notoya K, Yoshida K, Taketomi S, et al. Inhibitory effect of ipriflavone on pit formation in mouse unfractionated bone cells. Calc Tissue Int 1992; 51(suppl):3–6.
575. Morita I, Sakaguchi K, Kurachi T, Murota SI. Ipriflavone inhibits murine osteoclast formation in vitro. Calc Tissue Int 1992; 51(suppl):7–10.
576. Kakai Y, Kawase T, Nakano T, et al. Effect of ipriflavone and estrogen on the differentiation and proliferation of osteogenic cells. Calc Tissue Int 1992; 51 (suppl):11–15.
577. Notoya K, Tsukuda R, Yoshida K, Taketomi S. Stimulatory effect of ipriflavone on formation of bone-like tissue in raat bone marrow stromal cell culture. Calc Tissue Int 1992; 51(suppl):S16–20.
578. Ozawa H, Nakamura H, Irie K, Irie M. Histochemical and fine structural study of bone of ipriflavone-treated rats. Calc Tissue Int 1992; 51(suppl):21–26.
579. Watanabe K, Takekoshi S, Kakudo K. Effects of ipriflavone on calcitonin synthesis in C cells of the rat thyroid. Calc Tissue Int 1992; 51(suppl):27–29.
580. Nakamura S, Morimoto S, Takamoto S, et al. Effect of ipriflavone on bone mineral density and calcium-related factors in elderly females. Calc Tissue Int 1992; 51(suppl):30–34.
581. Suda A. Effect of parathyroid hormone on parietal bones of rats, and effect of ipriflavone. J Bone Miner Metab 1987; 5:5–56.
582. Yamazaki I, Shino A, Tsukuda R. Effect of ipriflavone on osteoporosis inducted by ovariectomy in rats. J Bone Miner Metab 1985; 3:205–210.
583. Orimo H, Nakai R, Itoh H, Shiraki M. Effectiveness and safety of TC-80 for osteoporosis. Preliminary double-blind trial. Prog Med 1985; 5:2943–2949.
584. Fujita T, Ono K, Inoue Y, et al. Dose finding study on TC-80 (ipriflavone) in osteoporosis. Prog Med 1985; 5:2959–2963.
585. Bonucci E, Ballanti P, Martelli A, et al. Ipriflavone inhibits osteoclast differentiation in parathyroid transplanted parietal bone of rats. Calcif Tissue Int 1992; 50:314–219.
586. Agnusdei D, Camporeale A, Zacchei F, et al. Effects of opriflavone on bone mass and bone remodeling in patients with established postmenopausal osteoporosis. Curr Ther Res 1992; 51:82–91.
587. Azria M, Behhar C, Cooper S. Lack of effect of ipriflavone on osteoclast motility and bone resorption in in vitro and ex vivo studies. Calcif Tissue Int 1993; 52:16–120.
588. Melis GB, Paoletti AM, Cagnacci A, et al. Lack of any estrogenic effect of ipriflavone in postmenopausal women. J Endocrinol Invest 1992; 15:755–761.
589. Hock JM, Gera I. Effects of continuous and intermittent administration and inhibi-

tion of resorption on the anabolic response of bone to parathyroid hormone. J Bone Miner Res 1992; 7:65–72.

590. Jerome CP, Gubler HP. Experimental determination of "the law of bone remodeling" and effect of rat parathyroid hormone (1–34) infusion on derived parameters. Calcif Tissue Int 1991; 49:398–402.
591. Kalu DN, Echon R, Hollis BW. Modulation of ovariectomy-related bone loss by parathyroid hormone in rats. Mech Ageing Dev 1990; 56:49–62.
592. Kimmel DB, Bozzato RP, Kronis KA, et al. The effect of recombinant humar (1-84) or synthetic human (1-34) parathyroid hormone on the skeleton of adult osteopenic ovariectomized rats. Endocrinology 1993; 132:1577–1584.
593. Liu CC, Kalu DN, Salerno E, et al. Preexisting bone loss associated with ovariectomy in rats is reversed by parathyroid hormone. J Bone Miner Res 1991; 6:1071–1080.
594. Mitlak BH, Williams DC, Bryant HU, et al. Intermittent administration of bovine PTH-(1-34) increases serum 1,20-dihydroxyvitamin D concentrations and spinal bone density in senile (23 month) rats. J Bone Miner Res 1992; 7:479–484.
595. Mosekilde L, Sogaard CH, Danielsen CC, et al. The anabolic effects of human parathyroid hormone (hPTH) on rat vertebral body mass are also reflected in the quality of bone, assessed by biomechanical testing: a comparison study between hPTH-(1-34) and hPTH-(1-84). Endocrinology 1991; 129:421–428.
596. Tada K, Yamamuro T, Okumura H, et al. Restoration of axial and appendicular bone volumes by h-pth(1-34) in parathyroidectomized and osteopenic rats. Bone 1990; 11: 163–169.
597. Wronski TJ, Yen CF, Qi H, Dann LM. Parathyroid hormone is more effective than estrogen or bisphosphonates for restoration of lost bone mass in ovariectomized rats. Endocrinology 1993; 32:823–831.
598. Hodsman AB, Steer BM, Fraher LJ, Drost JS. Bone densitometric and histomorphometric responses to sequential human parathyroid hormone (1-38) and salmon calcitonin in osteoporotic patients. Bone Miner 1991; 14:67–83.
599. Hodsman AB, Steer BM. Early histomorphometric changes in response to parathyroid hormone therapy in osteoporosis: evidence for de novo bone formation on quiescent cancellous surfaces. Bone 1993; 14:523–527.
600. Shen V, Dempster DW, Mellish RWE, et al. Effects of combined and separate intermittent administration of low-dose human parathyroid hormone fragment (1034) and 17β-estradiol on bone histomorphometry in ovariectomized rats with established osteopenia. Calcif Tissue Int 1992; 50:214–220.
601. Fenton AJ, Kemp BE, Kent GN, et al. A carboxylterminal peptide from the parathyroid hormone-related protein inhibits bone resorption by osteoblasts. Endocrinology 1991; 129:1762–1768.
602. Reeve J, Meunier PJ, Parsons JA, et al. Anabolic effect of human parathyroid hormone fragment on trabecular bone in involutional osteoporosis: a multicenter trial. Br Med J 1980; 280:1340–1344.
603. Reeve J, Davies UM, Hesp R, et al. Treatment of osteoporosis with human parathyroid peptide and observations on effect of sodium fluoride. Br Med J 1990; 301: 314–318.

604. Ejersted C, Andreassen TT, Oxlund H, et al. Human parathyroid hormone (1-34) and (1-84) increase the mechanical stength and thickness of cortical bone in rats. J Bone Miner Res 1993; 8:1097–1101.
605. Bradbeer JN, Arlot, ME Meunier PJ, Reeve J. Treatment of osteoporosis with parathyroid peptide (hPTH 1-34) and oestrogen: increase in volumetric density of iliac cancellous bone may depend on reduced trabecular spacing as well as increased thickness of packets of newly formed bone. Clin Endocrinol 1992; 37:282–289.
606. Reeve J, Bradbeer JN, Arlot M, et al. hPTH 1-34 treatment of osteoporosis with added hormone replacement therapy: biochemical, kinetic and histological responses. Osteoporos Int 1991; 1:162–170.
607. Reeve J, Arlot ME, Bradbeer JN, et al. Human parathyroid peptide treatment of vertebral osteoporosis. Osteoporos Int 3 1993; (suppl 1):S199–203.
608. Lindsay R, Cosman F, Nieves J, et al. A controlled clinical trial of the effects of 1-34hPTH in estrogen treated osteoporotic women. J Bone Miner Res 1993; 8(suppl 1):130.
609. Dempster DW, Cosman F, Parisien M, Shen V, Lindsay R. Anabolic actions of parathyroid hormone on bone. Endocrinol Rev 1993; 14:690–709.
610. Guldager B, Brixen KT, Jorgensen JS, et al. Effects of intravenous EDTA treatment on serum parathyroid hormone (1-84) and biochemical markers of bone turnover. Dan Med Bull 1993; 40:627–630.
611. Lindsay R, Nieves J, Henneman E, Shen V, Cosman F. Subcutaneous administration of the amino-terminal fragment of human parathyroid hormone-(1-34): kinetics and biochemical response in estrogenized osteoporotic patients. J Clin Endocrinol Metab 1993; 77:1535–1539.
612. Tyan ML. Effect of promethazine on lumbar vertebral bone mas in postmenopausal women. J Intern Med 1993; 234:143–148.
613. Riggs BL. Formation-stimulating regimens other than sodium fluoride. Am J Med 1993; 95(suppl 5A):62, 68.
614. Mosekilde L, Danielsen CC, Gasser J. The effect on vertebral bone mass and strength of long term treatment with antiresorptive agents (estrogen and calcitonin), human parathyroid hormone-(1-38), and combination therapy, assessed in aged ovariectomized rats. Endocrinology 1994; 134:2126–2134.
615. Mosekilde L, Sogaard CH, McOsker JE, Wronski TJ. PTH has a more pronounced effect on vertebral bone mass and biochemical competence than antiresorptive agents (estrogen and bisphosphonate)—assessed in sexually mature, ovariectomized rats. Bone 1994; 15:401–408.
616. Shea M, Tomita A, Battle MA, et al. Parathyroid hormone 1-84 increases morphologic properties and strength in ratbone. Presented at 40th Annual Meeting, Orthopaedic Research Society, New Orleans, La, 1994.
617. Mashiba T, Tanizawa T, Endo N, et al. Effect of human PTH1-34 on lumbar vertebra in young and mature rats. Presented at 40th Annual Meeting, Orthopaedic Research Society, New Orleans, La, 1994.
618. Jerome CP. Anabolic effect of high doses of human parathyroid hormone (1-38) in mature intact female rats. J Bone Miner Res 1994; 9:933–942.
619. Sogaard CH, Wronski TH, McOsker JE, Mosekilde L. The positive effect of para-

thyroid hormone on femoral neck bone strength in ovariectomized rats is more pronounced than that of estrogen or bisphosphonates. Endocrinology 1994; 134: 650–657.

620. Kaji H, Sugimoto T, Kanatani M, et al. Carboxyl-terminal parathyroid hormone fragments stimulate osteoclast-like cell formation and osteoclastic activity. Endocrinology 1994; 134:1897–1904.

621. Birkenhäger-Frenkel D et al. Effects of 1-hydroxyvitamin D_3 on various stages of predialysis renal bone disease. Bone Miner 1989; 6:311–322.

622. Orimo H, Shiraki M, Hayashi T, Nakamura T. Reduced occurrence of vertebral crush fractures in senile osteoporosis treated with 1(OH)-vitamin D_3. Bone Miner 1987; 3:47–52.

623. Shiraki M, Orimo H, Ito H, et al. Long-term treatment of postmenopausal osteoporosis with active vitamin D_3, 1-alpha-hydroxycholecalciferol (1OHD$_3$) and 1,24 dihydroxycholecalciferal (1,24(OH)$_2$D$_3$). Endocrinol Jpn 1985; 32:305–315.

624. Riggs BL, Nelson KI. Effect of long-term treatment with calcitriol on calcium absorption and mineral metabolism in postmenopausal osteoporosis. J Clin Endocrinol Metab 1985; 61:457–461.

625. Dabek JT, Robinson BHB, Naik RB, Al-Hiti K. Spinal calcium changes with 1-hydroxyvitamin D_3. Clin Endocrinol 1977; 7(suppl):147–150.

626. Caniggia A, Nuti R, Lore F, et al. Long-term treatment with calcitriol in postmenopausal osteoporosis. Metabolism 1990; 39(4):43–49.

627. Gallagher JC, Goldgar D, O'Neill J. Prevention of postmenopausal bone loss by 1,20-dihydroxyvitamin D_3 therapy in osteoporosis. In: Norman AW et al. (eds). Seventh Vitamin D Meeting. Chemical, Biochemical, and Clinical Update, 1990.

628. Aloia JF, Vaswani A, Yah JK. Calcitriol in the treatment of postmenopausal osteoporosis. Am J Med 1988; 84:401–408.

629. Ott SM, Chesnut CH. Calcitriol treatment is not effective in postmenopausal osteoporosis. Ann Intern Med 1989; 110:267–274.

630. Ott SM, Chesnut CH. Tolerance to dose of calcitriol is associated with improved bone density in women with postmenopausal osteoporosis. J Bone Miner Res 1990; 4(suppl 2):186.–

631. Schaadt OP, Bohr HH. Prednisone induced bone loss and Alfacalcidol. In: Ring EFJ, ed. Current Research in Osteoporosis and Bone Mineral Measurement. London: British Institute of Radiology, 1990:83–84.

632. Gallagher JC, Riggs BL, Recker RR, Goldgar D. The effect of calcitriol on patients with postmenopausal osteoporosis with special reference to fracture frequency. Proc Soc Exp Biol Med 1989; 191(3):287–292.

633. Tilyard MW. 1,20-Dihydroxlyvitamin D_3 vs calcium in the treatment of established postmenopausal osteoporosis. (Abstract.) J Bone Miner Res 1990; 5(2):275.

634. Gallagher J, Riggs B. Action of 1,20-dihydroxyvitamin D_3 on calcium balance and bone turnover and its effect on vertebral fracture rate. Metabolism 1990; 39(suppl 1):30–34.

635. Gallagher J, Goldgar D. Treatment of postmenopausal osteoporosis with high doses of synthetic calcitriol: a randomized controlled study. Ann Int Med 1990; 113: 649–655.

636. Aloia JF. Role of calcitriol in the treatment of postmenopausal osteoporosis. Metabolism 1990; 39(suppl 1):35–38.
637. Tilyard M. Low-dose calcitriol vs calcium in established postmenopausal osteoporosis. Metabolism 1990; 39(suppl 1):50–52.
638. Fujita T. Studies in osteoporosis in Japan. Metabolism 1990; 39(4):39–42.
639. Need A, Nordin B, Horowitz M, Morris H. Calcium and calcitriol therapy in osteoporotic postmenopausal women with impaired calcium absorption. Metabolism 1990; 39(suppl 1):53–54.
640. Nuti R, Martini G, Righi F, et al. Influence of intestinal calcium absorption on total body bone mineral content in postmenopausal osteoporotic women. In: Christiansen C, Overgaard K, eds. Osteoporosis. Copenhagen: Osteopress APS, 1990:895–897.
641. Lempert UG, Scharla SH, Minne HW, Ziegler R. Influence of parathyroidectomy, 1,20-dihydroxyvitamin D_3 and high dietary calcium intake on demineralized bone matrix powder-induced bone formation in the rat. Bone Miner 1991; 13:103–109.
642. Caniggia A, Nuti R, Galli M, et al. Effect of a long-term treatment with 1,20-dihydroxyvitamin D_3 on osteocalcin in postmenopausal osteoporosis. Calcif Tissue Int 1986; 38:328–332.
643. Hodsman AB, Toogood JH, Jennings B, Fraher LJ, Baskerville JC. Differential effects of inhaled budesonide and oral prednisolone on serum osteocalcin. J Clin Endocrinol Metab 1991; 72:530–540.
644. Eastell R, Yergey AL, Vieira NE, et al. Interrelationship among vitamin D metabolism, true calcium absorption, parathyroid function, and age in women: evidence of an age-related intestinal resistance to 1,20-dihydroxyvitamin D action. J Bone Miner Res 1991; 6:120–132.
645. Duda RJ, Kumar R, Nelson KI, et al. 1,20-Dihydroxyvitamin D stimulation test for osteoblast function in normal and osteoporotic postmenopausal women. J Clin Invest 1987; 79:1249–1203.
646. Egrise D, Martin D, Neve P, Verhas M, Schoutens A. Effects and interactions of 17β-estradiol, T_3 and $1,20(OH)_2D_3$ on cultured osteoblasts from mature rats. Bone Miner 1990; 11:273–283.
647. Fraser JD, Price PA: Induction of matrix Gla protein synthesis during prolonged 1,20-dihydroxyvitamin D_3 treatment of osteosarcoma cells. Calcif Tissue Int 1990; 46:270–279.
648. Nielsen HK, Brixen K, Kassem M, Mosekilde L. Acute effect of 1,20-dihydroxyvitamin D_3, prednisone, and 1,20-dihydroxyvitamin D_3 plus prednisone on serum osteocalcin in normal individuals. J Bone Miner Res 1991; 6:435–441.
649. Owen TA, Aronow MS, et al. Pleiotropic effects of vitamin D on osteoblast gene expression are related to the proliferative and differentiated state of the bone cell phenotype: dependency upon basal levels of gene expression, duration of exposure, and bone matrix competency in normal rate osteoblast cultures. Endocrinology 1991; 128:1496–1504.
650. Tilyard NW. 1,20-Dihydroxyvitamin D_3 vs calcium in the treatment of established postmenopausal osteoporosis. (Abstract.) J Bone Miner Res 1990; 5(2):275.
651. Fujita T. Vitamin D in the treatment of osteoporosis. Proc Soc Exp Biol Med 1992; 199:394–399.

652. Takizawa M, Fallon M, Stein B, Epstein S. The effect of a new vitamin D analog, 22-OXA-1(OH)$_2$D$_3$, on bone mineral metabolism in normal male rats. Calcif Tissue Int 1992; 50:521–523.
653. Sato F, Ouchi Y, Okamoto Y, et al. Effects of vitamin D$_3$ analogs on calcium metabolism in vitamin D–deficient rats and in MC3T3-E1 osteoblastic cells. Res Exp Med 1991; 191:235–242.
654. Erben RG, Weiser H, Sinowatz F, et al. Vitamin D metabolites prevent vertebral osteopenia in ovariectomized rats. Calcif Tissue Int 1992; 50:228–236.
655. Nakamura T, Nagai Y, Tamato H, et al. Regulation of bone turnover and prevention of bone atrophy in ovariectomized beagle dogs by the administration of 24R,20(OH)$_2$D$_3$. Calcif Tissue Int 1992; 50:221–227.
656. Nakamura T, Kurokawa T, Orimo H. Increased mechanical strength of the vitamin D–replete rat femur by the treatment with a large dose of 24R,20(OH)$_2$ D$_3$. Bone 1989; 10:117–123.
657. Suda T, Takahashi N, Abe E. Role of vitamin D in bone resorption. J Cell Biochem 1992; 49:53.
658. Nordin BEC, Morris HA. Osteoporosis and vitamin D. J Cell Biochem 1992; 49:19–20.
659. Kragballe K. Vitamin D analogues in the treatment of psoriasis. J Cell Biochem 1992; 49:46–52.
660. Okamura WH, Palenzuela JA, Plumet J, Midland MM. Vitamin D: structure-function analyses and the design of analogs. J Cell Biochem 1992; 19:10–18.
661. Lian JB, Stein GS. Transcriptional control of vitamin D–regulated proteins. J Cell Biochem 1992; 49:37–45.
662. Norman AW. Editorial: Vitamin D research frontiers. J Cell Biochem 1992; 49:1–3.
663. Nanjo M, Ichikawa F, Higuchi Y, et al. The mechanism of action, metabolism and distribution of 1-hydroxycholecalciferol in bone. Bone Miner 1992; 17(suppl 1):99.
664. Seimiya Y, Chen JT, Hirai Y, Shiraki M. Effect of active vitamin D$_3$ on reduction in bone mineral density after oophorectomy. Bone Miner 1992; 17(suppl 1):183.
665. McMurtry CT, Young SE, Downs RW, Adler RA. Mild vitamin D deficiency and secondary hyperparathyroidism in nursing home patients receiving adequate dietary vitamin D. J Am Geriatr Soc 1992; 40:343–347.
666. Walters MR, Kollenkirchen U, Fox J. What is vitamin D deficiency? Proc Soc Exp Biol Med 1992; 199:385–393.
667. Goldray D, Mizrahi-Sasson E, Merdler C, et al. Vitamin D deficiency in elderly patients in a general hospital. J Am Geriatr Soc 1989; 37:589–592.
668. Holick MF, Schnoes THK, DeLuca HF, Suda T, Cousins R. Isolation and identification of 1,20-dihydroxycholecalciferol, a metabolite of vitamin D active in intestine. J NIH Res 1992; 4:88–96.
669. Ebeling PR, Sandgren ME, Dimagno EP, et al. Evidence of an age-related decrease in intestinal responsiveness to vitamin D: relationship between serum 1,20-dihydroxyvitamin D$_3$ and intestinal vitamin D receptor concentrations in normal women. J Clin Endocrinol Metab 1992; 75:176–182.
670. Koren R, Ravid A, Liberman UA, et al. Responsiveness to 1,20-dihydroxyvitamin D$_3$ is reduced in lymphocytes from osteoporotic women. J Bone Miner Res 1992; 7: 1057–1061.

671. Quesada JM, Coopmans W, Ruiz B, et al. Influence of vitamin D on parathyroid function in the elderly. J Clin Endocrinol Metab 1992; 75:494–501.
672. Heikinheimo RJ, Inkovaara JA, Harju EJ, et al. Annual injection of vitamin D and fractures of aged bones. Calcif Tissue Int 1992; 51:105–110.
673. Dawson-Hughesa B, Dallal GE, Krall EA, et al. Effect of vitamin D supplementation on wintertime and overall bone loss in health postmenopausal women. Ann Intern Med 1991; 115:505–512.
674. Bikle DD. Clinical counterpoint: vitamin D: new actions, new analogs, new therapeutic potential. Endocrinol Rev 1992; 13:765–784.
675. DeLuca HF. New concepts of vitamin D functions. Ann NY Acad Sci 1992; 669: 59–69.
676. Walters MR. Newly identified actions of the vitamin D endocrine system. Endocrinol Rev 1992; 13:719–764.
677. Lukert B, Higgins J, Stoskopf M. Menopausal bone loss is partially regulated by dietary intake of vitamin D. Calcif Tissue Int 1992; 51:173–179.
678. Lidor C, Sagiv P, Amdur B, et al. Decrease in bone levels of 1,20-dihydroxyvitamin D in women with subcapital fracture of the femur. Calcif Tissue Int 1993; 52: 146–148.
679. Lind L, Wengle B, Sorensen OH, Ljunghall S. Serum levels of 1,20-$(OH)_2$-vitamin D are not altered by long-term supplementation with alhacalcidol (1-OH-vitamin D_3). Exp Clin Endocrinol 1992; 99:151–153.
680. Pouilles JM, Tremollieres F, Ribot C. Prevention of post-menopausal bone loss with 1-hydroxy vitamin D_3. A three-year prospective study. Clin Rheumatol 1992; 11:492–497.
681. Thavarajah M, Evans DB, Kanis JA. Differentiation of heterogeneous phenotypes in human osteoblast cultures in response to 1,20-dihydroxyvitamin D_3. Bone 1993; 14: 763–767.
682. Slatopolsky E, Berkoben M, Kelber J, Brown A, Delmez J. Effects of calcitriol and non-calcemic vitamin D analogs on secondary hyperparathyroidism. Kidney Int 1992; 42(suppl 38):43–49.
683. Van Schoubroeck V, Geusens P, Nijs J, et al. Treatment of bone loss after cardiac transplanation with one-alpha vitamin D_3 or cyclic etidronate. (Abstract.) Presented at Fourth International Symposium on Osteoporosis, Hong Kong, 1993:97.
684. Shiraki M. Treatment of osteoporosis with vitamin D_3. Osteoporos Int 1993; 3(suppl 1):176–180.
685. Shiraki M, Ito H, Orimo H. The ultra long-term treatment of senile osteoporosis with 1-hydroxyvitamin D_3. Bone Miner 1993; 20:223–234.
686. Gallagher JC. Prevention of bone loss in postmenopausal and senile osteoporosis with vitamin D analogues. Osteoporosis Int 1993; 3(suppl 1):172–175.
687. Caniggia A, Nuti R, Lore F, et al. Total body absorptiometry in postmenopausal osteoporosis patients treated with 1-hydroxylated vitamin D metabolites. Osteoporosis Int 1993; 3(suppl 1):181–185.
688. Kato T, Chen JT, Hasumi K, Ogata E, Shiraki M. Effect of 1-OH-vitamin D_3 on lumbar bone mineral density immediately after menopause. J Bone Miner Res 1993; 8(suppl 1):942.

689. Komar L, Nieves J, Cosman F, et al. Calcium homeostasis of an elderly population upon admission to a nursing home. J Am Geriatr Soc 1993; 41:1057–1064.
690. Need AG, Morris HA, Horowitz M, Nordin BEC. Effects of skin thickness, age body fat, and sunlight on serum 20-hydroxyvitamin D. Am J Clin Nutr 1993; 58:882–885.
691. Salamone LM, Dallal GE, Santos D, et al. Contributions of vitamin D intake and seasonal sunlight exposure to plasma 20-hydroxyvitamin D concentration in elderly women. Am J Clin Nutr 1993; 58:80–86.
692. Lamberg-Allardt C, Karkkainen M, et al. Low serum 20-hydroxyvitamin D concentrations and secondary hyperparathyroidism in middle-aged white strict vegetarians. Am J Clin Nutr 1993; 58:684–689.
693. Sambrook P, Birmingham J, Kelly P, et al. Prevention of corticosteroid bone loss. Osteoporos Int 1993; 3(suppl 1):141–143.
694. VanSchoubroeck I, Geusens P, Nijs J, et al. Treatment of bone loss after cardiac transplantation with one-alpha vitamin D_3 or cyclic etidronate. (Abstract.) Presented at Fourth International Symposium on Osteoporosis, Hong Kong, 1993:97.
695. Jones G, Calverley MJ. A dialogue on analogues. Newer vitamin D drugs for use in bone disease, psoriasis, and cancer. Trends Endocrinol Metab 1993; 4:297–303.
696. Morrison NA, Qi JC, Tokita A, et al. Prediction of bone density from vitamin D receptor alleles. Nature 1994; 367:284–287.
697. Anderson JJB, Toverud SU. Diet and vitamin D: a review with an emphasis on human function. J Nutr Biochem 1994; 5:58–65.
698. Iqbal SJ. Vitamin D metabolism and the clinical aspects of measuring metabolites. Ann Clin Biochem 1994; 31:109–124.
699. Tjellesen L. Metabolism and action of vitamin D in epileptic patients on anticonvulsive treatment and healthy adults. Dan Med Bull 1994; 41:139–150.
700. Reichel H, Szabo A, Uhl J, et al. Intermittent versus continuous administration of 1,20-dihydroxyvitamin D_3 in experimental renal hyperparathyroidism. Kidney Int 1993; 44:1209–1265.
701. Ruedin P, Rizzoli R, Slosman D, et al. Effects of oral calcitriol on bone mineral density in patients with end-stage renal failure. Kidney Int 45:245.
702. Shigematsu T, Kawaguchi Y, Unemura S, et al. Suppression of secondary hyperparathyroidism in chronic dialysis patients by single oral weekly dose of 1,20-dihydroxycholecalciterol. Intern Med 1993; 32:695–701.
703. Lewin E, Olgaard K. The in vivo effect of a new, in vitro, extremely potent vitamin D_3 analog KH1060 on the suppression of renal allograft rejection in the rat. Calcif Tissue Int 1994; 54:150–154.
704. Mellibovsky L, Diez A, Aubia J, et al. Long-standing remission after 20-OH D_3 treatment in a case of chronic myelomonocytic leukaemia. Br J Hematol 1993; 85: 811–812.
705. Pols HAP, Birkenhager JC, vanLeeuwen JPTM. Vitamin D analogues: from molecule to clinical application. Clin Endocrinol 1994; 40:285–291.
706. Thomasset M. Vitamine D et systeme immunitaire. Path Biol 1994; 42:163–172.
707. Mundy GR. Osteoporosis: Boning up on genes. Nature 1994; 367:216–217.
708. Orimo H, Shiraki M, Hayashi Y, et al. Effects of 1-(OH)-vitamin D_3. Bone Miner 1987; 3:47–52.

709. Orimo H, Shiraki M, Hayashi Y, et al. Effects of 1-hydroxyvitamin D_3 on lumbar bone mineral density and vertebral fratures in patients with postmenopausal osteoporosis. Calcif Tissue Int 1994; 54:370–376.
710. Menczel J, Foldes J, Steinberg R, et al. Alfacalcidol (alpha D_3) and calcium in osteoporosis. Clin Orthop 1994; 300:241–247.
711. O'Dowd KJ, Clemens TL, Kelsey JL, Lindsay R. Exogenous calciferol (vitamin D) and vitamin D endocrine status among elderly nursing home residents in the New York City area. J Am Geriatr Soc 1993; 41:414–421.
712. Hine TJ, Roberts NB: Seasonal variation in serum 20-hydroxyvitamin D_3 does not affect 1,20-dihydroxyvitamin D. Ann Clin Biochem 1994; 31:31–34.
713. Ravaglia G, Forti P, Pratelli L, et al. The association of ageing with calcium active hormone status in men. Age Ageing 1994; 23:127–131.
714. Khaw KT, Scragg R, Murphy S. Single-dose cholecalciferol suppresses the winter increase in parathyroid hormone concentrations in healthy older men and women: a randomized trial. Am J Clin Nutr 1994; 59:1040–1044.
715. Halabe A, Arie R, Mimran D, et al. Hypoparathyroidism—a long-term follow-up experience with 1-vitamin D_3 therapy. Clin Endocrinol 1994; 40:303–307.
716. Gallagher JC, Bishop CW, Knutson JC, et al. Effects of increasing doses of 1-hydroxyvitamin D_2 on calcium homeostasis in postmenopausal osteopenic women. J Bone Miner Res 1994; 9:607–614.
717. Tsurukami H, Nakamura T, Suzuki K, et al. A novel synthetic vitamin D analogue, 2-(3-hydroxypropoxy) 1,20-dihydroxyvitamin D_3 (ED-71), increases bone mass by stimulating the bone formation in normal and ovariectomized rats. Calcif Tissue Int 1994; 54:142–149.
718. Holick MF. McCollum award lecture: Vitamin D—new horizons for the 21st century. Am J Clin Nutr 1994; 60:619–630.
719. Rosen CJ, Morrison A, Zhou H, et al. Elderly women in northern New England exhibit seasonal changes in bone mineral density and calciotropic hormones. Bone Miner 1994; 20:83–92.
720. Martinez ME, del Campo MT, Sanchez-Cabezudo MJ, et al. Relations between calcidiol serum levels and bone mineral density in postmenopausal women with low bone density. Calcif Tissue Int 1994; 55:203–206.
721. Nieves J, Cosman F, Herbert J, Shen V, Lindsay R. High prevalence of vitamin D deficiency and reduced bone mass in multiple sclerosis. Neurology 1994; 44:1687–1692.
722. Ledger GA, Burritt MF, Keo PC, et al. Abnormalities of parathyroid hormone secretion in elderly women that are reversible by short term therapy with 1,20-dihydroxyvitamin D_3. J Clin Endocrinol Metab 1994; 70:211–216.
723. Ooms ME, Roos JC, Bezemer PD, Van der Vijgh JF, et al. Prevention of bone loss by vitamin D supplementation in elderly women: a randomized double-blind trial. J Clin Endocrinol Metab 1995; 80:1052–1058.
724. Kamel S, Brazier M, Picard C, et al. Urinary excretion of pyridinolines crosslinks measured by immunoassay and HPLC techniques in normal subjects and in elderly patients with vitamin D deficiency. Bone Miner 1994; 20:103–109.
725. Ng K, St John A, Bruce DG. Secondary hyperparathyroidism, vitamin D deficiency

and hip fracture: importance of sampling times after fracture. Bone Miner 1994; 20:103–109.

726. WHO Collaborating Centre for Metabolic Bone Diseases. Abstracts from the role of vitamin D and related compounds in the treatment of bone disease in the elderly. Bone 1994; 15:725–728.
727. Akesson K, Ljunghall S, Gardsell P, Sernbo L, Obrant KJ. Serum osteocalcin and fracture susceptibility in elderly women. Calcif Tissue Int 1993; 53:86–90.
728. Hodges JS, Akesson K, Vergnaud P, Obrant K, Delmas PD. Circulating levels of vitamins K_1 and K_2 decreased in elderly women with hip fracture. J Bone Miner Res 1993; 8:1241–1245.
729. Hodges JS, Pilkington MJ, Stamp TCB, et al. Depressed levels of circulating menaquinones in patients with osteoporotic fractures of the spine and femoral neck. Bone 1991; 12:387–389.
730. Szulc P, Chapuy MC, Meunier PJ, Delmas PD. Serum undercarboxylated osteocalcin is a marker of the risk of hip fracture in elderly women. J Clin Invest 1993; 91:1769–1774.
731. Pastoureau P, Vergnaud P, Meunier PJ, Delmas PD. Osteopenia and bone-remodeling abnormalities in warfarin-treated lambs. J Bone Miner Res 1993; 8:1417–1426.
732. Rosen HN, Maitland LA, Suttie JW, et al. Vitamin K and maintenance of skeletal integrity in adults. Am J Med 1993; 94:62–68.
733. Hara K, Akiyama Y, Ohkawa I, Tajima T. Effects of menatetrenone on prednisolone-induced bone loss in rats. Bone 1993; 14:812–818.
734. Orimo H, Shiraki M. Clinical evaluation of menatetrenone (vitamin K_2) in the treatment of involutional osteoporosis. In: Christiansen C, Riis B, eds. Proceedings of the Fourth international Symposium on Osteoporosis. Aaborg, Denmark, 1993: 148–149.
735. Michel BA, Bloch DA, Fires JF. Weight-bearing exercise, overexercise, and lumbar bone density over age 50 years. Arch Intern Med 1989; 149:2325–2329.

Index

About the Editor

DAVID J. SARTORIS is a Professor of Radiology in the Musculoskeletal Imaging Section at the University of California, San Diego, School of Medicine, and Chief of Quantitative Bone Densitometry at the University of California, San Diego, Medical Center. The author or coauthor of over 470 professional publications and nine books, Dr. Sartoris is a member of the American College of Radiology, the American Society for Bone and Mineral Research, the Radiological Society of North America, the International Skeletal Society, the National Osteoporosis Foundation, and the Society for Clinical Densitometry, among others. He received the B.S. degree (1976) in biology from Stanford University, California, and the M.D. degree (1980) from Stanford University School of Medicine, California.